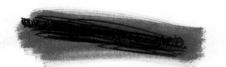

LACRIMAL
SURGERY

CONTEMPORARY ISSUES in OPHTHALMOLOGY VOLUME 5

SERIES EDITOR

George W. Weinstein, M.D.
Professor and Jane McDermott Shott Chairman
Department of Ophthalmology
West Virginia University School of Medicine
Morgantown, West Virginia

LACRIMAL SURGERY

Edited by

John V. Linberg, M.D.

Associate Professor
Department of Ophthalmology
West Virginia University School of Medicine
Morgantown, West Virginia

CHURCHILL LIVINGSTONE
NEW YORK, EDINBURGH, LONDON, MELBOURNE
1988

Library of Congress Cataloging-in-Publication Data

Lacrimal surgery.

  (Contemporary issues in ophthalmology ; v. 5)
  Includes bibliographies and index.
  1. Lacrimal organs—Surgery. 2. Lacrimal organs—
Diseases. I. Linberg, John V. II. Series. [DNLM:
1. Lacrimal Apparatus—surgery. W1 CO769MRM v.5 /
WW 208 L1456]
RE201.L327 1988   617.7'64059   88-14452
ISBN 0-443-08582-X

© **Churchill Livingstone Inc.** **1988**

Distributed in the United Kingdom by Churchill Livingstone, Robert Stevenson House, 1–3 Baxter's Place, Leith Walk, Edinburgh EH1 3AF, and by associated companies, branches, and representatives throughout the world.

Accurate indications, adverse reactions, and dosage schedules for drugs are provided in this book, but it is possible that they may change. The reader is urged to review the package information data of the manufacturers of the medications mentioned.

The Publishers have made every effort to trace the copyright holders for borrowed material. If they have inadvertently overlooked any, they will be pleased to make the necessary arrangements at the first opportunity.

Acquisitions Editor: *Kim Loretucci*
Copy Editor: *Margot Otway*
Production Designer: *Jill Little*
Production Supervisor: *Jocelyn Eckstein*

Printed in the United States of America

First published in 1988

To Dr. George Weinstein,
whose professional guidance
and personal support
made this work possible

Contributors

Kathleen F. Archer, M.D.
Clinical Instructor, Department of Ophthalmology, Oculoplastic and Reconstructive Surgery Service, University of Texas Medical School at San Antonio, San Antonio, Texas; Specialist, Oculoplastic and Reconstructive Surgery, Corpus Christi, Texas

Richard K. Dortzbach, M.D.
Clinical Professor, Department of Ophthalmology, University of Wisconsin Medical School, Madison, Wisconsin

Steven C. Dresner, M.D.
Assistant Clinical Professor, Department of Ophthalmology, Division of Ophthalmic Plastic and Reconstructive Surgery, Jules Stein Eye Institute, University of California, Los Angeles, UCLA School of Medicine, Los Angeles, California

Jonathan J. Dutton, M.D., Ph.D.
Associate Professor, Department of Ophthalmology, Duke University School of Medicine; Director, Oculoplastic and Orbital Surgery and Ophthalmic Oncology Service, Duke University Eye Center, Durham, North Carolina

Don S. Ellis, M.D.
Fellow, Ophthalmic Plastic, Reconstructive and Orbital Surgery, Department of Ophthalmology, Pacific Presbyterian Medical Center, San Francisco, California

Joseph C. Flanagan, M.D.
Professor, Department of Ophthalmology, Jefferson Medical College of Thomas Jefferson University; Director, Department of Oculoplastic Surgery, Wills Eye Hospital, Philadelphia, Pennsylvania

James W. Gigantelli, M.D.
Fellow, Department of Ophthalmology, Ophthalmic Plastic and Orbital Surgery Service, Cullen Eye Institute, Baylor College of Medicine, Houston, Texas

Michael J. Hawes, M.D.
Assistant Clinical Professor, Department of Ophthalmology, University of Colorado Health Sciences Center School of Medicine; Chief, Ophthalmology Service, Department of Surgery, Veterans Administration Hospital, Denver, Colorado

Richard C. Haydon, M.D.
Associate Professor, Department of Otolaryngology—Head and Neck Surgery, West Virginia University School of Medicine, Morgantown, West Virginia

LTC Donald A. Hollsten, M.D., M.C.
Chief, Department of Ophthalmology, Brooke Medical Center, San Antonio, Texas

Jeffrey J. Hurwitz, M.D., F.R.C.S.(C)
Associate Professor and Director, Oculoplastic Service, Department of Ophthalmology, University of Toronto Faculty of Medicine; Ophthalmologist-in-Chief, Department of Ophthalmology, Mount Sinai Hospital; Consultant, Oculoplastic Service, Department of Ophthalmology, Sunnybrook Medical Center, Toronto, Ontario, Canada

Bennie L. Jarvis, M.D.
Fellow, Department of Otolaryngology—Head and Neck Surgery, West Virginia University School of Medicine, Morgantown, West Virginia

James A. Katowitz, M.D.
Associate Professor, Department of Ophthalmology, Scheie Eye Institute, University of Pennsylvania School of Medicine; Director, Oculoplastic Surgery, The Center for Human Appearance, Hospital of the University of Pennsylvania; Director, Oculoplastic and Orbital Service, Division of Ophthalmology, The Children's Hospital of Philadelphia, Philadelphia, Pennsylvania

Peter S. Levin, M.D.
Fellow, Ophthalmic Plastic, Reconstructive and Orbital Surgery, Department of Ophthalmology, Pacific Presbyterian Medical Center, San Francisco, California

John V. Linberg, M.D.
Associate Professor, Department of Ophthalmology, West Virginia University School of Medicine, Morgantown, West Virginia

Steven A. McCormick, M.D.
Assistant Professor, Departments of Pathology and Ophthalmology, West Virginia University School of Medicine; Director, Autopsy Services and Ophthalmic Pathology Laboratory, West Virginia University Health Sciences Center, Morgantown, West Virginia

Jeffrey A. Nerad, M.D.
Assistant Professor and Director, Oculoplastic, Orbital, and Oncology Service, Department of Ophthalmology, University of Iowa College of Medicine, Iowa City, Iowa

J. Justin Older, M.D.
Associate Professor and Director, Oculoplastic Service, Department of Ophthalmology, University of South Florida College of Medicine, Tampa, Florida

James R. Patrinely, M.D.
Assistant Professor, Department of Ophthalmology, Ophthalmic Plastic and Orbital Surgery Service, Cullen Eye Institute, Baylor College of Medicine, Houston, Texas

Allen M. Putterman, M.D.
Professor of Clinical Ophthalmology, Department of Ophthalmology, and Chief, Oculoplastic Service, Eye and Ear Infirmary, University of Illinois College of Medicine at Chicago; Clinical Associate Professor, Department of Ophthalmology, University of Chicago Pritzker School of Medicine; Senior Attending Surgeon and Director, Oculoplastic Surgery, Michael Reese Hospital and Medical Center, Chicago, Illinois

William B. Stewart, M.D.
Director, Ophthalmic Plastic, Reconstructive and Orbital Surgery, Department of Ophthalmology, Pacific Presbyterian Medical Center, San Francisco, California

Roberto Javier Vásquez, M.D.
Fellow, Department of Ophthalmology, West Virginia University School of Medicine, Morgantown, West Virginia

Ralph E. Wesley, M.D.
Assistant Professor, Department of Ophthalmology, Meharry Medical College School of Medicine; Director, Ophthalmic Plastic and Reconstructive Surgery, Vanderbilt University Medical Center; Director, Ophthalmic Plastic and Orbital Surgery, Baptist Medical Center; Chief, Department of Ophthalmology, Park View Medical Center, Nashville, Tennessee

Christine L. Zolli, M.D.
Clinical Associate Professor, Department of Ophthalmology, University of Medicine and Dentistry of New Jersey, Newark, New Jersey; Associate Surgeon, Department of Oculoplastic Surgery, Wills Eye Hospital, Philadelphia, Pennsylvania

Preface

Lacrimal surgery has a written history dating back to the code of Hammurabi (2250 BC), and antedates most other types of ophthalmic surgery. This early attention to lacrimal surgery was probably motivated by the need to treat dacryocystitis, a life-threatening infection in the era before antibiotics. As techniques of surgery improved, the objectives of lacrimal surgery evolved from the simple elimination of infection to the reconstruction of a functional drainage pathway.

The practice of lacrimal surgery has been complicated by the division of ophthalmology and otorhinolaryngology into separate specialities. The ocular problems of lacrimal disease clearly place these patients under the care of the ophthalmologist, but surgical treatment often involves the nasal aspect of lacrimal anatomy. It is usually difficult for ophthalmologists to obtain instruction and training in the nasal techniques critical to successful lacrimal procedures. Thus, in this book we have made a special effort to include the relevant information on nasal anatomy, examination, and surgery in our descriptions of lacrimal surgery for the ophthalmologist.

The contributing authors have provided a broad but detailed survey of contemporary lacrimal surgery, ranging from the routine procedures familiar to every ophthalmologist to the most complex microsurgical reconstructions. The variety and ingenuity of these procedures is amazing when one considers that they address but a single facet of ophthalmic surgery. While this book focuses on lacrimal surgery, the text also discusses relevant aspects of anatomy, pathology, radiology, and multispecialty collaboration. Special emphasis has been given to the use of new materials and instruments.

It has been a real honor to serve such a distinguished and expert panel of contributing authors. We hope that this text will prove useful to every lacrimal surgeon, from the resident-in-training to the comprehensive ophthalmologist and oculoplastic subspecialist.

John V. Linberg, M.D.

Contents

1 | Surgical Anatomy of the Lacrimal System

John V. Linberg

A detailed knowledge of gross anatomy, crucial to proper technique in any surgical field, is particularly important in ophthalmic surgery. This principle assumes even more importance in lacrimal surgery because the anatomy involved is not learned during other types of ophthalmic surgery. For example, knowledge of extraocular muscle anatomy is used during retina surgery, strabismus surgery, and even cataract surgery. Experience and training in each of these areas will increase the surgeon's ability to identify and handle the extraocular muscles. By contrast, techniques of lacrimal surgery are quite specific and are generally distinct from the rest of ophthalmic surgery.

The ophthalmic surgeon who decides to perform lacrimal surgery must study the anatomy not only of the lacrimal system but also of the adjacent nasal and sinus structures. This chapter provides details of gross anatomy and establishes a basis for understanding the subsequent chapters on surgical technique.

THE LACRIMAL DRAINAGE SYSTEM

Tears in the marginal tear strip enter the lacrimal drainage system through the punctal openings of both eyelids. The puncta are located on the medial lid margin at the apex of small mounds of soft tissue, the papillae lacrimalis (Fig. 1-1). These papillae appear pale in contrast to the surrounding tissue (Fig. 1-2) because they contain more connective tissue and less vasculature. They are centered on the eyelid margin in line with the mucocutaneous junction. The upper papilla is located approximately 6 mm from the medial canthal angle, and the lower papilla is 6.5 mm from the medial canthus.[1] Medial to the papillae

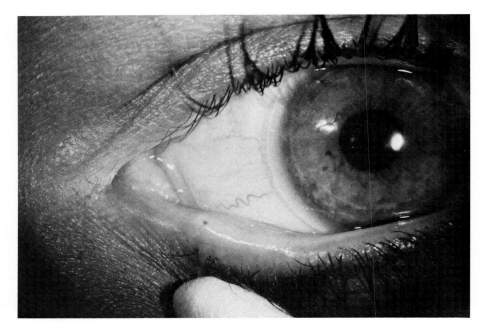

Fig. 1-1 Lower eyelid everted to show the lacrimal papilla and punctum. Note the absence of lashes medial to the punctum, and pale color of the papilla.

the eyelid margin has a rounded contour with few cilia, whereas laterally the lid margin is square in cross section and contains numerous cilia. There are no meibomian glands medial to the papillae, the last meibomian orifice being 0.5 to 1.0 mm lateral to the puncta. In cases of imperforate or stenotic puncta, the papillae may be identified by their pale color and localized by their relationships to the meibomian orifices, cilia, mucocutaneous junction, and canthal angle, as well as by the abrupt change in lid margin contour.

The punctal opening measures 0.2 to 0.3 mm in diameter and is surrounded by a ring of dense connective tissue that normally maintains a patent entrance. The aperture is round or oval in youth, but often collapses into a fishmouth or slit configuration with age. The puncta are normally directed somewhat posteriorly toward the globe and do not become visible unless the lid is slightly everted (Fig. 1-1). In primary gaze the papillae rest in the groove between the globe and the plica semilunaris, at the medial end of the marginal tear strip (Fig. 1-2).

The delicate mucosal ducts that convey tears from the puncta to the lacrimal sac are known as canaliculi, and measure about 10 mm in length (Fig. 1-3). The initial 2 mm segment of each canaliculus passes into the lid perpendicular to the lid margin. The base of each vertical segment dilates to form an irregular sac or ampulla, 2 mm in diameter, that collects tears between blinks. From each ampulla the canaliculi make a right-angle turn and pass medially,

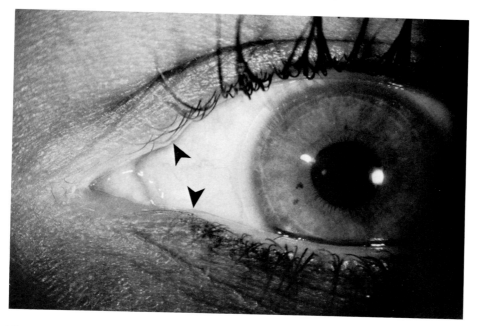

Fig. 1-2   Normal eye. Arrows indicate location of lacrimal papillae, resting against the globe.

parallel to the lid margin. These horizontal segments are narrower, perhaps 0.5 to 1.0 mm in diameter. The canaliculi and ampulla are surrounded by fibers of the pretarsal orbicularis oculi muscle, which compress and shorten the canaliculi during the closure phase of each blink.

At the medial canthal angle both the upper and lower canaliculus pass behind the stout medial canthal tendon. In 90 percent of cases[2] the two canaliculi meet at an angle of about 25 degrees[3] to form a common canaliculus before draining into the lacrimal sac. In the other 10 percent of cases, the two canaliculi enter the lacrimal sac separately. The common canaliculus measures 3 to 5 mm in length and dilates just before penetrating the lacrimal sac fascia. This dilation, termed the sinus of Maier, is seen by some anatomists as a diverticulum of the lacrimal sac.[1] The opening of the common canaliculus into the lacrimal sac is superior and posterior to the middle of the lateral wall, and 2 to 3 mm behind the medial canthal tendon. Within the sac, the canalicular ostium is guarded by a fold of mucosa known as the valve of Rosenmüller. This arrangement normally prevents the reflux of fluid or air from the sac into the canaliculi. It is not a constant finding, and absence of the valve does not seem to produce epiphora.[4] The valve of Rosenmüller plays a more important role in the physiology of the lacrimal sac when a pathologic obstruction of the distal nasolacrimal duct is present. The sac is often distended by secretions or byproducts of infection, causing the valve to press firmly against the ostium

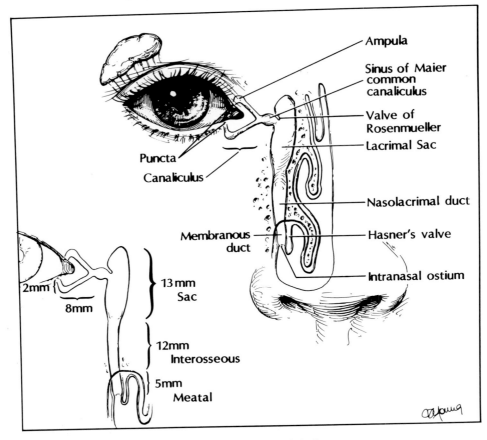

Fig. 1-3 Diagram of the lacrimal drainage system.

of the common canaliculus. Gentle probing with a blunt tip may be sufficient to displace the valve and allow decompression of the sac. This maneuver will relieve pain and assist in the control of infection. In some cases it will be necessary to decompress the sac by percutaneous needle aspiration before the valve can be displaced and opened.

The lacrimal sac rests in a shallow osseous groove of the medial orbital wall, the fossa sacci lacrimalis (Fig. 1-4). This depression runs up the foremost aspect of the medial orbital wall, just behind the orbital rim. The fossa varies considerably in depth and shape, but average dimensions are 15 mm high, 4 to 8 mm wide, and 2 mm deep. The lacrimal bone and nasal process of the maxilla contribute roughly equal portions of the fossa, with a suture line running up the center of the groove along its long axis. Rarely, the maxilla may form the entire lacrimal sac fossa.[5]

The front edge of the lacrimal sac fossa is formed by the anterior lacrimal crest, which is contiguous with the inferior orbital rim. A distinct narrow groove

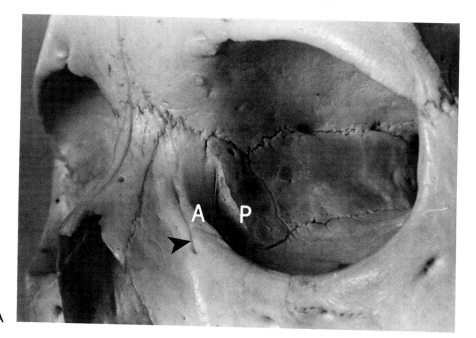

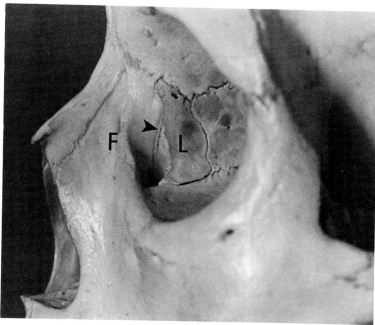

Fig. 1-4 **(A)** Lacrimal sac fossa, oblique view. A, anterior lacrimal crest; P, posterior lacrimal crest. Arrowhead indicates the sutura notha, a groove formed by a nutrient artery. **(B)** Lacrimal sac fossa, lateral view. L, lacrimal bone; F, frontal process of maxilla. Arrowhead indicates suture line between lacrimal bone and frontal process of maxilla bone.

caused by a nutrient artery is found 2 to 3 mm anterior to the anterior lacrimal crest (Fig. 1-4A). The groove is called the *sutura notha* in older texts, although in fact it is not a suture line. The sutura notha is a valuable landmark during dacryocystorhinostomy. As the surgeon begins to elevate periosteum toward the lacrimal sac, the groove serves as a warning that the anterior crest is being approached, and the surgeon should take increased care to avoid lacerating the lacrimal sac. The nutrient artery in this false suture sometimes causes troublesome bleeding that must be controlled with bone wax.

The bone of the nasal process of the maxilla, and particularly the anterior lacrimal crest, is thick and strong (Fig. 1-5), a circumstance that protects the lacrimal sac from trauma. Even when the nasal pyramid fractures, the fracture lines tend to run above or below the sac.[6] In contrast, the floor of the fossa formed by the lacrimal bone is eggshell thin (Fig. 1-5). The dacryocystorhinostomy surgeon therefore finds it much easier to penetrate the lacrimal fossa behind the suture line between the lacrimal bone and maxilla. The posterior edge of the lacrimal sac fossa, referred to as the posterior lacrimal crest, is more prominent. This ridge on the lacrimal bone terminates inferiorly at the opening of the nasolacrimal duct, where the process hamalaris of the lacrimal bone articulates in the lacrimal notch of the orbital surface of the maxillary

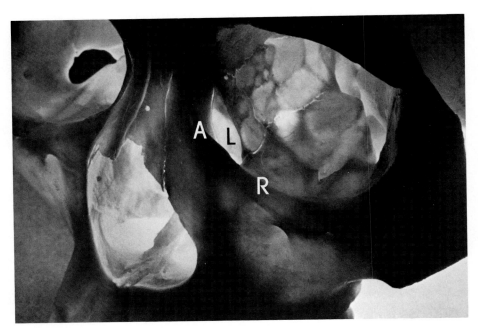

Fig. 1-5 Skull shown with retroillumination (compare with Fig. 1-4A) to demonstrate thickness of bone. Note the strength of the anterior lacrimal crest (A) and inferior orbital rim (R). Observe thinness of lacrimal bone (L) forming the posterior lacrimal fossa, which overlies the anterior ethmoid air cells.

bone (Fig. 1-4B). Inferiorly, the lacrimal sac fossa deepens and becomes more oval in cross section as it approaches the nasolacrimal duct. Superiorly, the lacrimal sac fossa shallows and becomes inconspicuous without a definite margin, but is limited by the angular process of the frontal bone (Fig. 1-4).

The lacrimal sac fossa is adjacent to the middle meatus of the nasal cavity (Fig. 1-6). In almost all individuals the superior and posterior portions of the fossa are separated from the nasal cavity by ethmoid air cells (Fig. 1-5). In some cases large ethmoid air cells (agar nasi) may extend under the entire fossa, and thus involve the frontal, ethmoid, lacrimal, and maxillary bones. These variable air cells can confuse the dacryocystorhinostomy surgeon intent upon resecting bone between the lacrimal sac and nasal mucosa. In some individuals the removal of bone comprising the lacrimal sac fossa will only open the anterior compartment of ethmoid air cells and fail to expose nasal mucosa. In this anatomic situation the potential exists for a serious mistake, because the lacrimal sac can be opened into the ethmoid compartment rather than the nasal cavity. In order to avoid confusion, the lacrimal surgeon must be able to distinguish the gross appearance of ethmoid versus nasal mucosa. The mucosa of ethmoid air cells is thin, gray and friable in contrast to the thick, red mucoperiosteum of the nasal cavity. Fortunately these differences are quite reliable, and the surgeon should encounter no real difficulty.

The mucosal lacrimal sac resting in its fossa is surrounded by a dense layer of fascia. The medial canthal tendon, orbicularis oculi muscle, and periorbita of the medial orbital wall all contribute to this envelope. At the posterior lacrimal crest the periorbita splits into two leaves, the thinner layer passing into the fossa under the lacrimal sac. The thicker layer passes over the lateral aspect of the sac to insert on the anterior crest. This span of connective tissue is reinforced by the medial canthal tendon. As the tendon approaches the lacrimal sac it divides into anterior and posterior leaves. The posterior leaf inserts on the posterior lacrimal crest and is reinforced by the deep heads of the pretarsal orbicularis muscle (Horner's muscles) and the preseptal orbicularis muscle (Jones' muscles). The anterior leaf of the medial canthal tendon passes over the anterior lacrimal crest to insert several millimeters further medial on the nasal process of the maxilla. Superiorly, the medial canthal tendon fans out to cover the fundus of the sac with dense fascia.[7]

The inferior edge of the medial canthal tendon presents a well-defined free margin. Below this line the lacrimal sac is covered only by septum, orbicularis muscle, and skin. Mechanically this is the weakest area in the covering of the lacrimal sac, and therefore is the area where fistulas develop in untreated dacryocystitis. It is rare for infection of the sac to fistulize into the orbit.

By definition, any tissue posterior to the orbital septum and within the osseous orbital walls is intraorbital. Clinically, the lacrimal sac behaves as a separate compartment, distinct both from the face and the orbit. One clinical result of this anatomic situation is the syndrome of acute dacryocystitis, in which infected and edematous tissues within the lacrimal compartment cannot expand into either the orbit or the face. Instead, the lacrimal fascia is placed under extreme tension that results in the severe pain typical of acute dacry-

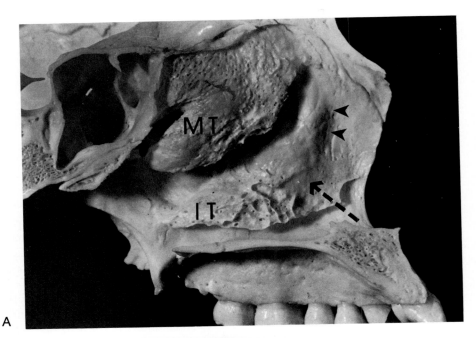

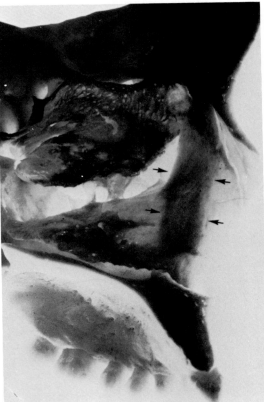

Fig. 1-6 (A) Sagittal view of lateral nasal wall. Observe the middle turbinate (MT) and inferior turbinate (IT). Arrowheads mark the bulge over the nasal wall of the lacrimal sac fossa. This area, just anterior to the tip of the middle turbinate, is resected during dacryocystorhinostomy. The opening of the nasolacrimal canal is hidden under the inferior turbinate (broken arrow). (B) Same view as Fig. A but shown with retroillumination. Arrows outline the nasolacrimal canal.

ocystitis. Immediate relief may be provided by incising the anterior lacrimal fascia, thus decompressing the compartment.

The actual mucosa of the lacrimal sac is thin, with a moist, gray, irregular surface. It is separated from the lacrimal fascia by a layer of loose connective tissue containing a plexus of veins. Inferiorly, the plexus assumes the microscopic appearance of the erectile tissue of the inferior turbinate. Because of this intervening layer, lacrimal sac mucosa is only loosely adherent to the surrounding fascia. The potential cleavage plane between lacrimal fascia and mucosa may present problems during dacryocystorhinostomy. An incision through the lacrimal sac fascia may only displace the mucosa and not open the sac. Obviously, this difficulty must be recognized and the mucosa opened separately if successful drainage into the nasal cavity is to be accomplished.

The shape of the lacrimal sac is often represented as a smooth cylindrical tube with a rounded apex. In fact, the sac is typically flattened and irregular in contour. The superior fundus is roughly triangular in outline with a sharp margin at the apex. The anterior edge tends to be sharp because of the less prominent character of the anterior lacrimal crest. The posterior margin is usually thicker and rounded because of the greater prominence of the posterior crest (Fig. 1-4). The lumen is normally collapsed unless pathologically distended by fluid, tumor, or dacryolith. Dacryocystography of normal subjects often shows a narrowing of the lumen just above the opening of the osseous nasolacrimal canal.[8] This may result from the superficial and deep heads of the inferior preseptal orbicularis muscle as the sac passes between them to enter the nasolacrimal canal.

The opening of the nasolacrimal canal is round to oval in cross section, 3 mm in diameter, and located at the anterior medial corner of the orbital floor. The osseous canal is approximately 12 mm long, and is formed by the lacrimal, maxillary, and ethmoid bones. The maxilla usually contributes the anterior, lateral, and posterior walls of the duct, with some variation.[5] Superiorly, the medial wall is formed by the lacrimal bone. Inferiorly, the concha of the inferior turbinate (ethmoid bone) covers the medial aspect of the canal. The bulge of the canal may be seen on the lateral wall of the nose running up from the tip of the inferior turbinate across the area in front of the middle turbinate (Fig. 1-6B). The nasolacrimal canal ostium is located under the inferior turbinate, 15 mm from the tip, emptying into the inferior meatus.

A membranous or mucosal segment of the duct extends under the inferior turbinate for 3 to 5 mm before opening at the ostium lacrimalis (Fig. 1-3). The mucosal ostium is found 30 to 35 mm from the external nares. The opening presents a variety of shapes and locations, and may even be multiple.[9] These variations account for some of the difficulties involved with the Jones dye tests. The flap of mucosa forming the medial wall of the membranous duct, referred to as Hasner's valve, normally acts as a one-way valve, preventing reflux of air into the lacrimal drainage passages.

In adults the lacrimal fossa and nasolacrimal canal form a more or less continuous straight line that angles back 15 degrees from the frontal plane of the face. The canal also angles slightly lateral from the midline, depending upon the intercanthal distance and width of the nasal cavity. Busse[10] observed that one-third of neonates have an angulation at the junction of the sac and duct. Further, he found that the distal nasolacrimal duct bends medially in an irregular J shape. The curved shape of the infantile nasolacrimal duct may account for some of the difficulties encountered during probing; thus, a flexible probe is helpful in following the path of the duct. The age at which this infantile pattern changes to the straight adult configuration has not been documented.

Vascular Supply

The medial canthal area contains numerous anastamoses between the internal and external carotid system, assuring adequate blood supply to the lacrimal drainage system. The inferior and superior medial palpebral arteries, as well as the supraorbital artery, are terminal branches of the ophthalmic artery and internal carotid system. The external carotid supplies blood through the infraorbital artery, a branch of the internal maxillary, as well as through the angular artery, the terminal portion of the external maxillary artery. The external maxillary artery exits from under the mandible to become the facial artery, which passes diagonally across the face to the nasolabial fold. The vessel continues up between the levator labia superioris and the levator ala nasi muscles to form the angular artery.[11] The final segment of the angular artery is consistently located against the periosteum of the nasal process of the maxilla, just at the insertion of the medial canthal tendon. The angular artery and vein are covered only by skin in this location and are often visible to external inspection. Blood flow in the angular vein normally passes downward to the neck, but connections exist to both the superior and inferior ophthalmic veins. Lymphatic drainage from the lacrimal sac and duct passes to the submaxillary, retropharyngeal, and deep cervical glands.

Innervation

Sensory innervation to the lacrimal sac and duct is provided by an infratrochlear branch of the nasociliary nerve as well as anterior superior alveolar nerves.

Physiology

No discussion of lacrimal drainage anatomy would be complete without reference to the controversy over the tear pump. It is clear to clinicians that some active mechanism of tear transport must exist, since patients with seventh nerve (facial) palsy have epiphora. Mild facial palsy produces tearing even in the presence of a patent and anatomically normal drainage system.

Based almost entirely on static anatomic observations, Jones suggested a twofold lacrimal pump mechanism[2,12,13] powered by orbicularis oculi contraction. First, he speculated that contraction of pretarsal fibers surrounding the canaliculi would compress and shorten these ducts, and therefore pump tears toward the sac. Secondly, he believed that the pull of the deep heads of the pretarsal and preseptal muscle on the lacrimal fascia would create a negative pressure within the sac during eyelid closure. Because of this mechanism, he suggested that the fascia covering the lacrimal sac be referred to as the lacrimal diaphragm.

The canalicular pump mechanism has been confirmed by intubation and manometric studies that documented a positive pressure peak in the canaliculus with each blink.[14-16] Unfortunately, similar intubation studies in the lacrimal sac did not demonstrate the negative pressure phase predicted by Jones. Instead, positive pressure peaks were documented within the sac. A recent high-speed cinematic study of blinking[17] suggests that a negative pressure phase may exist in the lacrimal drainage system at the end of each blink. Tears were observed to rush into the canalicular system just after lid opening, a phenomenon that may persist for several seconds.[17]

It seems clear from clinical evidence that pressure changes in the lacrimal sac cannot be very important, since dacryocystorhinostomy works so well. During this surgical procedure the lacrimal sac is widely opened into the nasal cavity. It would be impossible to generate any pressure variations within the sac after dacryocystorhinostomy surgery, yet patients show no problem with tear transport. The canalicular pump mechanism has been well documented, and would appear to be the important mechanism of tear transport.

LACRIMAL SECRETORY SYSTEM

The lacrimal gland is a flattened oval mass weighing about 78 g[18] that fills the space between the globe and orbital roof in the superior temporal quadrant. The superior convex surface of the gland rests in the fossa glandulae lacrimalis, a shallow depression in the anterior lateral aspect of the frontal bone (Fig. 1-7). This fossa, not to be confused with the fossa of the lacrimal sac, may be seen on plain radiographs as a smooth line arching over the superior temporal orbital rim. The inferior surface of the gland is molded by the globe into a mildly concave form. The lateral edge of the levator palpebrae aponeurosis creates a deep cleft in the anterior aspect of the gland, dividing it into two lobes that remain contiguous in their posterior extent. In life, the surface of the gland is grayish-pink, with a lobulated pattern that readily distinguishes it from surrounding orbital fat. A thin pseudocapsule of connective tissue surrounds the gland and is continuous with the connective tissue between the glandular lobules. While not a true capsule, this layer is surgically quite distinct and important in the management of some lacrimal neoplasms.[19,20]

The superior or orbital lobe measures 20 × 12 × 5 mm and is two to three times larger than the inferior palpebral lobe. The posterior edge of the orbital lobe is in the approximate coronal plane of the posterior pole of the globe. The

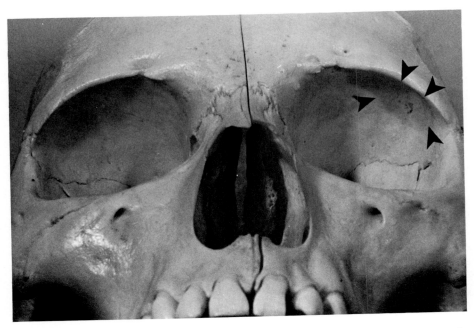

Fig. 1-7   Approximate area of lacrimal gland fossa is outlined by arrows. The entire fossa is formed by the frontal bone.

anterior margin rests on the superior surface of the levator aponeurosis, covered by orbital septum, orbicularis oculi muscle, and skin. The anterior medial edge also rests on the levator aponeurosis in the preaponeurotic fat pocket, while more posteriorly the medial edge approximates the lateral margin of the superior rectus muscle. The lateral edge extends as far inferiorly as the superior margin of the lateral rectus muscle.[1] The much smaller palpebral lobe is under the levator aponeurosis just above the superior lateral conjunctival fornix. In many individuals it will prolapse into view when the upper lid is everted.

The lacrimal gland is said to be supported by four different fascial structures,[21] although the actual significance of each is difficult to evaluate. The superior surface is weakly adherent to the periosteum of the lacrimal fossa by fine trabecular ligaments sometimes referred to as Sommering's ligaments. The edge of the levator aponeurosis and its lateral horn provide some support as they press into the lacrimal gland. The superior transverse ligament,[22] also known as Whitnall's ligament,[23] probably provides the greatest support. The lateral expansion of this ligament sends a small slip to insert on Whitnall's tubercle, but most of the fibers pass under and through the orbital lobe of the lacrimal gland to insert on the orbital roof.[23] Finally, a small band of fascia associated with the lacrimal artery and nerve passes under the posterior lip of the gland, and is called the inferior ligament of Schwalbe.

The anterior margin of the inferior ligament of Schwalbe and the free (lateral) margin of the levator aponeurosis defines a roughly oval opening, the lacrimal foramen.[21] Through the lacrimal foramen the orbital and palpebral lobes are continuous and the two to six ductules of the orbital lobe pass down into the palpebral lobe. The ductules from the orbital lobe mingle with those of the palpebral lobe and a total of 10 to 12 ducts penetrate the conjunctiva of the lateral superior fornix. These openings are usually found 4 to 5 mm above the superior margin of the upper tarsus, and sometimes extend as far as the lateral canthus.

The palpebral lobe occasionally prolapses with age, presenting an unsightly bulge in the upper lid. Resection of the palpebral lobe for cosmetic improvement or to reduce lacrimal secretion has been suggested, but clearly runs the risk of obliterating all lacrimal ducts. Some authorities have suggested that the reflex secretion of the main lacrimal gland is not normally necessary for the health of the eye,[24] but keratitis sicca has been reported as a complication of lacrimal gland resection.[25] Prolapse of the lacrimal gland may be corrected without resection of ductules or gland,[26] an approach that avoids the risk of keratitis sicca.

The accessory lacrimal glands have a histologic structure identical to that of the main lacrimal glands, except that they are smaller and distributed over the upper conjunctival fornix. Approximately 20 accessory glands, called the glands of Krause, are located along the apex of the superior conjunctival fornix (Fig. 1-8). The glands of Wolfring (Fig. 1-8), less numerous, are located just above the superior edge of the upper tarsus, sometimes invading the tarsal tissue. Hawes was unable to identify any accessory lacrimal glands in the lower eyelid.[27] No innervation to the accessory lacrimal glands has been identified; therefore, some authorities conclude that the accessory glands provide basal tear secretion while the main gland produces reflex secretion.[21] Other experimental work indicates that all lacrimal secretion is under reflex control.[27,28]

The deep mucin layer of the tear film is predominantly supplied by unicellular goblet cells of the conjunctiva. Most of these cells are concentrated in the conjunctival fornix, and in adults the bulbar conjunctiva contains very few goblet cells. Mucin is also provided by the complex crypts of Henle, located in palpebral conjunctiva near the peripheral tarsal margin. In perilimbal conjunctiva, humans have a few complex mucin glands named after Manz, who first described them in animals.

The superficial lipid layer of the tear film is mainly secreted by the meibomian glands, with a lesser amount contributed by the accessory glands of Zeiss and Moll. The meibomian glands are linear, running perpendicular to the eyelid margin in the connective tissue of the tarsus. Twenty-five to 30 glands are located in the upper tarsus and 15 to 20 in the lower tarsus. Each gland contains a single longitudinal duct that empties at the posterior lid margin. The meibomian orifices are arranged in a single regularly spaced row just behind the mucocutaneous junction. Meibomian glands are classified as sebaceous—characterized by a process of secretion whereby mature cells disintegrate to release their contents into the excretory duct. Elsewhere in the body sebaceous glands are associated with a pilosebaceous apparatus, and the meibomian

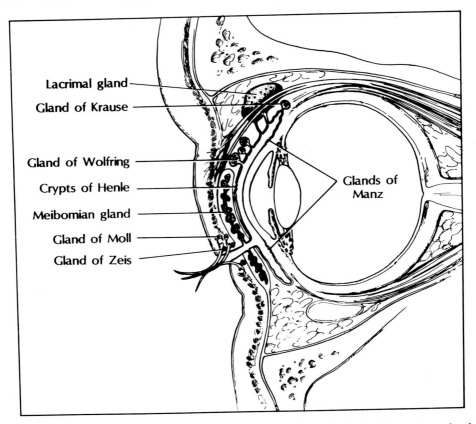

Lacrimal gland

Gland of Krause

Gland of Wolfring

Crypts of Henle

Meibomian gland

Gland of Moll

Gland of Zeis

Glands of Manz

Fig. 1-8   Cross section of the eye and ocular adnexa, showing lacrimal secretory glands.

glands probably represent a further specialization of this unit. Under stress, the meibomian glands are capable of an atavistic regressive metaplasia that results in the production of a hair shaft.[29] Thus, in inflammatory conditions such as Stevens-Johnson syndrome, a second row of acquired lashes may emerge from the row of meibomian orifices.

The glands of Zeiss are also sebaceous, and two lobules are found in association with each cilia follicle. These accessory glands discharge their secretions around the hair shaft. A single eccrine gland of Moll is also found associated with each follicle, which also discharges its secretions around the hair shaft. Eccrine secretion takes place by the decapitation of cytoplasm from the apical end of cuboidal secretory cells.

Innervation

The parasympathetic motor innervation to the lacrimal glands runs a complicated route (Fig. 1-9). Fibers originate from the lacrimal nucleus in the pons, close to the salivary nucleus.[30] Because the nucleus is so distinct, some authors

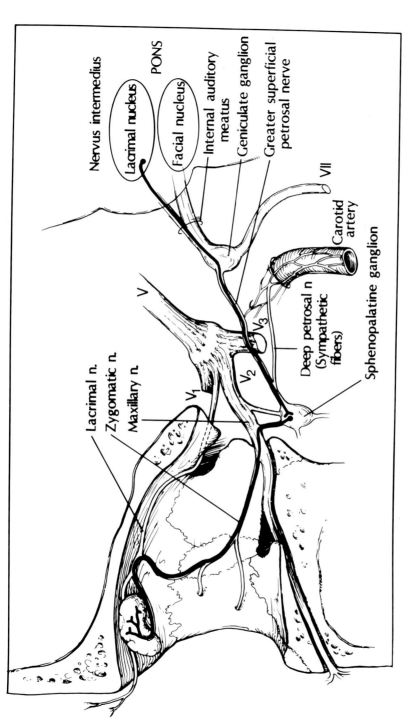

Fig. 1-9 Pathway of parasympathetic innervation to the main lacrimal gland. The pathway depicted from the sphenopalatine ganglion to the gland is widely accepted but has not been definitively proven.

have suggested that it be considered a separate cranial nerve.[22] Fibers exit the pons in the ventrolateral aspect of the cerebellopontine angle as the nervus intermedius. This fine nerve runs between the motor root of the seventh (facial) and eighth (acoustic) cranial nerves as it enters the internal auditory meatus. The fibers pass through the geniculate ganglion without synapsing, and turn away from the facial nerve as the greater superficial petrosal nerve. This nerve runs in a groove on the front of the petrous temporal bone. Under the gasserian ganglion it joins the deep petrosal nerve (sympathetic fibers from the internal carotid plexus) to form the vidian nerve in the cartilage over the foramen lacerum.[1]

The vidian nerve passes the pterygoid canal to the sphenopalatine ganglion, also referred to as Meckel's ganglion or pterygopalatine ganglion. This roughly triangular mass of cells, about 5 mm across, is located in the pterygopalatine fossa, just under the maxillary nerve. The ganglion is attached to the maxillary nerve by several short pterygopalatine nerves. The parasympathetic pathway from the pterygopalatine ganglion to the lacrimal gland has not been definitively demonstrated.[28] After synapsing in the ganglion, parasympathetic lacrimal fibers pass back to the maxillary nerve through the pterygopalatine nerves and enter the orbit with the zygomatic nerve. In the infraorbital groove the zygomatic nerve sends a branch up the lateral orbital wall to join the lacrimal nerve before it enters the gland. This branch probably contains the fibers to the lacrimal gland. The lacrimal nerve usually bifurcates as it enters the posterior edge of the gland, and the branch containing fibers to the lacrimal gland penetrates to the hilus. Fibers then pass peripherally with the ductules to innervate individual lobules of acini. The other branch of the lacrimal nerve passes forward, providing sensory innervation to the upper lid and superior conjunctival fornix. Sympathetic innervation is known to reach the lacrimal gland by at least two routes. Sympathetic fibers of the internal carotid sheath join the parasympathetic fibers to form the vidian nerve, and follow a common pathway to the lacrimal gland. Other sympathetic fibers pass into the orbit with the ophthalmic artery and follow the lacrimal artery to the main lacrimal gland. The role of sympathetic innervation in the control of lacrimal secretion remains unknown.

Vascular Supply

Blood supply to the lacrimal gland is provided mainly by the lacrimal artery, a branch of the ophthalmic artery and, therefore, of the internal carotid system. The lacrimal artery usually anastomoses with the anterior division of the middle meningeal artery, a branch of the external carotid system, through the distal tip of the superior orbital fissure. Terminal branches of the lacrimal artery also anastomose in the lids with the anterior deep temporal artery, another artery of the external carotid system. Occasionally, the infraorbital artery sends a branch to the lacrimal gland, establishing a third potential anastomosis between the internal and external carotid system in the vascular supply to the gland. Venous return from the lacrimal gland drains into the superior ophthalmic vein. Lymphatic drainage passes with the conjunctival system to the preauricular nodes.

CONCLUSION

The discussion of surgical anatomy is complemented by a review of normal histology in Chapter 10. Further instruction on gross anatomy of the nasal passages is contained in Dr. Haydon's description of nasal examination techniques (Chapter 3).

The student of lacrimal surgery who invests time in the reading of anatomy and dissection of cadavers will be rewarded in the operating room. Successful procedures accomplished with a minimum of blood loss, scarring, or complication are the result of anatomic knowledge.

ACKNOWLEDGMENT

This work was supported in part by an unrestricted departmental grant from Research to Prevent Blindness, Inc., New York, NY.

REFERENCES

1. Wolff E: The Anatomy of the Eye and Orbit. 4th Ed. Blakiston, New York, 1954
2. Jones LT: An anatomical approach to problems of the eyelids and lacrimal apparatus. Arch Ophthalmol 66:111, 1961
3. Werb A: The anatomy of the lacrimal system. In Milder B, Wei BO (eds): The Lacrimal System. Appleton-Century-Crofts, Norwalk, Conn, 1982
4. Bailey JH: Surgical anatomy of the lacrimal sac. Am J Ophthalmol 6:665, 1923
5. Whitnall SE: The nasolacrimal canal: The extent to which it is influenced by the maxilla and the influence on its caliber. Ophthalmoscope 10:557, 1912
6. Stranc MF: The pattern of lacrimal injuries in nasoethmoid fractures. Br J Plast Surg 23:339, 1970
7. Anderson RL: Medial canthal tendon branches out. Arch Ophthalmol 95:2051, 1977
8. Campbell W: The radiology of the lacrimal system. Br J Radiol 37:1, 1964
9. Schaeffer JP: Types of ostia nasolacrimalis in man and their genetic significance. Am J Anat 13:183, 1913
10. Busse H, Muller KM, Kroll P: Radiologic and histologic findings of the lacrimal passages of newborns. Arch Ophthalmol 9:528, 1980
11. Lemke BN: Lacrimal anatomy. In Bosniak SL (ed): Advances in Ophthalmic Plastic and Reconstructive Surgery: The Lacrimal System. Vol. 3. Pergamon Press, New York, 1984
12. Jones LT: Epiphora II. Its relationship to the anatomic structures and surgery of the medial canthal region. Am J Ophthalmol 43:203, 1957
13. Kuribayshi Y: Observations of the opening of the nasolacrimal duct. Report 2. Jpn J Ophthalmol 1:96, 1957

14. Rosengren B: On lacrimal drainage. Ophthalmologica 164:409, 1972
15. Maurice DM: The dynamics and drainage of tears. Int Ophthalmol Clin 13:103,1973
16. Hill JC, Bethell W, Smirmaul HJ: Lacrimal drainage—a dynamic evaluation. Can J Ophthalmol 9:411, 1974
17. Doane MG: Blinking and the mechanics of the lacrimal drainage system. Ophthalmology 88:844, 1981
18. Whitnall SE: The Anatomy of the Human Orbit and Accessory Organs of Vision. 2nd Ed. Oxford University Press, London, 1932
19. Stewart WB, Krohel GB, Wright J: Lacrimal gland and fossa lesions. Ophthalmology 86:886, 1979
20. Jakobiec FA, Yeo JH, Trokel SL: Combined clinical and computed tomographic diagnosis of primary lacrimal fossa lesions. Am J Ophthalmol 94:785, 1982
21. Jones LT, Wobig JL: Surgery of the Eyelids and Lacrimal System. Aesculapius, Birmingham, AL, 1976
22. Doxanas M, Anderson, RL: Clinical Orbital Anatomy. Williams & Wilkins, Baltimore, MD 1984
23. Anderson RL, Dixon RS: Role of Whitnall's ligament in ptosis surgery. Arch Ophthalmol 97:705, 1979
24. Jones LT: The lacrimal tear system and its treatment. Am J Ophthalmol 62:47, 1966
25. Scherz W, Dohlman CH: Is the lacrimal gland dispensable? Arch Ophthalmol 93:281, 1975
26. Smith B, Petrelli R: Surgical repair of prolapsed lacrimal gland. Arch Ophthalmol 96:113, 1978
27. Hawes MJ, Dortzbach RK: The microscopic anatomy of the lower eyelid retractors. Arch Ophthalmol 100:1313, 1982
27. Jordan A, Baum J: Basic tear flow. Does it exist? Ophthalmology 87:920, 1980
28. Linberg JV, Slade S: Lacrimal secretion after sphenopalatine ganglion block. Ophthalmic Plast Reconstr Surg 2:97, 1986
29. Anderson RL, Harvey JT: Lid splitting and posterior lamella cryosurgery for congenital and acquired distichiasis. Arch Ophthalmol 99:631, 1981
30. Crosby EC, Humphrey T, Lauer EW: Correlative Anatomy of the Nervous System. Macmillan, New York, 1962

2 | Diagnostic Tests and Imaging Techniques

Jonathan J. Dutton

The lacrimal drainage system is an intricate mucous membrane-lined conduit the function of which depends on a complex interplay of anatomy and physiology. Appropriate drainage of tears depends on a large variety of factors, including the volume of tear production, eyelid position, normal pump mechanisms, anatomic status of the drainage passages, gravity, and nasal air convection currents. The patient with symptomatic epiphora may have a normal anatomic system overwhelmed by an oversecretion syndrome, or a drainage system that is anatomically compromised and unable to handle normal tear production. On the other hand, a patient with partial drainage obstruction may have a concomitant reduction in tear production and therefore be completely asymptomatic. Patients with demonstrably reduced drainage function but simultaneous marked impairment of tear production may even suffer from symptomatic dry eye syndrome. The clinical picture of bothersome epiphora thus depends on the balance between tear production and tear drainage, not on the absolute functional status of either one.

The etiologies of lacrimal drainage dysfunction can be divided into two categories. *Anatomic obstruction* refers to a gross structural abnormality of the drainage system. This may be a complete obstruction, such as punctal occlusion, canalicular blockage, or nasolacrimal duct fibrosis, or a partial obstruction caused by punctal or canalicular stenosis, inflammatory narrowing of the duct, or mechanical obstruction within the lacrimal sac (e.g., by a stone or tumor).

In patients with *physiologic dysfunction*, epiphora results not from anatomic blockage, but from a failure of functional mechanisms. These may be caused by anatomic deformity, such as punctal eversion or other eyelid malpositions, but can also result from lacrimal pump inadequacy caused by poor

19

orbicularis muscle tone or eyelid laxity. The clinical distinction between anatomic and physiologic dysfunction, and determination of the exact location of the anatomic block, are essential if appropriate therapy is to be offered.

The clinical evaluation of gross lacrimal function is not difficult, and the diagnosis of epiphora can be made largely on history alone. However, determination of its etiology may be extremely difficult and often requires a variety of diagnostic procedures. There is no single test that will pinpoint the anatomic site or physiologic basis for tear production/drainage imbalance. A host of clinical tests have been described, many of which must be used together in order to diagnose specific disease processes adequately. In this chapter, we briefly describe the most important tests and imaging techniques and discuss their clinical significance.

CLINICAL DIAGNOSTIC TESTS

The following diagnostic tests have been devised to evaluate the tear production and lacrimal drainage systems. These include some simple clinical procedures that should be a routine part of every evaluation, as well as more complex radiographic and echographic examinations that are used in selected patients. In most cases of epiphora, a number of tests must be employed to determine the specific etiology and to plan appropriate therapy.

Clinical History

Clinical history is one of the most important aspects in the evaluation of the patient with epiphora, yet it is frequently glossed over or completely overlooked. Epiphora in a child with a history of tearing since birth is almost always the result of an imperforate Hasner's membrane, whereas acquired epiphora in a child may have a very different etiology such as canalicular obstruction. The use of ophthalmic drops (i.e., phospholine iodide) should lead the clinician to suspect canalicular occlusion, and a history of facial trauma should prompt radiographic examination of the nasolacrimal bony canal. Previous sinus surgery, particularly intranasal antrostomy or ethmoidectomy, should alert us to the possibility of duct injury. Epiphora associated with nasal obstruction or bleeding from the puncta or nose should raise the suspicion of a nasal, sinus, or sac malignancy. Intermittent acquired epiphora in an adult usually results from early inflammation of the membranous duct, but may be seen also with allergic rhinitis. A history of recurrent severe dacryocystitis not only suggests lower nasolacrimal duct obstruction, but potential stenosis of the proximal system as well.

External Examination

Evaluation of epiphora begins with a careful examination of the external ocular surface and eyelid structures. Conjunctival or corneal irritation, either inflammatory or mechanical, may cause hypersecretion with resultant epiphora, even in the presence of a normally draining system. Marginal blepharitis is a common condition associated with increased lacrimation. Eyelid malpositions such as entropion produce corneal irritation and secondary reflex epiphora. Lid laxity with ectropion may lead to corneal exposure and reflex lacrimal oversecretion or to physiological dysfunction due to a weakened orbicularis pump mechanism or punctal eversion. Mass lesions in the medial canthal region may mechanically obstruct tear drainage function. Careful palpation of the lacrimal sac will reveal the presence of a sac mucocele, and pressure behind the anterior lacrimal crest may produce reflux of mucopurulent material suggestive of lower system obstruction. A careful examination of the nasal vestibule must be made, since hypertrophic mucosa or the presence of polyps can obstruct the nasolacrimal ostium. Such findings during external examination will direct the clinician toward further specific diagnostic tests.

Schirmer Tests

In 1903, Schirmer described this technique for evaluation of tear production.[1] Since that time the Schirmer tests have become an important clinical tool for the diagnosis of dry eye and hypersecretion syndromes. The Schirmer I test is used to evaluate gross tear production. It is usually performed without topical anesthetic. A strip of #41 Whatman filter paper, 50 mm long and 5 mm wide, is folded 5 mm from one end, and the small folded end is placed into the inferior conjunctival fornix at the junction of the lateral and middle thirds of the lower eyelid. The amount of wetting on the filter paper is measured at 5 minutes. The test should be performed in subdued lighting, and both eyes must be tested simultaneously. This test measures the aqueous component of the tear film and does not distinguish between basic and reflex tear production. It gives only a very crude estimate of true tear flow. The paper itself may stimulate the reflex component. If the investigator is not careful to wipe the tear lake from the conjunctiva before inserting the paper strips, an excessive degree of wetting will be recorded. If the tear drainage system is functioning, a significant volume of tear flow passes into the puncta without being recorded. The fractional volume lost is in proportion to the adequacy of the drainage system and may be significantly more than the volume recorded.[2] Average wetting is between 10 and 30 mm in 5 minutes and varies with age, being greater than 25 mm in individuals 0 to 30 years old, and 10 mm or less in persons over age 60.[3]

If the Schirmer I test is abnormal, the test may be modified to separate the reflex component from basic secretion. A drop of topical anesthetic is instilled into the eye and the test is repeated. This test must be performed in the dark, since light can stimulate reflex tearing. Any combination of basic and reflex tearing may be found in patients complaining of dry eyes or epiphora, and the volume of this aqueous flow alone is not an indication of tear function.

When the Schirmer I test results are below normal, the Schirmer II test will give some indication of stressed reflex capability. Topical anesthetic is used in the eye, and the nasal mucosa is stimulated mechanically with a cotton swab or chemically with ammonium chloride. The amount by which the Schirmer II test exceeds basic production represents stressed reflex secretion.[3]

Rose Bengal Staining

Rose Bengal is a chloride-substituted iodinated fluorescein dye that stains devitalized epithelial cells. Increased conjunctival staining is a sensitive indicator of inadequate tear function, regardless of gross aqueous tear flow determined by the Schirmer test. In the patient with epiphora and significant staining, reflex hypersecretion and inadequacy of tear physiology should be suspected.

Tear Break-Up Time

Stability of the normal tear film depends upon its basal mucin layer, which increases the hydrophilic quality of epithelial cells, allowing uniform wetting of the corneal surface. When this mucin component is reduced, the tear film will bead up on the relatively more hydrophobic corneal surface. The tear break-up time is a simple clinical test for evaluation of this component of tear function. One drop of fluorescein is placed in the eye and the patient is instructed to blink once. Observing the corneal surface under slit-lamp magnification with cobalt blue illumination, the observer notes at what time dry spots appear in the tear film. Normal tear break-up time is between 15 and 30 seconds. A tear break-up time of less than 10 seconds indicates a probable mucin deficiency, which may result not only in the symptoms of dry eye syndrome but in reflex hypersecretion of the aqueous component and in epiphora.

Dye Disappearance Test

The dye disappearance test is usually performed as part of the primary Jones dye test (Jones I test). It is a crude measurement of the rate of tear flow out of the conjunctival sac. One drop of 2 percent fluorescein is placed in the lower conjunctival fornix and the amount remaining at 5 minutes is estimated on a 0 to 4+ scale where 0 represents no dye remaining in the tear lake and 4+ represents all the dye remaining. The test is most meaningful when both sides are compared simultaneously. Little or no fluorescein remaining in the conjunctival sac (positive test) indicates probable normal drainage outflow, whereas most or all of the dye remaining (negative test) indicates partial or complete obstruction, or pump failure. Care must be taken to note any lid overflow. Also, a significant amount of dye may disappear in the presence of a large dilated sac mucocele and distal obstruction. The test cannot distinguish between physiologic and anatomic causes of drainage dysfunction, nor can it localize the site of mechanical blockage. The dye disappearance test has been shown to be positive in 95 percent of asymptomatic normal individuals and may be more sensitive than the primary Jones test.[4] Unlike the latter, it does not appear to be dependent upon gross tear flow as measured by the Schirmer test.

Primary Jones Dye Test

In 1961, Jones[5] described a simple test of lacrimal drainage function that has become one of the most used procedures in the evaluation of epiphora. The primary Jones dye test (Jones I) is a true functional test and should be carried out in as nearly physiologic conditions as possible. The patient should be in an upright position, and should blink normally; topical anesthetic should not be used. For comfort, the nose is usually sprayed with 4 percent cocaine, although this probably somewhat alters normal nasal mucosal physiology. Two percent fluorescein is instilled into the conjunctival sac and a fine cotton-tipped applicator is passed beneath the inferior turbinate to the level of the nasolacrimal ostium after 2 minutes and again at 5 minutes. The test is positive if dye is recovered, and indicates patent anatomy and adequate physiological function. However, the dye may be difficult to recover, and false-negative results may be seen in up to 22 percent of normal individuals and in up to 42 percent of asymptomatic eyes in patients with unilateral epiphora.[6] Transit time for the dye to reach the nose is quite variable and shows a significant correlation with the Schirmer test. Even in eyes without epiphora, passage of dye into the nose may take considerably longer than the 5 minutes allowed for this test. Testing conditions may alter results since transit time is influenced by factors such as blink rate, gravity, and fluorescein volume.[7] Although a positive test strongly suggests a normal system, it does not completely rule out physiological dysfunction or mild anatomic obstruction. More significantly, a negative test alone does not necessarily indicate abnormal drainage.

The fluorescein appearance test, described by Flach,[8] is a modification of the primary Jones dye test. It is designed to avoid the difficulty and variability involved in recovering dye from the inferior nasal meatus. Two percent fluorescein is placed in the conjunctival sac and the oropharynx is examined with ultraviolet light, beginning at 5 minutes and continuing up to 1 hour if necessary. With this technique 90 percent of normal individuals are said to show oropharyngeal fluorescence within 30 minutes, and 100 percent within 60 minutes. This procedure is best used as a supplement to a negative primary Jones test; it should be used to examine the oropharynx 20 to 30 minutes later. Because of the persistence of fluorescence, only one eye can be tested by this technique during a single office visit.

In 1973, Hornblass[9] elaborated on a variation of the primary Jones dye test originally mentioned by Lipsius.[10] In this version 0.4 ml of 1 percent sterile solution of sodium saccharin is instilled into the conjunctival sac and the patient is asked to report when he or she tastes the solution. Hornblass found a mean transit time to the nose of 3.5 minutes, with 65 percent of normal individuals reporting a positive test within 6 minutes, and 90 percent reporting positive within 15 minutes. Transit times in excess of 15 minutes suggest partial nasolacrimal duct obstruction. The test depends on a subjective response from the patient, and before the solution can be tasted it must pass into the pharynx, where threshold taste sensitivity is quite variable. Lipsius noted that 3 percent of normal individuals were incapable of tasting saccharin.

Secondary Jones Dye Test

A negative primary Jones dye test suggests delayed transit time through the lacrimal drainage system; this may result from either physiologic dysfunction or anatomic obstruction. The secondary Jones dye test (Jones II) evaluates anatomic patency of the system in such cases. Residual fluorescein is flushed from the conjunctival sac and a topical anesthetic is instilled. The patient sits with head tilted forward while clear saline is irrigated into one canaliculus through a cannula, and is instructed to blow or spit any fluid that passes into the nose or pharynx onto a clean tissue. The presence of any fluid in the nose indicates gross anatomic patency of the nasolacrimal passages (Table 2-1). In this situation, complete obstruction is not present since saline did traverse the

Table 2-1. Interpretation of Clinical Tests in the Evaluation of Epiphora

Dye Disappearance Test	Jones I Test	Jones II Test	Probing	Palpation	Diagnosis
Rapid	+	+	Normal	−	Probable oversecretion
+	+	+	Normal	−	Normal vs functional
+	−	+	Normal	−	Normal vs functional vs mild NLD obstruction
+	−	+	Normal	+	Partial NLD obstruction & dilated sac
Slow	−	+	Normal	−	Mild NLD obstruction vs functional
Slow or −	−	+	Normal	+	Partial NLD obstruction
−	−	−	Normal	+	Complete NLD obstruction
−	−	+	Stenotic	−	Partial canalicular obstruction
−	−	−	Stenotic	+	Combined NLD & canalicular obstruction
−	−	−	Blocked	−	Complete canalicular obstruction

Abbreviations: +, positive; −, negative; NLD, nasolacrimal duct.

system under pressure. Recovery of dye-stained saline demonstrates normal punctal and canalicular anatomy, since the dye must have passed freely into the sac during the previous Jones I test. Such a result is compatible with a partial anatomic block at the level of the lower sac or duct. Recovery of clear saline without fluorescein suggests punctal or canalicular stenosis, with failure of dye from the primary Jones test to enter the lacrimal sac. If fluid does not reach the nose at all but regurgitates from the opposite punctum, a high-grade obstruction is likely. Regurgitation of dye-stained fluid suggests blockage at the level of the lower sac or duct, with residual dye in the sac being flushed out by the irrigation. Very rarely, a dilated canalicular mucocele may retain sufficient dye to produce similar results. Regurgitation of clear saline from the opposite punctum suggests obstruction at the level of the distal common canaliculus or upper sac with no residual dye from the primary Jones test. When clear saline regurgitates from the same punctum that is being irrigated without flow from the opposite punctum, a proximal obstruction in that canaliculus is likely.

During the irrigation of saline, distension of the lacrimal sac to palpation confirms the presence of lower nasolacrimal duct obstruction. Under such conditions a palpable sac without fluid passing into the nose suggests complete nasolacrimal duct blockage, whereas a palpable sac with fluid passing into the nose implies a partial obstruction.[11] However, a sac that is contracted and fibrotic because of chronic inflammation may not dilate under these conditions.

The secondary Jones dye test evaluates anatomic patency under increased hydrostatic pressure. When positive, it does not differentiate between epiphora caused by physiological dysfunction and epiphora resulting from partial anatomic obstruction. When a primary Jones test is positive, the secondary Jones test should always be positive as well, and is therefore unnecessary. With a negative primary test, a positive secondary test would be consistent with physiologic or partial anatomic dysfunction, but would rule out complete blockage. Negative results on both the primary and secondary tests confirm high grade obstruction (Table 2-2).

Probing

When the secondary Jones test indicates canalicular obstruction, the canaliculus in question should be probed gently to the lacrimal sac. The punctum may first be dilated by pulling the lid laterally to prevent canalicular kinking and inserting a pointed dilator. The distance of the stenosis or blockage from the punctum is noted in millimeters by measuring directly on the probe. In most individuals, a short common canaliculus is present 6 to 9 mm from the puncta. The canalicular system should not be probed without prior indication of possible obstruction because of the risk of inadvertent injury and subsequent fibrosis.

Table 2-2. Results of Primary and Secondary Jones Tests and Probable Sites of Lacrimal System Obstruction

Jones I Test	Jones II Test	Probable Site of Obstruction
+	+, Dye in nose	Patent system; normal vs low-grade partial obstruction vs functional; nonlocalizing
−	+, Dye in nose	Partial nasolacrimal duct obstruction vs functional
−	+, Saline in nose	Partial canalicular obstruction vs functional
−	−, Regurgitation from opposite punctum with dye	Complete nasolacrimal duct obstruction
−	−, Regurgitation from opposite punctum without dye	Complete common canaliculus obstruction
−	−, Regurgitation from same punctum with dye	Complete opposite canalicular obstruction with nasolacrimal duct obstruction
−	−, Regurgitation from same punctum without dye	Complete canalicular obstruction

DIAGNOSTIC IMAGING TECHNIQUES

Diagnostic Ultrasonography

The techniques of A- and B-mode ultrasonography provide a simple, non-invasive method of evaluating gross anatomic abnormalities of the lacrimal drainage system.[12,13] Physiological dysfunction cannot be evaluated, nor can the precise site of anatomic obstruction be localized. However, a dilated lacrimal sac can easily be distinguished from one of normal dimensions, and mucus within the sac can be differentiated from air or concretions.[14,15] Lacrimal sac neoplasms can also be detected.

With the B-mode probe oriented vertically, placed in the medial canthus, and aimed toward the lacrimal sac fossa, an oblique longitudinal cross section of the lacrimal sac and upper duct is obtained (Fig. 2-1A). The canaliculi cannot usually be visualized unless they are dilated.[15] The diameter of the sac and upper duct may be evaluated; thickness of the walls can often be appreciated; diverticula may be seen (Fig. 2-2A); and a variety of echogenic densities within the system such as inflammatory membranes and exudate (Fig. 2-3A) and tumors can be detected.[14] The position and size of a surgically created lacrimal-nasal ostium may also be imaged with this technique, although its patency cannot be evaluated (Fig. 2-4).

For precise measurements of the sac and evaluation of the internal reflectivity of sac contents, A-mode scanning must be used. The probe is first oriented as for a periocular orbital study, but with the beam aimed just behind the anterior lacrimal crest toward the sac fossa. An oblique anterolateral-posteromedial cut of the sac is thus obtained. If the sac is filled with air it appears as an echolucent defect bounded by sharply defined vertical anterior and posterior sac walls (Fig. 2-1B). Often the presence of dilated diverticula can be detected (Fig. 2-2B). Mucus in the sac produces uniform, homogeneous, low-

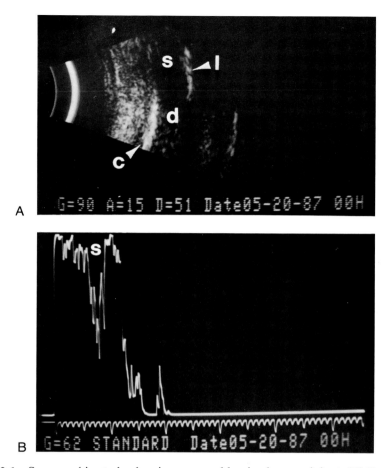

Fig. 2-1 Sonographic study showing a normal lacrimal sac and duct. **(A)** B-mode scan showing normal lacrimal sac (s) and upper duct (d). The anterior lacrimal crest (c) and the lacrimal bone (l) are easily identifiable landmarks. **(B)** A-mode scan showing normal appearance of the lacrimal sac. The sac (s) appears as a defect with sharply demarcated anterior and posterior walls.

density internal echoes, and inflammatory exudate and membranes show stronger, more irregular echoes (Fig. 2-3B). Multiple high-density, irregular echoes with infiltration of the sac walls suggest a sac tumor. A transocular A-mode image of the sac is obtained with the probe held above the lateral canthus and directed toward the lacrimal sac fossa. This technique gives an approximate horizontal cross section of the sac. The average dimensions of the sac in normal individuals is 2.5 mm (SD = 0.95 mm) in horizontal diameter and 4.0 mm (SD = 1.49 mm) in anteroposterior extent.[16] A sac more than 4.5 mm wide or 7.0 mm deep should be considered abnormally dilated.

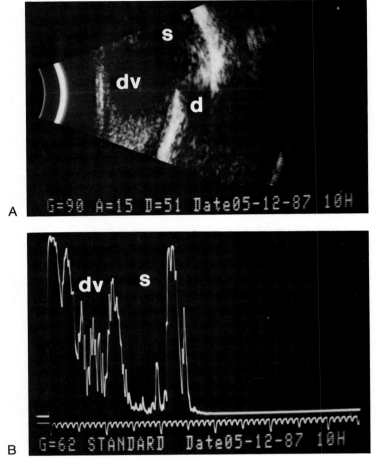

Fig. 2-2 Sonographic examination of the lacrimal sac in a patient with dacryocystitis. (**A**) B-mode scan showing a dilated lacrimal sac (s) and a massive anterior diverticulum (dv). Inflammatory thickening of the sac wall can be seen just above the entrance to the duct (d). (**B**) A-mode scan of the same patient showing the lacrimal sac (s) dilated to 8 mm and an anterior diverticulum (dv) filled with low to medium density echoes representing mucopurulent material.

Contrast Dacryocystography

The first attempt to visualize the lacrimal drainage system radiographically was made by Ewing in 1909.[17] He used bismuth paste for retrograde filling of the nasolacrimal duct. Such early attempts proved unsatisfactory, and the technique was used infrequently until the introduction of better aqueous contrast media such as Sinografin and Angiografin, and especially the low-viscosity

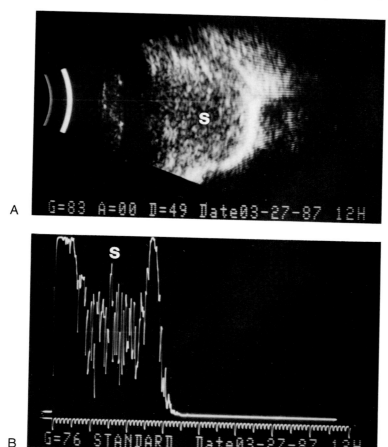

A   G=83 A=00 D=49 Date03-27-87 12H

B   G=76 STANDARD Date03-27-87 12H

Fig. 2-3 A patient with acute dacryocystitis. (**A**) B-mode scan aimed anterior to the lacrimal crest. A massively dilated sac (s) is seen with thickened walls and filled with medium-density inflammatory exudate. (**B**) A-mode scan of the same patient showing a sac (s) dilated to 15 mm filled with regular to irregular internal echoes of medium density.

iodized oils such as Pantopaque, Ethiodol, and ultrafluid Lipiodol. In a standard dacryocystography (DCG) study, contrast material is injected separately into one canaliculus on each side and films are taken immediately in Caldwell's posteroanterior frontal projection and in both lateral projections. Repeat films are obtained at 5 and 15 minutes.

A magnified image of the lacrimal system is obtained using Campbell's technique,[18] in which a microfocusing tube is used and the film plane is situated some distance from the positioning table. An extended Caldwell's view projects the petrous pyramids to the floor of the antrum and images the lacrimal system

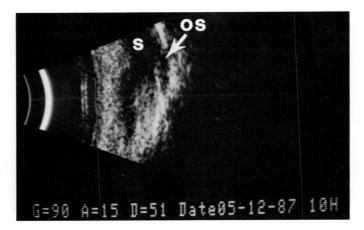

Fig. 2-4 Post-dacryocystorhinostomy B-mode scan showing the position of a surgically created lacrimal-nasal ostium (os). The lacrimal sac (s) is somewhat dilated because of soft tissue closure of the ostium.

against the ethmoid and maxillary sinuses. It also aligns the nasolacrimal canal approximately parallel to the film plane.

In 1968, Iba and Hanafee[19] described the technique of distension dacryocystography, first used by Barrie Jones in 1959. Here, films are taken during injection of 0.5 to 1.0 ml of contrast so that the lacrimal system is imaged in the distended state. Both sides are studied simultaneously and injection is accomplished through the placement of canalicular indwelling tapered Teflon catheters.[20] This method provides maximum visualization of the anatomic structure of the system and, because of the back pressure, gives good filling of the canaliculi. It is the best technique for demonstration of fistulae, diverticulae, supernumerary canaliculi, and the presence of stones and sac tumors.[21] However, it does not reveal sac and duct dimensions under normal physiologic conditions.

Improved imaging can be obtained with a technique adopted from subtraction angiography that eliminates confusing bony shadows. A scout film is taken before injecting contrast material and is used to produce bone-free images of the dacryocystogram.[22] More sophisticated computer-assisted digital subtraction images can be produced using fluoroscopically controlled angiographic equipment and an image intensifier.[23]

The dacryocystogram of a normal lacrimal drainage system will usually show the canaliculi when less viscous aqueous contrast media are used. The sac appears as a smooth, straight or gently curved passage with the concavity facing laterally (Fig. 2-5 to 2-7). The anteroposterior dimension is wider than the transverse. There is usually a constriction at the sac-duct junction caused by the split fascia of the orbicularis muscle as it passes around the system.[18] The duct widens at the level of the bony rim and the surface becomes more

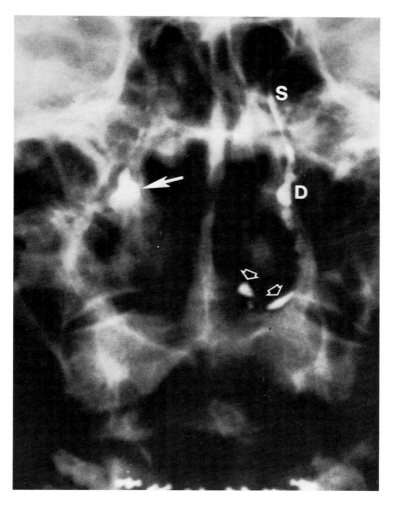

Fig. 2-5 Contrast dacryocystogram in a patient with unilateral epiphora on the right side imaged in Caldwell's anteroposterior projection immediately after injection of contrast material. The right lacrimal sac is dilated (large arrow), and an obstruction is noted at the sac-duct junction. The left system shows a normal caliber sac (S) and duct (D), and contrast agent is seen flowing into the nose (small arrows).

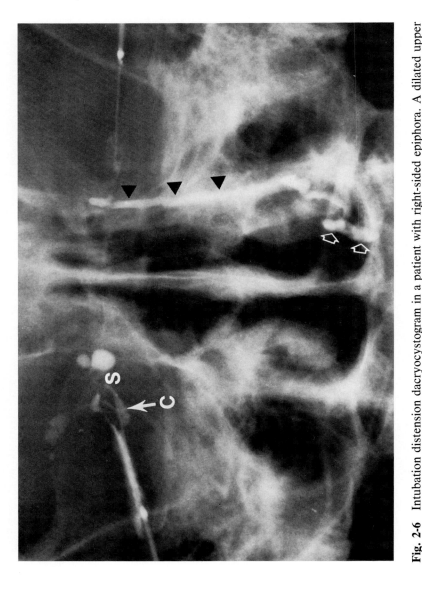

Fig. 2-6 Intubation distension dacryocystogram in a patient with right-sided epiphora. A dilated upper sac (S) and inferior canaliculus (C) are seen on the right side where an obstruction is present at the midportion of the sac. The left system shows an anatomically normal sac and duct (arrowheads) with contrast material present in the inferior nasal meatus (open arrows).

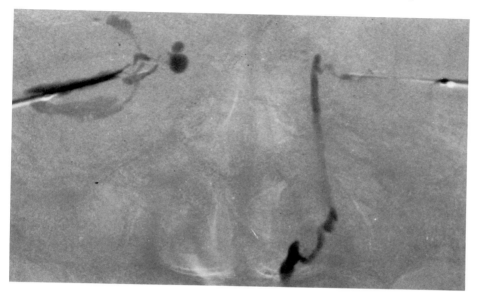

Fig. 2-7 Subtraction dacryocystogram of the same patient as in Fig. 2-6, with photographic elimination of overlying bony shadows.

irregular because of the presence of mucosal folds.[24] Such folds may be exceptionally well developed in younger children (Fig. 2-8). Further constrictions are seen in the duct's mid-portion in the region of Hytle's and Taillefer's valves. Finally, in its lower third, the duct widens again. Visualization by DCG reveals considerable variation in the structure of the sac and duct among normal individuals. Atypical narrowing and widening of the sac and duct, as well as unusual angulations and diverticula, may all be seen in the absence of clinical symptoms.[25]

A combination of subtraction, distension, and macrodacryocystography provides the best visualization of the anatomic structure of the lacrimal drainage system. This approach will provide accurate localization of any anatomic obstruction in approximately 86 percent of cases.[26] Imaging of the canaliculi with dye failing to pass into the sac or duct implies obstruction at the common canaliculus. Obstruction at the sac-duct junction usually results in a dilated sac with no dye reaching the duct or nose, even on late films. Obstruction at the level of the nasolacrimal duct will show dilatation of the sac, with dye in the duct, but not reaching the nose. A patent dacryocystorhinosotomy ostium is easily demonstrated by passage of contrast into the nose at the level of the middle meatus (Fig. 2-9). Demonstration of patent lacrimal passages by DCG in the face of epiphora suggest physiological dysfunction or a mild incomplete anatomic block.

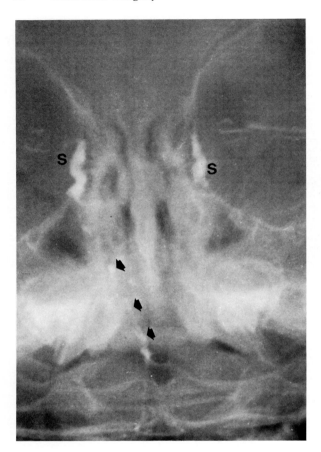

Fig. 2-8 Dacryocystogram of a child with congenital epiphora. Both lacrimal sacs (s) appear dilated. On the right side contrast material is seen passing into the nose under pressure (arrows), but the duct is not clearly outlined. On the left side the contrast fluid does not reach the lower duct. Deep mucosal folds are present bilaterally.

Radionuclide Dacryoscintigraphy

The first use of radionuclide tracer to image the lacrimal drainage system was by Bozoky and Korchmaros,[27] who used radioactive ^{198}Au and measured the buildup of activity over the sac and duct. Ursing[28] measured the disappearance of ^{22}Na from the conjunctival sac in rabbits. Rossomondo et al[29] introduced the first modern nuclear imaging technique for the lacrimal drainage system. They instilled a drop of saline with sodium [^{99m}Tc]pertechnetate, and imaged the system with a gamma camera. In the first clinical evaluation of the technique, Carlton et al[30] demonstrated its value in visualizing the lacrimal system, and in measuring some physiological parameters of tear flow. In their study of 28 asymptomatic volunteers they recorded a transit time for the nuclide of 4 to 43 seconds to the sac, and 4 to 323 seconds to the nose. There is a high degree of correlation between dacryoscintigraphy and contrast dacryocystography; the former is more sensitive to incomplete blocks, especially in the upper system.

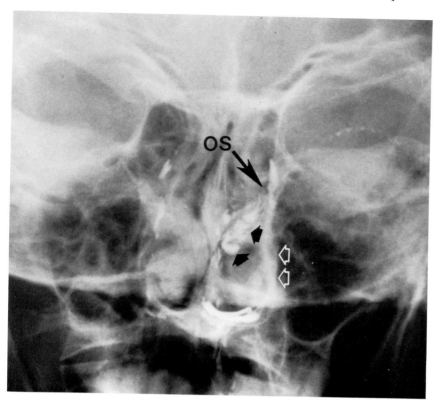

Fig. 2-9   Contrast dacryocystogram following a surgical dacryocystorhinostomy. Note contrast material flowing into the nose (short black arrows) through the patent lacrimal-nasal ostium (OS). Some contrast oil passes through the partially obstructed nasolacrimal duct (open arrows).

The technique commonly employed today uses [^{99m}Tc]pertechnetate in saline or technetium sulfur colloid delivered as a 10 μl drop to the lateral conjunctival sac by micropipette. The specific activity of this dose is in the range of 50 to 150 μCi, and results in radiation exposure to the lens of less than 2 percent of that for a complete contrast dacryocystogram.[31] The tracer is imaged by a gamma camera fitted with a 1 mm micropinhole collimator projected to the inner canthus. A sequence of images is recorded over a 15- to 20-minute period.

Dacryoscintigraphy does not provide the detailed anatomic visualization available with contrast DCG. In standard nuclear studies the proximal canalicular system is usually poorly imaged unless dilated. The sac and duct are usually well outlined (Fig. 2-10). Complete blocks in the sac or duct can be detected, although precise localization of the obstruction may be difficult (Fig. 2-11). However, the procedure can yield considerable information concerning

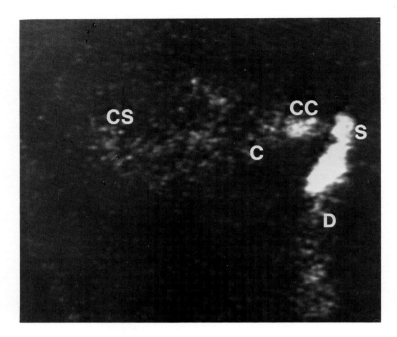

Fig. 2-10   Normal dacryoscintigram showing residual tracer in the conjunctival sac (CS) and canaliculi (C). Tracer is concentrated in the common canaliculus (CC) and lacrimal sac (S), and is seen filling the lower duct (D).

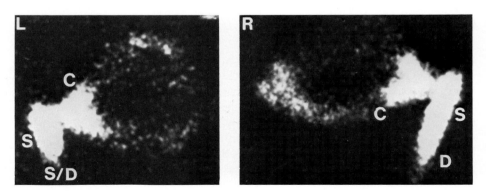

Fig. 2-11   Dacryoscintigraphy in a patient with unilateral epiphora on the left side. The right lacrimal drainage system fills normally, with tracer concentrated in the canaliculi (C), sac (S), and duct (D). The left system shows no tracer below the sac-duct junction (S/D).

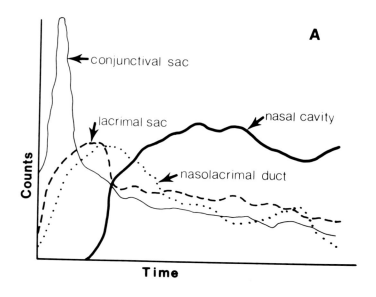

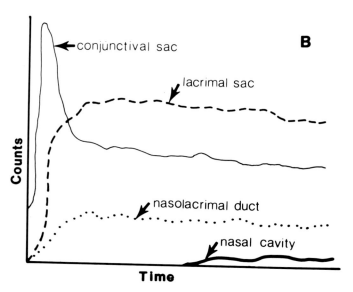

Fig. 2-12 Dynamic flow curves obtained from quantitative dacryoscintigraphy for four regions of interest in the lacrimal drainage system. (**A**) Normal curves obtained from the asymptomatic eye in a patient with unilateral epiphora. (**B**) Abnormal curves generated in a patient with partial nasolacrimal duct obstruction. (Drawn from data in Amanat LA, Hilditch TE, Kwok CS: Lacrimal scintigraphy. II. Its role in the diagnosis of epiphora. Br J Ophthalmol 67:720, 1983.)

physiological function. Generation of dynamic activity curves for specific regions of interest (conjunctival sac, lacrimal sac, duct, and nose) will demonstrate incomplete anatomic obstructions as well as rather subtle degree of functional impairment (Fig. 2-12).[7,32,33] This technique is most accurate and reproducible for the upper lacrimal system. Transit times become quite variable for the lower system, with 25 to 32 percent of asymptomatic individuals showing no tracer in the nose after 12 minutes. This is consistent with findings on the primary Jones dye test. By using more sophisticated rapid sequence display and computer interfacing for image optimization by contrast enhancement, background subtraction, and frame arithmetic, quantitative evaluation of tracer movement provides the most revealing interpretation of lacrimal function and tear flow dynamics currently available.[34,35]

Computed Tomography

In selected cases,[36] computed tomography (CT) of the lacrimal system can be extremely useful in the evaluation of epiphora. In axial scans through the lower orbit, the lacrimal sac fossa appears as a depression in the anteromedial wall (Fig. 2-13). In successively lower sections, the duct appears as a round-to-oval defect in the frontal process of the maxillary bone at the anteromedial corner of the antrum (Fig. 2-14). The duct may be filled with air or fluid. As

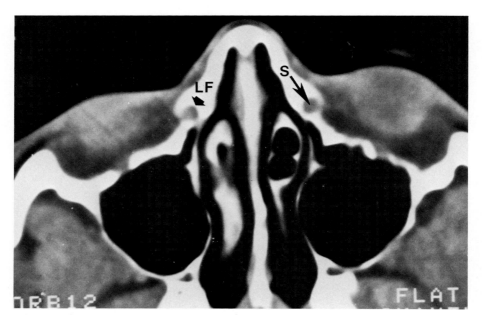

Fig. 2-13 Computed axial tomographic scan of a normal lacrimal system. The plane of section is through the lower orbit and shows the lacrimal sac (S). The lacrimal fossa (LF) appears as a depression in the anteromedial orbital wall. The sac is filled with mucus.

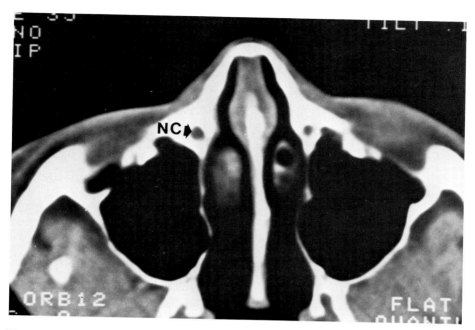

Fig. 2-14 Axial CT scan at the level of the nasolacrimal canal. The canal appears as a round defect (NC) in the orbital process of the maxillary bone at the anteromedial corner of the antrum.

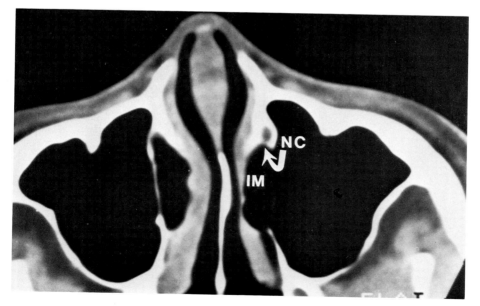

Fig. 2-15 Low section CT scan of the lacrimal drainage system demonstrating the normal nasolacrimal canal (NC) opening into the inferior nasal meatus (IM).

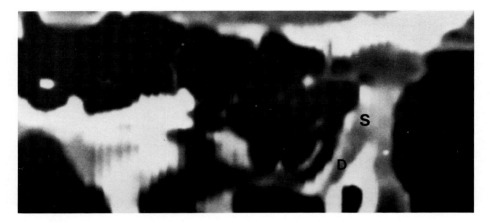

Fig. 2-16   Parasagittal reformatted CT image demonstrating a longitudinal cross section of the lacrimal sac (S) and duct (D).

the duct is traced inferiorly, it can be seen to open beneath the inferior turbinate (Fig. 2-15). Cross sections of the system are seen in coronal reformatted images since the line of section is oriented downward and obliquely backward. Parasagittal reformatted images will reveal the entire length of the system in longitudinal section (Fig. 2-16).

Although dilatation of the sac and dacryocystitis can be seen, these are

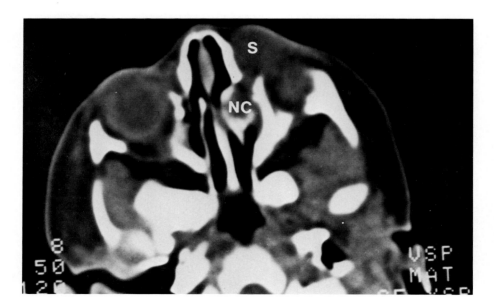

Fig. 2-17   Infant with a congenital cystic mass at the left medial canthus. CT scan shows an amniocele with a dilated lacrimal sac (S) and duct. The bony nasolacrimal canal (NC) is markedly enlarged.

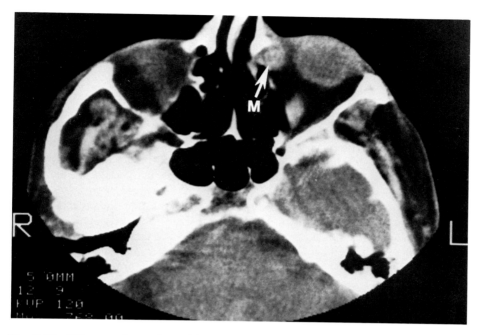

Fig. 2-18   CT scan of a patient with a four-month history of painless bloody discharge from the left lacrimal system. A mass (M) is seen in the left lacrimal sac. There is no bony destruction. Biopsy revealed a squamous cell carcinoma. (Spira R, Mondshine R: Demonstration of nasolacrimal duct carcinoma by computed tomography. Ophthalmic Plast Reconstr Surg 2:159, 1986).

more easily and inexpensively studied by other techniques. When epiphora follows trauma and subsequent clinical studies indicate nasolacrimal duct obstruction, CT may reveal orbital rim or maxillary fractures compressing the sac or duct. In cases of congenital lacrimal amniocele, CT will reveal the dilated duct, often associated with bony changes. It is essential to differentiate this soft, near-midline dilated sac from a meningocele (Fig. 2-17). In all cases of suspected malignancy, especially if there is a history of bloody epiphora or pain, a CT scan will demonstrate soft tissue masses of the sac or adjacent paranasal sinuses (Fig. 2-18).

OTHER DIAGNOSTIC TECHNIQUES

Percutaneous Contrast Dacryocystography

Radiographic imaging of the site of blockage in patients with epiphora has demonstrated a high incidence of common canaliculus obstruction.[16,32,37] When such blockages are complete, routine DCG is not possible, and the concomitant presence of lower sac or duct pathology cannot be easily demonstrated unless echography is used to detect a dilated sac. In 1972, Putterman[38] described a technique of percutaneous injection of aqueous contrast material directly into the lacrimal sac to bypass the occluded common canaliculus. In his small series of four patients there were no complications and results were good.

Chemiluminescence

Chemiluminescent material has proved a feasible nonradiologic technique for demonstrating the outline of the lacrimal drainage system and verifying its patency.[39,40] The luminescent agents are dimethylphthalate and tertiary butyl alcohol activated by dibutylphthalate, which produce an intense cold light. (The product is commercially used as a safety light.) When these agents are injected into the lacrimal system, the glow is visible through the skin and clearly outlines the upper system.[41] The lower duct is not readily demonstrated. The compounds are safe and nontoxic, if confined within the lacrimal system, but extravasation into tissues or onto the globe can produce severe complications of corneal scarring and vascularization, purulent infection, granuloma formation, and fibrosis.[42] Chemiluminescence has not yet been used extensively enough to evaluate its clinical effectiveness as an alternative or adjunct to other procedures.

Lacrimal Thermography

The canaliculi and lacrimal sac have been visualized by thermography, using an infrared scanner and color monitor with a resolution of 0.5° C.[43] The lacrimal system is easily differentiated from surrounding tissues by irrigation with cold water, and decreased temperature in the nose demonstrates patency. A large dilated sac can be visualized, and persistent inflammation will produce increased temperature within the sac. The duct is not demonstrated with this method.

In a related technique, a mini-thermocouple probe has been used to detect temperature differences within the lacrimal sac.[44] Increased temperatures are seen with vascularity and inflammation, and decreased temperatures with hemorrhage and mucocele formation. Nasolacrimal duct obstruction without associated inflammation shows no difference in temperature compared with the contralateral uninvolved side.

Dacryocystoscopy

Cohen et al[45] described a 1-mm diameter rigid endoscope for direct visualization of the lacrimal drainage system, as a supplement to other diagnostic tests. No clinical evaluation of the instrument has been presented, and its reliability in evaluating nasolacrimal obstruction remains to be demonstrated.

INTERPRETATION OF DIAGNOSTIC TESTS

Like many diagnostic tests in medicine, most of those described above require some subjective interpretation in order to determine the probable etiology of epiphora. Some knowledge of the variability in patient response, as well as of the reliability of the specific tests in suggesting pathology, are needed before meaningful conclusions can be drawn. The mere demonstration of lacrimal system pathology, either anatomic or physiological, does not indicate lacrimal dysfunction. Patients with significant degrees of partial or even complete outflow obstruction may be entirely asymptomatic as long as tear production and drainage balance are maintained.

Not every test mentioned here must be performed on each patient with epiphora. In most cases, a relatively simple clinical evaluation in the office will adequately demonstrate the cause of tearing and allow appropriate therapeutic decisions. Some cases, however, will present more difficult diagnostic challenges, particularly those with proximal system anatomic stenoses and physiologic dysfunctions. Here, more elaborate procedures, including radiographic studies, may be required.

In the face of a normal Schirmer test of basic and reflex tear response, the dye disappearance test can be a sensitive, though subjective, indicator of gross drainage. With a normally draining system, fluorescein should be almost gone within 5 minutes. Epiphora due to physiologic dysfunction or partial anatomic obstruction will show prolonged presence of dye in the conjunctival sac, whereas epiphora resulting from oversecretion syndrome with normal drainage should yield normal or even rapid disappearance of dye. It is important to realize that the rate of dye clearance through the lacrimal system is strongly influenced by the pressure head from above. Even in the presence of decreased drainage function, a large volume of fluorescein augmented by increased reflex tear secretion from conjunctival irritation may result in an artifactually rapid dye disappearance. It is therefore important to administer this test under conditions as nearly physiologic as possible, with the patient in an upright position, blinking normally, and receiving only one drop of fluorescein.

When the dye disappearance test is abnormal or the history strongly suggests inadequate drainage, the primary Jones dye test is usually performed next. In interpreting the results of this test it is essential to keep in mind that in up to one-third of asymptomatic individuals, dye will not be recovered in the nose after 5 minutes. It is also important to remember that this test strongly correlates with the results of the Schirmer test and therefore with the volume of fluorescein placed into the conjunctival sac. Like the dye disappearance test, an artifactually positive Jones I test may result from volume overload even when epiphora is present under normal physiological conditions. To be meaningful, the test must be conducted under as close to normal physiological function as possible. Only a small volume of dye should be used, the patient should be in an upright position, and blinking should be normal. Variants of the Jones I test, such as the saccharin taste test, add little, and, because of the often lengthy delay in patient response, are even more difficult to interpret. When the primary Jones dye test is positive, one may conclude that the system is grossly patent, although minor stenoses and physiological dysfunctions cannot be ruled out. When the test is negative, it is likely that significant anatomic or physiological pathology exists, but this test alone is not sufficient to document this conclusion.

When both the dye disappearance test is prolonged and the primary Jones dye test is negative, the probability of drainage dysfunction is greater than would be indicated by a negative primary Jones dye test alone. The secondary Jones dye test is then performed and, if negative, will demonstrate complete obstruction in the system. The results of the test will indicate the location of the block. When the secondary test is negative and saline irrigated through one punctum causes dye to regurgitate from the opposite punctum, then the blockage is probably at the level of the lower sac or duct, since the dye in the sac must be left over from the primary Jones test. If only clear saline regurgitates from the opposite punctum, the block is probably at the common canaliculus. Probing should encounter an obstruction at the distal canaliculus 6 to 9 mm from the puncta. If an obstruction or stenosis is not found, the test should be repeated with care. However, if there is a lengthy delay between the primary and secondary tests, there may be too little dye remaining in the sac to stain the regurgitating fluid.

When the secondary Jones test is positive, a low-grade partial obstruction or stenosis may be present that can be overcome by increased hydrostatic pressure, or failure of the lacrimal pump mechanism may be responsible for the negative primary Jones test and delayed dye disappearance test. Recovery of clear saline alone in the nose suggests partial canalicular obstruction since no dye entered the sac during the primary test. Appearance of dye-stained saline in the nose demonstrates free flow of fluorescein to the sac during the primary test and therefore an open canalicular system. The partial block is probably present in the distal system at the lower sac or duct. Retrograde flow out of the canaliculi may be seen even with a partially open duct if injection pressures are above 100 mmHg.[46] A negative primary Jones test and positive secondary test could also be compatible with intact canalicular capillary action, but with pump failure in propulsion through the lower system.

When hypersecretion syndrome has been ruled out and the dye disappearance test and primary and secondary Jones tests are all negative, a complete anatomic blockage is present somewhere along the nasolacrimal system. The results of the secondary Jones test will usually indicate if the block is proximal, requiring canalicular repair or bypass, or distal enough to be corrected with a dacryocystorhinostomy. If the results are equivocal, there is either a history of trauma, suspicion of tumor, recurrent epiphora following surgery, or persistent chronic dacryocystitis, then radiographic evaluation may be indicated to image the anatomic structure of the system and to pinpoint the site of obstruction. Dacryocystography clearly outlines the patent conduit of the lacrimal drainage system, but may not demonstrate low-grade stenoses that are easily opened when the distension technique is employed. Variations in normal anatomy include widened or narrowed sac or duct, diverticula, angulations of the system, or occlusions of one canaliculus,[25] all of which may give false-positive indications of pathology. The test does not easily visualize the canalicular system without intubation distension and subtraction, and gives no information concerning physiological function. Nevertheless, DCG gives the most reliable anatomic information available.

When the primary Jones test is negative and the secondary test positive, one must distinguish between physiological dysfunction and partial anatomic obstruction. In the absence of obvious eyelid or punctal deformity or atonic orbicularis muscle, the problem is most likely anatomic, and the secondary Jones test should indicate whether it is proximal or distal. Nevertheless, minor degrees of stenosis and functional failure due to eyelid laxity, a dilated sac, a diverticulum or a calculus cannot be differentiated with the above tests. Dacryocystography will usually demonstrate the presence of a stenotic segment.

If clinical and radiographic evaluation fail to show an anatomic blockage, physiological dysfunction is probably responsible for the epiphora. Radionuclide dacryoscintigraphy is indicated here, especially when used with computer interfacing for qualitative evaluation of function. Subtle functional abnormalities may be uncovered, particularly in the proximal system. However, the physiology of lacrimal drainage is poorly understood. The function of Rosenmüller's and Hasner's valves is complex, their competency varies with age, and their patency is influenced by hydrostatic pressure and volume.[46,47] The results of dacroscintigraphy are influenced by head position, blinking, and volume overload. A significant number of asymptomatic individuals will show some dysfunction with this test, making interpretation in patients with epiphora more difficult.

In summary, most patients with epiphora can be evaluated adequately with a few relatively simple office procedures. A small number of cases will require more sophisticated studies to confirm the site of anatomic block or region of physiological dysfunction. With the range of tests available, appropriate medical or surgical management can be determined in the vast majority of patients with tear production and drainage imbalance.

EDITOR'S COMMENT

Patients who complain of epiphora but have a patent lacrimal drainage system to gentle irrigation are a challenge to our diagnostic evaluation. If hypersecretion, eyelid malposition, pump failure, and proximal obstruction have been eliminated, then the patient is thought to have a partial or "functional" obstruction of the nasolacrimal duct. The ophthalmologist is now faced with a most difficult decision: will surgery be beneficial to the patient? After all, irrigation has demonstrated a patent communication with the nose, and the patient's complaints of intermittent epiphora may not be entirely convincing.

In this situation the editor has found that a dacryocystogram with a late film is very useful. A normal lacrimal drainage system will not retain radiopaque dye (Hypaque at body temperature) in the lacrimal sac for more than a few seconds. If significant dye is retained in the sac on a 30-minute delayed film, the real obstruction of the nasolacrimal duct has been objectively demonstrated.[48] In my experience, these patients report improvement with lacrimal surgery.

Since only the late film is of interest in these cases, the process of obtaining a dacryocystogram may be greatly simplified. I often inject the dye in my outpatient clinic, and then send the patient up for a single posteroanterior Water's view film. This approach avoids the need for separate appointments with radiology and the expense of a full dacryocystogram.

At least two surgical options are available for the treatment of these patients with functional obstruction of the nasolacrimal duct. Formerly, I performed a standard dacryocystorhinostomy, and it must be admitted that results were good. In recent years, I have been persuaded by reports in the literature, that silicone intubation is an effective procedure with less morbidity.[49] My initial experience with silicone intubation has been good.

The histopathology of the nasolacrimal duct in cases of early acquired obstruction (functional) has shown an intense lymphocytic inflammation (Chapter 10). For this reason, I have also added topical steroid drops to the treatment of patients with functional obstruction.

REFERENCES

1. Schirmer O: Studien zur Phisiologie und Pathologie der Tranenabsonderung und Tranenabfuhr. Arch fur Ophthalmol 56:197, 1903
2. Norn MS: Lacrimal apparatus tests. Acta Ophthalmol 43:557, 1965
3. Milder B: Diagnostic tests of lacrimal function. p. 71. In Milder B, Weil BA (eds): The Lacrimal System. Appleton-Century-Crofts, Norwalk, CT, 1983
4. Zappia RJ, Milder B: Lacrimal drainage function. 2. The fluorescein dye disappearance test. Am J Ophthalmol 74:160, 1972
5. Jones LT: An anatomical approach to problems of the eyelids and lacrimal apparatus. Arch Ophthalmol 66:111, 1961
6. Zappia RJ, Milder B: Lacrimal drainage function. 1. The Jones fluorescein test. Am J Ophthalmol 74:154, 1972
7. Chavis RM, Welham AN, Maisey MN: Quantitative lacrimal scintillography. Arch Ophthalmol 96:2066, 1978
8. Flach A: The fluorescein appearance test for lacrimal obstruction. Ann Ophthalmol 11:237, 1979
9. Hornblass A: A simple taste test for lacrimal obstruction. Arch Ophthalmol 90:435, 1973
10. Lipsius EI: Sodium saccharin for testing the patency of the lacrimal passages. Am J Ophthalmol 41:320, 1956
11. Frueh BR: The role of lacrimal sac palpation in evaluation of lacrimal drainage problems. Ophthalmic Surg 16:576, 1985
12. Rochels R, Hackelbusch R: B-Bild-Echographie bei Erkrankungen der ableitenden Tranenwege. Klin Monatsbl Augenheilkd 181:181, 1982
13. Ossoinig KC: Echography of orbital disorders. In de Vlieger M (ed): Handbook of Clinical Ultrasound. Wiley Press, New York, 1978

14. Rochels R, Lieb W, Nover A: Echographische Diagnostik bei Erkrankungen der ableitenden Tranenwege. Klin Monatsbl Augenheilkd 185:243, 1984
15. Montanara A, Mannino G, Contestabile M: Macrodacryocystography and echography in diagnosis of disorders of the lacrimal pathways. Surv Ophthalmol 28:33, 1983
16. Malik SRK, Gupta AK, Chaterjee S, et al.: Dacryocystography of normal and pathological lacrimal passages. Br J Ophthalmol 53:174, 1969
17. Ewing AE: Roentgen ray demonstration of the lacrimal abscess cavity. Am J Ophthalmol 24:1, 1909
18. Campbell W: The radiology of the lacrimal system. Br J Radiol 37:1, 1964
19. Iba GB, Hanafee WN: Distention dacryocystography. Radiology 90:1020, 1968
20. Lloyd GAS, Jones BR, Welham RAN: Intubation macrodacryocystography. Br J Ophthalmol 56:600, 1972
21. Hurwitz JJ, Welham RAN, Lloyd GAS: The role of intubation macro-dacryocystography in the management of problems of the lacrimal system. Can J Ophthalmol 10:361, 1975
22. Lloyd GAS, Welham RAN: Subtraction macrodacryocystography. Br J Radiol 47:379, 1974
23. Galloway JE, Kavic TA, Raflo GT: Digital subtraction macrodacryocystography. Ophthalmology 91:956, 1984
24. Milder B: Dacryocystography. p. 79. In Milder B, Weil BA (eds): The Lacrimal System. Appleton-Century-Crofts, Norwalk, CT, 1983
25. Rodrigeuz HP, Kittleson AC: Distension dacryocystography. Radiology 109:317, 1973
26. Keast-Butler J, Lloyd GAS, Welham RAN: Analysis of intubation macrodacryocystography with surgical correlations. Trans Ophthalmol Soc UK 93:593, 1973
27. Bozoky L, Korchmaros I: Uber die Untersuchung der Tranenableitung mittels radioaktiver Isotope. Zbl ges Ophthalmol 87:185, 1967
28. Ursing J: On the disappearance of radiosodium ions from conjunctival and subconjunctival deposits in the rabbit. A methodological study. Berlingska Boktryckeriet, Lund, 1967, p. 70
29. Rossomondo RM, Carlton WH, Trueblood JH, Thomas RP: A new method of evaluating lacrimal drainage. Arch Ophthalmol 88:523, 1972
30. Carlton WH, Trueblood JH, Rossomondo RM: Clinical evaluation of microscintigraphy of the lacrimal drainage apparatus. J Nucl Med 14:89, 1973
31. Brown M, El Gammal TAM, Luxenberg MN, Eubig C: Dacryocystography. Semin Nucl Med 11:250, 1981
32. Amanat LA, Hilditch TE, Kwok CS: Lacrimal scintigraphy. II. Its role in the diagnosis of epiphora. Br J Ophthalmol 67:720, 1983
33. Hilditch TE, Kwok CS, Amanat LA: Lacrimal scintigraphy. I. Compartmental analysis of data. Br J Ophthalmol 67:713, 1983
34. Hurwitz JJ, Maisey MN, Welham RAN: Quantitative lacrimal scintillography. I. Method and physiological application. Br J Ophthalmol 59:308, 1975
35. Doucet TW, Hurwitz JJ, Chin-Sang H: Lacrimal scintillography: Advances and functional applications. Surv Ophthalmol 27:105, 1982
36. Russell EJ, Czervionke L, Huckman M, et al.: CT of the inferomedial orbit and the lacrimal drainage apparatus: normal and pathologic anatomy. Am J Radiol 145:1147, 1985
37. Hurwitz JJ, Welham RAN: Radiography in functional lacrimal testing. Br J Ophthalmol 59:323, 1975

38. Putterman AM: Dacryocystography with occluded common canaliculus. Am J Ophthalmol 76:1010, 1973
39. Raflo GT, Hurwitz JJ: Chemiluminescent evaluation of the human lacrimal outflow system. Can J Ophthalmol 16:30, 1981
40. Cohen SW, Sherman M, Schwartz GG: Lacrimal outflow patency demonstrated by chemiluminescence. Arch Ophthalmol 98:126, 1980
41. Raflo GT, Hurwitz JJ: Assessment of the efficacy of chemiluminescent evaluation of the human lacrimal drainage system. Ophthalmic Surg 13:36, 1982
42. Vettese T, Hurwitz JJ: Toxicity of the chemiluminescent material Cyalume in anatomic assessment of the nasolacrimal system. Can J Ophthalmol 18:131, 1983
43. Raflo GT, Chart P, Hurwitz JJ: Thermographic evaluation of the human lacrimal drainage system. Ophthalmic Surg 13:119, 1982
44. Billington BM, Hurwitz JJ, Galbraith DJ, Gentles W: Miniprobe for lacrimal sac temperature measurement. Ophthalmic Surg 15:680, 1984
45. Cohen S, Prescott R, Sherman M, Banko W, Castillejos ME: Dacryoscopy. Ophthalmic Surg 10:57, 1979
46. Callahan WP, Forbath PG, Besser WDS: A method of determining the patency of the nasolacrimal apparatus. Am J Ophthalmol 60:475, 1965
47. Amanat LA, Hilditch TE, Kwok CS: Lacrimal scintigraphy. III. Physiological aspects of lacrimal drainage. Br J Ophthalmol 67:729, 1983
48. Milder B: Dacryocystography. p 79–88. In Milder B, Weil BA (eds): The Lacrimal System. Appleton-Century-Crofts, Norwalk, CT, 1983
49. Agrist RC, Dortzbach RK: Silicone intubation for partial and total nasolacrimal duct obstruction in adults. Ophthalmic Plastic Reconstr Surg 1:51, 1985

3 | Examination of the Nose and Paranasal Sinuses

Bennie L. Jarvis
Richard C. Haydon

Preoperative evaluation for lacrimal surgery includes examination of the nose and paranasal sinuses. The surgeon must assess mucosal health, the presence of associated infection, and most importantly, the presence of other pathology that may be responsible for intranasal obstruction of the nasolacrimal duct. Correction of such factors as hypertrophied inferior turbinates, nasal polyps, and malignancy may obviate the need for lacrimal surgery in some patients. Intranasal manipulations such as stent placement or control of hemorrhage may be required in the course of lacrimal procedures; familiarity with relevant anatomy will aid in the process.

ANATOMY OF THE NOSE AND PARANASAL SINUSES

Primarily formed of bone with an anterior cartilaginous component, the nasal cavity is lined with respiratory epithelium and divided into roughly equal halves by the nasal septum. Bony, mucosa-lined nasal conchae or turbinates hang from each lateral nasal wall. While the superior and middle turbinates arise from the ethmoid bone, the inferior turbinate develops separately. The inferior turbinate functions primarily to control the nasal airstream; the stroma of the inferior turbinate contains numerous vascular lakes which periodically engorge, causing alternate swelling and shrinking of the inferior turbinate and subsequent variation in size of the nasal airway.

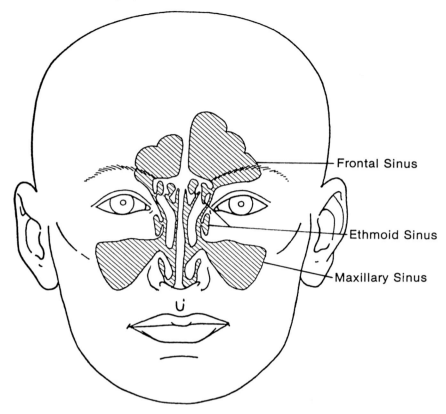

Frontal Sinus

Ethmoid Sinus

Maxillary Sinus

Fig. 3-1 Locations of the paranasal sinuses. The sphenoid sinus (not shown) is located posterior to the nasopharynx in the sphenoid bone.

Within the facial bones, air-filled cavities called the paranasal sinuses (frontal, ethmoid, sphenoid, and maxillary) communicate with the nasal cavity via openings beneath each turbinate (Fig. 3-1). Inferior and lateral to each turbinate lies a corresponding meatus or space, containing the ostia of the various paranasal structures (Fig. 3-2). The nasolacrimal duct opens directly beneath the inferior turbinate into the inferior meatus. The middle meatus contains a fissure known as the *hiatus semilunaris* into which the frontonasal duct and the maxillary sinus ostium open. The anterior ethmoid sinus, a group of interconnected air cells, communicates with the nose via the middle meatus, while the posterior ethmoid air cells open into the superior meatus.

The sphenoid sinus opens directly into the nasopharynx from the sphenoid bone at the level of the superior turbinate. A fourth supreme turbinate may arise above the superior turbinate. Olfactory mucosa extends from the cribriform plate to line the uppermost portion of the nose.

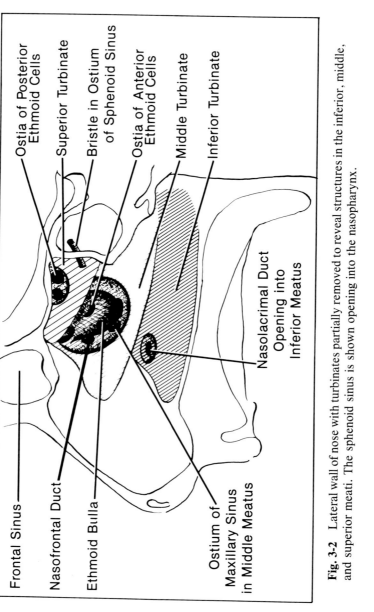

Frontal Sinus

Nasofrontal Duct

Ethmoid Bulla

Ostium of
Maxillary Sinus
in Middle Meatus

Ostia of Posterior
Ethmoid Cells

Superior Turbinate

Bristle in Ostium
of Sphenoid Sinus

Ostia of Anterior
Ethmoid Cells

Middle Turbinate

Inferior Turbinate

Nasolacrimal Duct
Opening into
Inferior Meatus

Fig. 3-2 Lateral wall of nose with turbinates partially removed to reveal structures in the inferior, middle, and superior meati. The sphenoid sinus is shown opening into the nasopharynx.

HISTORY

Any examination should begin with a thorough history. Important points to be addressed in the patient with epiphora include[1]:

1.   Unilateral versus bilateral blockage—while unilateral tearing is associated primarily with ductal obstruction, bilateral tearing often indicates a secretory problem
2.   Response to environmental irritants—pollen, dry air, smoke, etc.
3.   Associated allergic rhinitis or sinusitis
4.   History of recurrent dacryocystitis—recurrent dacryocystitis usually results from ductal obstruction
5.   History of facial or nasal trauma

TECHNIQUE OF NASAL EXAMINATION

Proper patient positioning is the key to successful examination (Fig. 3-3). Patients tend to slump in the chair with the head against the headrest, which makes the nose nearly impossible to reach or reposition. The patient must be

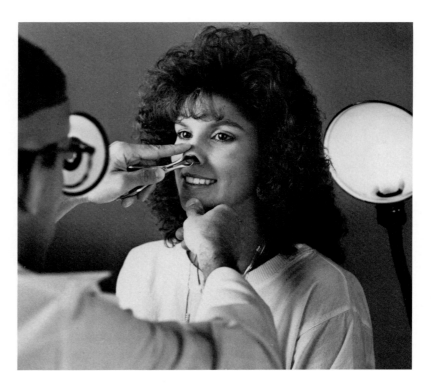

Fig. 3-3 Technique of nasal examination.

instructed to sit fully erect with hips back, knees together, and back away from the chair. The examiner sits close to the patient's left side with the patient's nose at eye level, and uses the right hand to adjust the patient's head position as needed.

Basic equipment for intranasal examination consists of a strong focused light source and a Vienna nasal speculum. The nasal passage may be likened to a long dark tunnel; an adequate light source is essential for seeing beyond

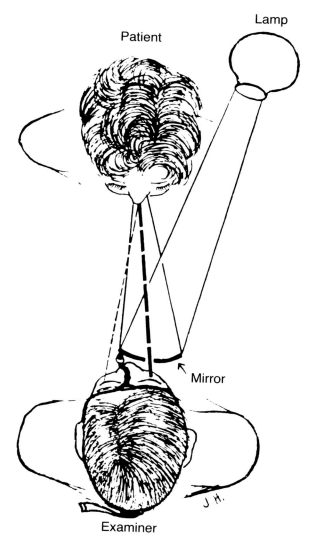

Fig. 3-4 Correct position for using the head mirror. Note right eye looking through mirror at focal point of reflected light. (Foxen EH: Lecture Notes on Diseases of the Ear, Nose, and Throat. 5th Ed. Blackwell, Oxford, 1980, p. 85.)

its entrance. With practice, a strong light focused on a head mirror provides superior visualization. The right-handed examiner places the head mirror over his or her right eye, with the back of the mirror touching the examiner's face or glasses (Fig. 3-4). A strong light shines from behind the patient's left shoulder, and the examiner positions the mirror to reflect the beam to a bright narrow point on the patient's face. Stereoscopic vision is possible only when the right eye actually *looks through* the mirror's central opening; to accomplish this, the examining physician closes the left eye and adjusts the mirror so that the reflected light on the patient's nose may be seen through the mirror.[2] It is not possible to examine all areas from one vantage point; repeated readjustment of the patient's head position is necessary.

Despite its superiority as a light source, the head mirror requires practice and has fallen out of general use; either a fiberoptic headlight or an indirect ophthalmoscope provides a useful alternative. It is *not* sufficient to peer into the nasal vestibule with a hand-held otoscope; neither adequate examination nor manipulation are possible with this instrument.

The right-handed examiner holds the nasal speculum with the last three fingers of the left hand, using the index finger to steady the hand against the nose (Fig. 3-5). The right hand is used for instrumentation and to readjust the patient's head as required. The speculum is gently inserted into the nasal vestibule and opened widely without exerting medial pressure on the highly sensitive nasal septum (Fig. 3-3). Children are often frightened by the speculum and become difficult to examine; turning the tip of the nose up and back with

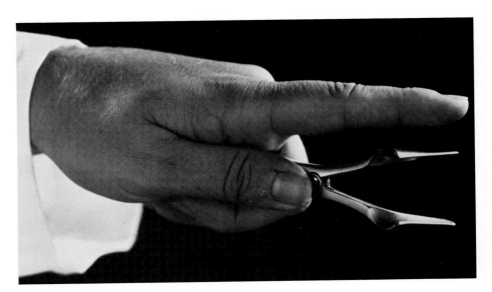

Fig. 3-5 Correct method of holding the nasal speculum. Extended forefinger will rest on patient's nasal tip to steady the hand.

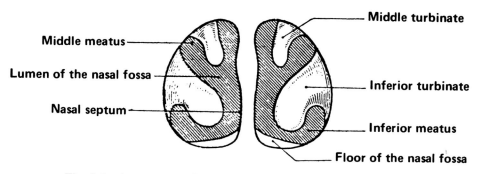

Middle meatus

Lumen of the nasal fossa

Nasal septum

Middle turbinate

Inferior turbinate

Inferior meatus

Floor of the nasal fossa

Fig. 3-6   Appearance of the nasal cavity on anterior rhinoscopy.

the examiner's thumb may afford adequate visualization in very young patients.[3]

Examination proceeds in a systematic fashion by looking first at the vestibule, then down at the nasal floor, inferior turbinate and lower septum, and finally upward at the middle meatus, middle turbinate, and superior septum (Fig. 3-6). The nose should be examined before and after vasoconstriction with 0.25 percent phenylephrine hydrochloride or 1 percent ephedrine hydrochloride spray.

Common errors[4] include:

1. Using inadequate lighting or failing to keep the light sharply focused
2. Improper patient positioning
3. Using a nasal speculum that is too large or too small to allow adequate visualization
4. Failing to open the speculum wide (a wide-open speculum will not compromise patient comfort if the examiner takes care to avoid pressing against the septum)
5. Failing to begin the examination with the patient's head in a neutral position (the nasal floor and turbinates extend backward at right angles to the patient's face, not upward along the bridge of the nose; thus, the inferior turbinate and nasal floor are best seen with the head erect)
6. Failing to adjust the patient's head position in order to see all parts of the nose
7. Neglecting to use vasoconstrictors

PHYSICAL FINDINGS

External Nose

Examine the external nose for structural deformity or indications of old trauma such as a crooked dorsum or displaced nasal bones. Also note any crusting, ulceration, or granular lesions.

Vestibule

The vestibule, which is rarely involved in intranasal disease, is lined with skin rather than mucosa. It is often more easily examined without the nasal speculum.

Mucosa

The remainder of the nasal cavity except for the olfactory area is lined with respiratory epithelium, which is normally moist and deep pink in color. Mucosal changes are generally most marked on the inferior and middle turbinates; inflammation results in erythema and edema, while the mucosa in allergic disease generally appears pale gray and boggy. Dry, atrophic mucosa with crusting suggests atrophic rhinitis.

Nasal Floor

Foreign bodies are often missed if the examiner fails to look directly down and along the floor of the nose. Ulcerations or masses in this area may arise from the oral cavity.[3]

Septum

The nasal septum is rarely perfectly straight; only deviations severe enough to obstruct the airway are considered significant. Examine the septum along its length for crusting, ulcerations, and mass lesions. Crusting and bleeding may occur at the site of a nasal septal deviation; another common site of bleeding is Keisselbach's plexus of blood vessels on the anterior septum. Septal perforations are often asymptomatic, but may cause problems with crusting, bleeding, or whistling sounds. Ulceration may occur secondary to trauma, atrophic rhinitis, malignancy, or granulomatous disease. Adhesions between the septum and turbinates may also occur, usually as a result of trauma or surgery.

Lateral Wall

The inferior turbinate, the largest turbinate, lies along the inferior portion of the lateral wall of the nose. The inferior turbinates alternately swell and decongest as part of the normal nasal cycle, so that they are rarely equal in size. When the septum deviates to one side, the opposite turbinate may enlarge to fill the concavity; turbinate hypertrophy also results from allergic or inflammatory disease. Hypertrophy or lateral displacement of the inferior turbinate may lead to obstruction of the nasolacrimal duct, which opens just beneath the overhanging turbinate in the anterior inferior meatus. Examination before and after vasoconstriction may help determine underlying pathology and delineate mucosal changes such as the pale, boggy mucosa of allergic disease.

The middle turbinate arises superiorly and posteriorly on the lateral wall of the nose, sometimes partially hidden by a deviated septum. Though not composed of erectile tissue, the middle turbinate may be enlarged by the presence of an anterior ethmoid air cell. Polypoid changes in the middle turbinate mucosa commonly occur in chronic inflammatory or allergic states.

The ostia of the frontal, maxillary, and anterior ethmoid sinuses drain beneath the middle turbinate into the middle meatus; erythematous nasal mucosa and purulent discharge in the middle meatus may be seen in sinusitis.[4] Nasal polyps appear as glistening, smooth, cystic masses originating high in the nose, usually from the middle meatus; they are fairly mobile, not tender, and do not bleed easily. Though sometimes confused with neoplasms, nasal polyps actually represent extensions of diseased mucosa from the maxillary or ethmoid sinuses, usually in patients with uncontrolled allergic disease.[5] The superior turbinate, superior meatus, and olfactory area are not seen via anterior rhinoscopy.

Neoplasms

Intranasal neoplasms often cause unilateral nasal obstruction, and epiphora may be noted secondary to occlusion of the nasolacrimal duct. Papilloma, the most common benign tumor of the sinonasal tract, appears as an elevated keratotic mass with a fine granular surface. Fifty percent of these neoplasms originate on the septum. These are usually asymptomatic; however, inverting papilloma, arising from the lateral nasal wall or antrum, may be locally invasive.

Squamous cell carcinomas represent 50 to 80 percent of intranasal malignancies. They usually arise from the lateral nasal wall. Most of these lesions demonstrate bony invasion by the time of diagnosis. A rare variant, verrucous carcinoma, is often mistaken for papilloma.

Malignant melanoma, the second most common intranasal malignancy, appears as a pigmented necrotic mass with obvious bony destruction. Other neuroectodermal tumors such as schwannomas, neurofibromas or meningiomas may also present as intranasal masses, often resembling benign nasal polyps.[6]

EXAMINATION OF THE PARANASAL SINUSES

The continuity of nasal and sinus mucosa results in intimate interrelation of nasal and sinus pathology; nasal examination, therefore, must include evaluation of the paranasal sinuses. As described, anterior rhinoscopy may reveal purulent discharge from the sinus ostia as well as intranasal extension of a mass or polyp. Palpation may elicit tenderness over the anterior maxillary wall in maxillary sinusitis, over the medial orbital rim in ethmoid sinusitis and upward toward the medial aspect of the superior orbital rim in frontal sinusitis. Infection, mucocele, or malignancy may result in visible edema or fullness over the various sinuses; asymmetric findings provide the most useful information. It is not possible to evaluate the sphenoid sinus directly via physical examination; diagnosis of sphenoid sinus disease relies on radiography and invasive procedures.

Transillumination of the maxillary and frontal sinuses rests upon the principle that abnormalities such as fluid or thickened mucosa will alter transmission of light through the hollow sinus cavity. Maxillary sinus transillumination is performed in a darkened room by having the patient hold a bright light in the mouth with the lips closed; normally the pupils appear red, the sinuses glow, and crescents of light are seen under the eyes (Fig. 3-7). Transillumination aids in diagnosis only if one sinus transilluminates more clearly than the other, since the amount of light transmitted varies widely among patients. Because of the frequency of asymmetric development, transillumination of the frontal sinus is not usually helpful.[4]

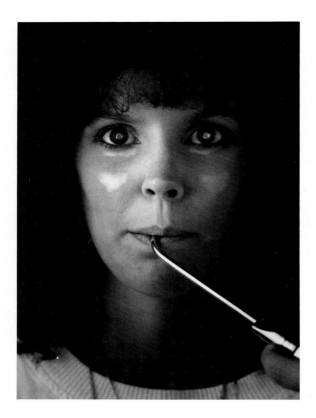

Fig. 3-7 Transillumination of the maxillary sinus, showing areas of normal transillumination.

REFERENCES

1. Moazed KT, Cooper WC: Dacryocystorhinostomy. p. 224. In Blitzer A, Lawson W, Friedman WH (eds): Surgery of the Paranasal Sinuses. WB Saunders, Philadelphia, 1985

2. Foxen EH: Lecture Notes on Diseases of the Ear, Nose and Throat. 5th Ed. Blackwell, Oxford, 1980, p. 85

3. Jones RM: Examination of the nose. p. 1. In Ballantyne J, Groves J (eds): Scott-Brown's Diseases of the Ear, Nose and Throat. 3rd Ed. Vol. 3. Butterworths, London, 1971

4. DeWeese DD, Saunders WM: Textbook of Otolaryngology, 5th Ed. CV Mosby, St. Louis, 1977

5. English GM: Nasal polyposis. Ch. 19. In English GM: Otolaryngology. Vol. 2. Harper & Row, Philadelphia, 1987

6. Hyams VJ: Pathology of the nose and paranasal sinuses. Ch. 8. In English GM: Otolaryngology. Vol. 2. Harper & Row, Philadelphia, 1987

4 | Eyelid Malpositions

Jeffrey A. Nerad

The relationship between eyelid malpositions and tearing has been recognized for thousands of years. The first major medical work, the "Papyrus Ebers" (ca. 1500 BC) described ectropion, entropion, and trichiasis. Written accounts of ectropion may be found in the Bible. In 1474, Grassus hypothesized that an "excess of phlegmatic humor" (lacrimal secretions) was the cause, rather than the result, of ectropion. At the beginning of the nineteenth century Scarpa recognized that ectropion led to "continual discharge of tears onto the cheek, aridity of the eyeball, chronic ophthalmia, intolerance to light and eventually ulceration of the cornea."[1] Over the following two centuries the etiologies of eyelid malformations have been more clearly identified. A myriad of operations and modifications have been described to relieve epiphora and related eye conditions attributed to lid malpositions.

When evaluating the patient with epiphora, the surgeon must recognize and treat any eyelid abnormalities before recommending surgery on the lacrimal sac or nasolacrimal duct. Changes in the eyelid anatomy and function as a result of aging or trauma may affect the normal drainage of tears. Subtle scarring or paralysis may alter the function of the lacrimal pump. Ectropion of the punctum or entire eyelid may prevent tears from reaching the canaliculi. Entropion and trichiasis can cause ocular irritation and reflex tearing that will surpass the capacity for normal tear drainage. Identification and appropriate treatment of these eyelid problems will correct the patient's epiphora.

THE LACRIMAL PUMP

Tear drainage depends on normal eyelid anatomy and function as well as on an intact nasolacrimal sac and duct. The orbicularis muscle is intimately related to the lacrimal sac through fascial and tendinous connections around the sac known as the "lacrimal diaphragm." It has been suggested that move-

61

ments of the eyelids by orbicularis contraction serve as a "lacrimal pump" that opens and closes the sac. Jones[2] identified two parts of the palpebral orbicularis muscle; the pretarsal and preseptal portions. The origins of these muscles are at the medial canthus, and each has two heads, superficial and deep. Each pretarsal muscle is formed by the junction of Horner's muscle (deep head) with the superficial head from the anterior limb of the medial canthal tendon. The deep head of the pretarsal muscle (Horner's muscle) originates on the posterior lacrimal crest and inserts around the ampulla of each canaliculus. The superficial head arises from the anterior limb of the medial canthal tendon and inserts on the tarsal plate. Each preseptal muscle consists of a deep head (Jones' muscle) that arises from the lacrimal fascia, and a superficial head that arises from the medial canthal tendon.

The pretarsal muscles, preseptal muscles, and lacrimal diaphragm have been termed the "lacrimal pump." Jones[2] wrote that as the orbicularis contracted the sac opened, causing a negative pressure in the sac, which helped to suck tears away from the eye. The action is summarized as follows:

1.   With the lids open, capillary action draws tears from the tear lake into the open ampulla of the canaliculus. The sac is collapsed.
2.   Eyelid closure causes a medial movement of the canaliculi (via Horner's muscle) accompanied by closure of the puncta. Continued contraction shortens the canaliculus, and tears are forced medially.
3.   The deep heads of the preseptal muscles simultaneously pull the lacrimal diaphragm laterally, creating a negative pressure in the tear sac.
4.   As the lids open, the sac collapses and tears are forced into the nasolacrimal duct. Tears collect in the canaliculus, and the cycle repeats.

There is much debate over the validity of the details of this theory; however, it is clear that normal eyelid function is essential for tear drainage. Eyelid malpositions, paralysis of the lids, or abnormal stiffness or contracture of the eyelids affect the integrity of the lacrimal pump and the drainage of tears.

ECTROPION

Ectropion of the eyelid is characterized by a turning of the eyelid margin away from the eyeball. A separation of the eyelid from the globe is usually associated with the turning of the lid. As the eyelid turns outward, conjunctival exposure occurs and the patient complains of a red eyelid margin often accompanied by tearing. As exposure becomes chronic, metaplastic changes in the palpebral conjunctiva lead to keratinization (Fig. 4-1). Corneal exposure results in inferior punctate keratopathy and, rarely, in corneal ulceration. Epiphora increases because exposure causes increased reflex tearing. Rubbing the eyes and wiping away the tears exacerbate the problem. The tear meniscus enlarges, and excess tears are squeezed out of the eye onto the face. Often patients complain that their vision is disturbed as though they are looking

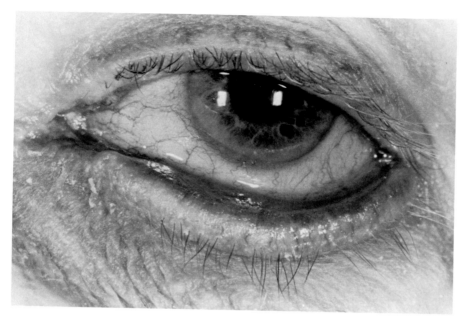

Fig. 4-1 Ectropion of lower lid. There is keratinization of the palpebral conjunctiva.

through water. Mucus and particulate matter in the tear lake may cause intermittent blurring of vision.

In 1713, Peter Kennedy gave one of the first descriptions of the etiology of ectropion.[1] He attributed ectropion ("lower eyelid falling down or inside out") to the "relaxation and weakness of the orbicular muscle of the inferior eyelid." In essence, Kennedy's thoughts remain correct today. Lid laxity or horizontal lid elongation is an etiologic factor in all types of ectropion.

In the beginning of the nineteenth century Scarpa divided ectropion into two broad categories: a "pretarsal tumefaction of the palpebrae" (involutional etiology) and a shortening of the skin that covers the eyelid (cicatricial etiology).[1] A third etiology of ectropion is recognized today, the paralytic form. Absence of innervation to the orbicularis, generally in association with lid laxity, may cause ectropion.

Involutional Ectropion

By far the most common form of lower lid ectropion is the involutional form. The primary mechanism is laxity of the eyelid associated with stretching of the canthal tendons. The tarsal plate is thought to remain unchanged.

The onset of involutional ectropion is gradual. Often the first sign of lid laxity will appear medially as a *punctal eversion*. On slit lamp examination,

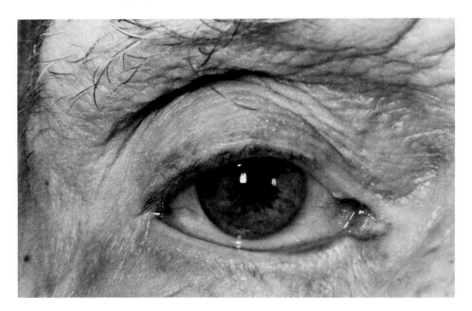

Fig. 4-2   Medial ectropion. Punctum is not apposed to eyeball.

the punctum should appose the globe and not be visible without pulling the lid downward. If the punctum is pointing straight up or outward, there is punctal eversion. As the lid laxity increases, the medial portion of the lid will turn outwards. *Medial ectropion* (Fig. 4-2) is more common than a localized lateral ectropion; however, ectropion may occur anywhere on the lid. Often, gradual worsening of the condition will lead to ectropion of the entire lid.

Lid laxity may be demonstrated by the *pinch test*.[3] (Fig. 4-3) If the lower lid can be distracted more than 6 mm from the globe, the lid is lax. An approximation of eyelid elasticity can be made by pulling the lid down from the globe and allowing it to snap back into place.[4] (Fig. 4-4) If the lid returns to normal position without blinking, lid laxity is absent. If one or more blinks are required to place the lid into normal position, laxity is present. Measurements are seldom made with these tests, but a qualitative estimation of the eyelid support can be obtained easily.

Lid laxity associated with involutional ectropion is thought to be caused by stretching of the canthal tendons rather than elongation of the tarsal plate. Older patients may complain that their eyes appear smaller than when they were young. Narrowing of the vertical measurements of the palpebral fissures occurs because of stretching or dehiscence of the levator aponeurosis and lower lid retractors. Similarly, the horizontal dimensions of the palpebral fissures narrow because of canthal tendon lengthening. Lateral tendon laxity will be evident by rounding or blunting of the lateral canthus. Medial canthal tendon

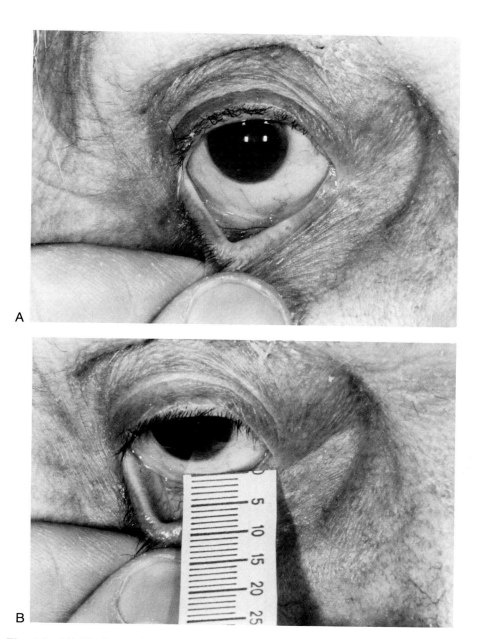

Fig. 4-3 (A) Pinch test demonstrating lid laxity. (B) More than 6 mm of distraction is abnormal.

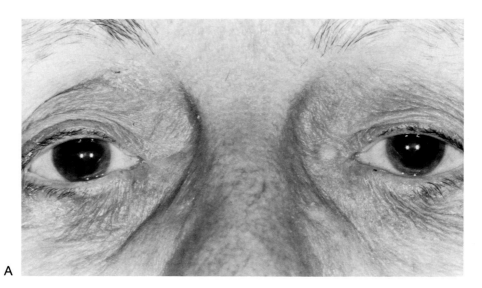

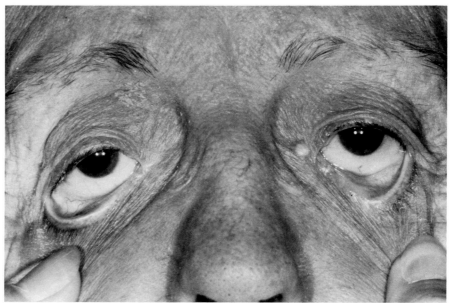

Fig. 4-4 Snap test. (**A**) Eyelids resting in the normal position. (**B**) The eyelids are retracted. (*Figure continues.*)

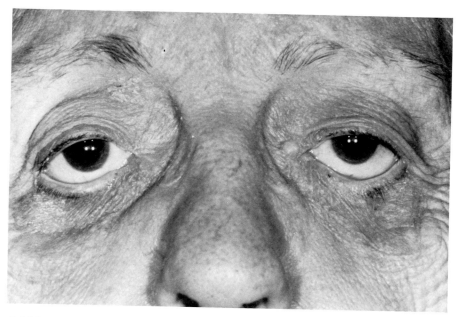

C

Fig. 4-4 (*Continued*). (**C**) When released, the eyelids do not immediately return to normal resting position. (Note: Left lower lid punctum is marked.)

laxity is demonstrated when stretching the lid temporally causes the punctum to be pulled at or lateral to the nasal limbus (Fig. 4-5).

The treatment of involutional ectropion is directed at repair of the lid laxity by shortening the lower lid. Numerous operations have been devised over the years to accomplish this goal. In 1812, Adams described a V-shaped wedge resection of central conjunctiva, tarsus, and later full-thickness lid as a treatment of ectropion. Initially, the defects were allowed to granulate closed. Later, Adams advocated a single-suture closure to reunite the lid margin. In 1831, Von Amon described a lateral V-shaped full-thickness eyelid resection of ectropion.[1] Bick[5] described essentially the same procedure in 1966, emphasizing that the medial margin of eyelid resection should be attached to the stump of lateral canthal tendon and the wound closed carefully to avoid notching.

In 1883, Kuhnt[6] split the lid at the gray line and removed a wedge of posterior lamella. Although this closure avoided previous problems of eyelid margin healing, it caused an unsightly pucker of the anterior lamella. In 1870, Szymanowski[7] described an anterior lamellar resection at the lateral canthus which Meller (in 1953)[1] combined with Kuhnt's posterior lamella excision. Horizontal lid shortening via resection of the posterior lamella centrally and anterior lamella laterally became known as the Kuhnt-Szymanowski operation. Smith[8] suggested using a subciliary incision rather than a gray line incision for this operation. The Bick procedure and Smith's modification of the Kuhnt-Szymanowski operation are used by many surgeons for correction of ectropion.

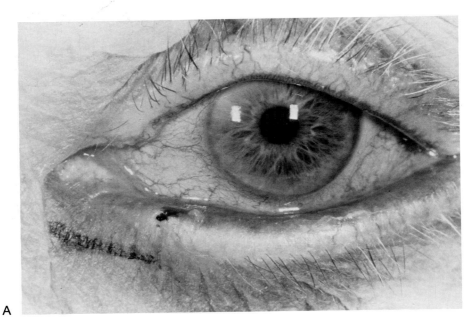

A

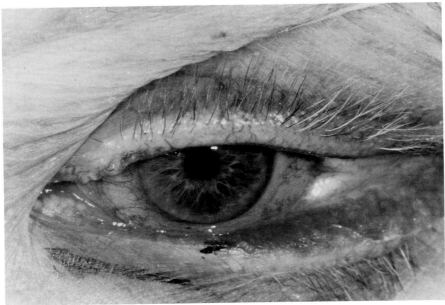

B

Fig. 4-5 Medial canthal tendon laxity. Punctum is marked. **(A)** Medial ectropion in resting position. **(B)** Canthal lid traction pulls punctum under pupil.

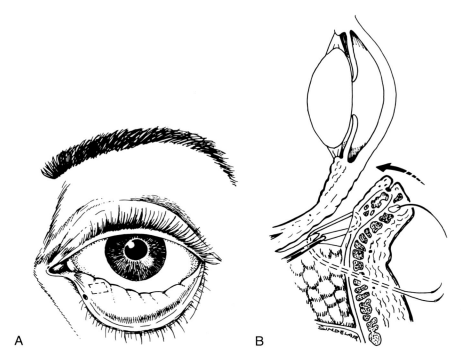

Fig. 4-6   The medial spindle operation. (**A**) A diamond of conjunctiva is excised. (**B**) Double-armed suture shortens diamond vertically and mechanically inverts lid.

Our treatment plan is based on the location of the ectropion, the degree of laxity, and the position of the laxity. In cases of punctal eversion or minimal medial ectropion, little lid laxity may be present. In these cases, a posterior lamellar shortening procedure, the *medial spindle operation,* will reappose the punctum[9,10] to the globe without need for lid shortening. A diamond of conjunctiva and tarsus below the punctum is excised. The lower lid retractors (often difficult to identify) are grasped, and a horizontal mattress suture is placed using a double-armed 4-0 chromic suture. The sutures are passed through the upper apex of the diamond from tarsus to conjunctiva and then through the conjunctiva of the lower apex of the diamond to continue through the eyelid. The arms of the suture are tied on themselves, titrating the degree of inward turning of the punctum (Fig. 4-6). A small overcorrection or punctal inversion is desirable at the end of the operation. If the punctum is stenosed, a punctoplasty may be performed. If cicatricial changes are the cause of punctal eversion, the medial spindle may not be effective and often will cause the medial aspect of the lid to be slightly retracted.

If lid laxity is present with medial laxity, as is most often the case, a horizontal lid shortening operation is performed. The degree of success in reapposing the punctum can be anticipated at the slit lamp. As the lid is drawn temporally, the punctum should revert to its normal position. If complete apposition is not accomplished with this maneuver, a medial spindle operation is combined with a horizontal lid shortening procedure. When combined, the medial spindle operation must be performed before the lid shortening.

For generalized lower lid involutional ectropion, horizontal lid shortening at the lateral canthus is performed. Although pentagonal resections of the lid as in the Bick procedure and Kuhnt-Szymanowski operation will tighten the lid, they unnecessarily shorten the tarsus and do not correct the lateral canthal blunting associated with elongation of the lateral canthal tendon. Similarly the "lazy-T"[11] operation for medial ectropion, which combines a diamond resection of posterior lamella with a pentagonal wedge resection of tarsus, does not attack the problem of lid laxity at its origin, the canthal tendons.

Tenzel[12,13] described the lateral canthal tendon sling for repair of the ectropion. Anderson and Gordy modified this procedure and termed it the tarsal strip procedure.[14] This operation is very effective in correcting ectropion and is our choice for horizontal lid shortening because it does not shorten the normal tarsus. Rather, it restores a normal canthal configuration.

The tarsal strip operation is performed as an outpatient procedure using 2 percent lidocaine with 1:100,000 mg/ml epinephrine mixed with an equal part of 0.75 percent Marcaine. The local anesthetic solution is injected into the lateral canthus and then into the periosteum near the attachment of the lateral canthal tendon at Whitnall's tubercle. Additional local anesthetic is injected subconjunctivally in the lateral lower conjunctival cul-de-sac. A small canthotomy is performed and then the deep tissues are incised to expose the lateral orbital rim. The white periosteum should be visible. The eyelid is grasped and lateral traction is applied. Strumming the inferior limb of the canthal tendon and the septum with scissors identifies tissues that are cut when a cantholysis is performed. The cantholysis should be adequate to allow the lid to pull temporally, but not so large as to allow fat prolapse through the cut septum. The inferior edge of the tarsus and conjunctiva is cut parallel to the lid margin for the estimated length of lid shortening desired. The mucocutaneous lid margin is trimmed off. The conjunctiva is scraped off the back of the tarsus using a scalpel blade. The strip is then sutured to the medial aspect of the lateral rim, at or slightly above mid-pupil height, with a 4-0 Vicryl suture. A small half-circle needle (P-2 Ethicon) is essential. A slight overcorrection in height is desired. A slight undercorrection in shortening is recommended because excessive shortening may cause the lid to slide inferiorly on the globe. Excess anterior lamella, including lashes, is trimmed off, and a minimal number of canthal sutures using 7-0 Vicryl or fast-absorbing 6-0 gut are placed to close the canthotomy (Fig. 4-7).

As mentioned earlier, a medial spindle may be combined with the tarsal strip operation. A severe form of ectropion occurs in which the entire lid is everted and the tarsus is essentially upside down. Fox termed this "tarsal ectropion."[15] It may be seen in young or old persons, sometimes in the absence of horizontal lid laxity, perhaps associated with a retractor disinsertion (Fig. 4-8). Wesley described[16] conjunctival excision beneath the tarsal border with

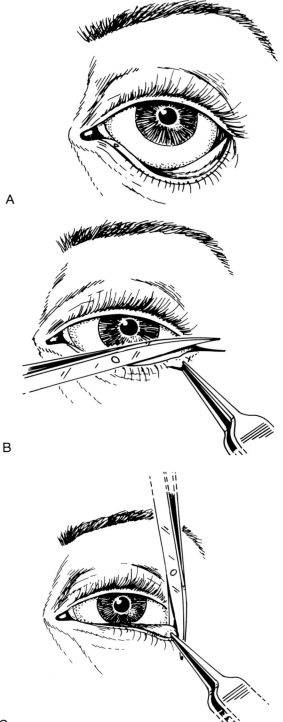

Fig. 4-7 The lateral tarsal strip operation. (**A**) Lower lid ectropion. (**B**) A small lateral canthotomy is performed. (**C**) A cantholysis is performed, severing the inferior crus of the lateral canthal tendon, the lower lid retractors, and the orbital septum. (*Figure continues.*)

A

B

C

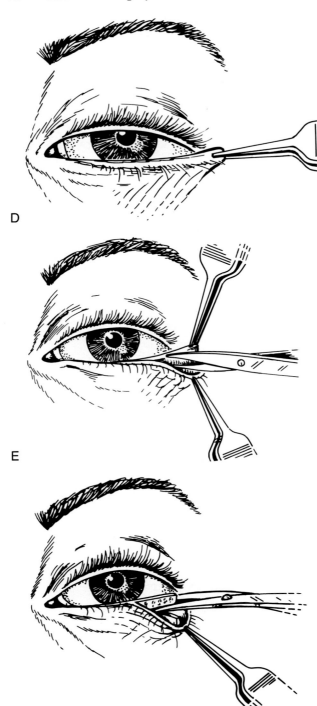

D

E

F

Fig. 4-7 (*Continued*). (**D**) The lid is pulled laterally to estimate amount of shortening. (**E**) The anterior and posterior lamellae are split. (**F**) A strip of tarsus is formed. (*Figure continues.*)

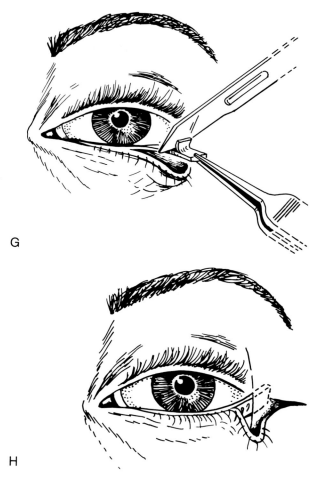

Fig. 4-7 (*Continued*). (**G**) The mucosa is scraped off the lid margin and posterior surface. (**H**) The "tarsal strip" is sutured to periosteum on the inner aspect of the lateral orbital rim using two passes of 4-0 Vicryl on a P-2 needle. (*Figure continues.*)

G

H

closure including the retractors. An alternate treatment is to use medial, central, and lateral diamond resections as described in the medial spindle procedure in combination with horizontal lid shortening.

The correction of horizontal lid laxity due to medial canthal tendon laxity is difficult. A medial canthal tendon plication operation can be performed, but often results are unsatisfactory because of bunching of the canaliculus and distraction of lid from the globe. These problems occur because only the anterior limb of the medial canthal tendon is shortened. We prefer not to perform medial canthal tendon plication operations.

In the face of mild to moderate medial canthal tendon laxity, horizontal lid shortening is performed laterally. A wedge resection medial to the punctum and canalicular reanastomosis over silicone stents is used if severe medial canthal tendon laxity is present, as suggested by McCord.[15,17]

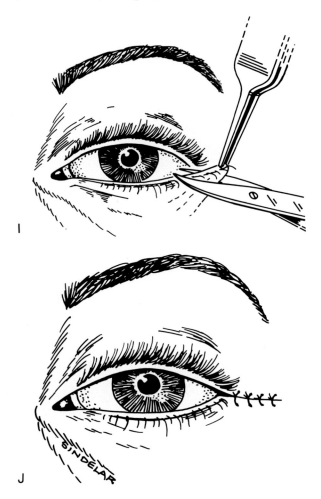

Fig. 4-7 (*Continued*). (**I**) Redundant anterior lamella is trimmed. (**J**) The canthotomy is closed with interrupted 7-0 Vicryl sutures.

Cicatricial Ectropion

Shortening of the anterior lamella of the eyelid may cause a cicatricial ectropion. The onset of the symptoms and signs may be gradual in disease conditions affecting the skin or may be sudden, following surgery or accidental trauma. Shortening of the skin and muscle may result from irradiation, burns, tumors, chemical injury, and cicatricial skin diseases, and may follow skin removal for skin cancer excision, xanthelasma removal, or blepharoplasty. In most cases an element of lid laxity accompanies the ectropion.

If possible, the original cause should be treated. In cicatrizing skin disease, topical steroid lotion may be helpful. If scarring is permanent, as is often the case, the shortened skin must be replaced. Often no local tissue is available to use as a flap, and a full-thickness skin grafting is necessary.

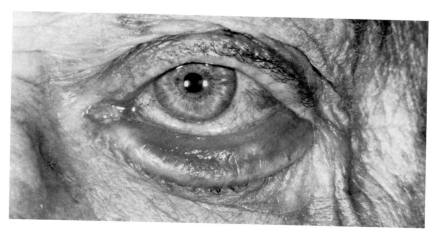

Fig. 4-8 Tarsal ectropion.

The best source for skin is from the upper lid skin fold. Eyelid skin is the thinnest and most flexible on the body. Only skin from another lid will match in texture and mobility. A flap for correcting cicatricial medial ectropion of the lower lid can be made by mobilizing skin and muscle from above the upper lid skin crease and hinging it at the medial canthus.[18] Alternative sources for a full-thickness graft are the retroauricular or preauricular skin.[19] We prefer to use preauricular skin (Fig. 4-9) because of its convenience. A piece 15 mm × 40 mm can be obtained and is generally the correct size and shape for correcting cicatricial changes in the lower lid. The facial nerve is easy to avoid since it is deep to the parotid fascia.

Our full-thickness skin grafting technique starts with two transmarginal lid traction sutures, placed temporally and medially to the limbus. The scar bands are cut and the lid is allowed to fall back into normal position against the globe. A template is made and transferred to the graft donor site. The graft is harvested and thinned of subcutaneous fat. Cardinal sutures tack the graft in place and then the wound is closed with a running suture. A bolster of surgical sponge is tied into position using the long ends of the cardinal sutures. The traction sutures are taped to the brow. A firm eye patch is placed for 1 week. Post-operatively there is generally a moderate overcorrection that reduces spontaneously.

Paralytic Ectropion

Paralysis of the orbicularis, usually due to facial nerve palsy, will cause loss of support to the tarsoligamentous sling of the lower lid. In elderly individuals with an element of lid laxity, a paralytic ectropion will develop. In younger individuals with tight lids, ectropion is often not a consequence of the

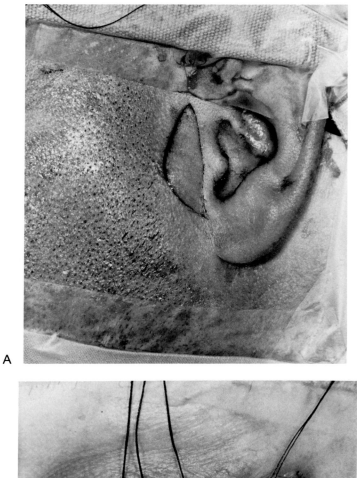

A

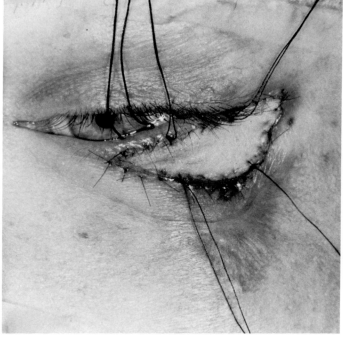

B

Fig. 4-9 (A) Preauricular skin harvested for repair of cicatricial ectropion. (B) Preauricular graft sewn into position.

paralysis; however, abnormalities in the lacrimal pump may cause exposure and tearing.

Facial nerve paralysis may occur as a result of trauma, tumor growth, tumor resection, or inflammatory conditions. Paralysis secondary to tumor growth or resection or trauma is often permanent and severe. Removal of cerebellopontine angle tumors such as acoustic neuromas may cause trigeminal nerve damage as well as facial nerve paralysis because of the proximity of these structures to the eighth nerve. Ectropion secondary to facial nerve paralysis in association with an anesthetic cornea is a particularly dangerous situation because exposure may progress to ulceration without the patient's knowledge. Bell's palsy or idiopathic facial palsy is the most common inflammatory condition affecting the facial nerve. Viral, inflammatory, and immune factors have been implicated. Approximately 70 to 80 percent of patients with Bell's palsy have a complete or satisfactory return of function.[17]

Signs and symptoms of facial nerve paralysis are varied. A subtle brow ptosis, an incomplete blink, and a shallowing of the nasolabial fold may be the only signs of a mild or nearly resolved facial nerve paralysis. Other patients may develop a complete facial paralysis with severe ectropion, brow ptosis obscuring the vision, and difficulty speaking because of orbicularis oris involvement (Fig. 4-10). Eye findings vary from minimal inferior epithelial keratopathy to frank corneal ulceration. Tearing may result from inadequate lacrimal pump function, punctal eversion, or ectropion.

Mild cases often resolve and can be managed conservatively with lubricants. Nonincisional tarsorrhaphy with temporary 5-0 prolene sutures may be helpful.[20] Temporary tarsorrhaphy is possible by simply denuding the eyelid margins.[17] We generally split the anterior and posterior lamellae and then suture the exposed tarsal edges together with mattress sutures of 5-0 Vicryl. This serves as either a temporary or permanent tarsorrhaphy. Many other permanent tarsorrhaphies have been described.[17] Medial and lateral tarsorrhaphies are useful in combination when a lateral tarsorrhaphy alone is not sufficient to prevent exposure. Ectropion can be corrected using the tarsal strip operation, sometimes in association with a medial spindle procedure.

A variety of mechanical devices have been suggested as a substitute for orbicularis function. Upper lid gold weights have been used.[21,22] Muhlbauer described palpebral magnets whose attraction aided in eyelid closure.[23] Arion[24] suggested using a silicone band encircling the lids in the pretarsal space as an aid to lid closure (Arion sling). Morel et al.[25] devised a palpebral spring that would push the upper eyelid closed as the levator muscle relaxed. The Arion sling and the palpebral spring are useful devices, but with time they often extrude.

Reinnervation and reanimation procedures have been described.[26] Direct nerve suturing or facial nerve grafting is useful in cases of laceration or iatrogenic injury to peripheral facial nerve. Where facial paralysis results from intracranial lesions or disorders of the temporal bone, and no spontaneous recovery is observed, nerve crossovers employing the glossopharyngeal, accessory, phrenic, or hyoglossal nerves or the contralateral facial nerve may be useful. Muscle transpositions with intact nerve supply have been performed

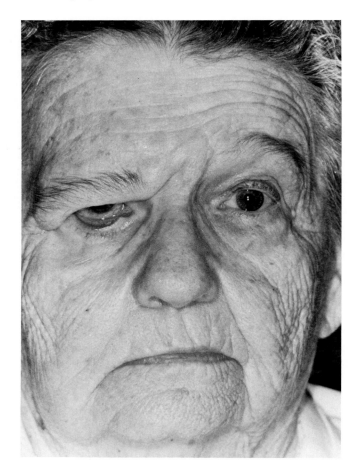

Fig. 4-10 Paralytic ectropion secondary to facial nerve paralysis. Note complete facial paralysis, ectropion, and brow ptosis.

with the temporalis and masseter muscles. When patients are carefully selected, good results have been obtained in a high percentage of cases.

ENTROPION

Entropion of the eyelid is characterized by turning of the eyelid margin toward the eyeball (Fig. 4-11). Lashes and keratinized lid skin rub against the eye, causing a foreign body sensation and corneal exposure problems. Once irritation begins, lid spasm follows, and a vicious cycle of increasing entropion may result. Because of pain and irritation, patients with entropion tend to seek medical attention sooner than patients with ectropion. Epiphora due to reflux

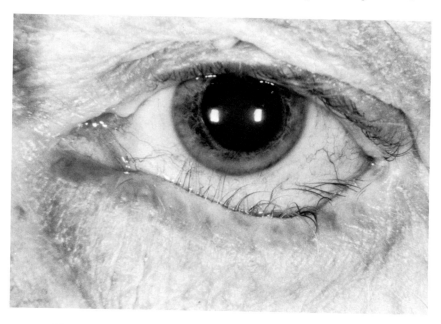

Fig. 4-11   Entropion of lower lid. Note lid margin is inverted.

tearing is often a symptom of entropion. The entropion may be intermittent, and therefore cause intermittent epiphora.

Epiblepharon and forms of trichiasis, including distichiasis and misdirected lashes, are often confused with entropion. Similarities exist; lashes abrade the cornea in all of these conditions and may be the source of irritation and tearing. However, the eyelid margin remains in normal anatomic position with epiblepharon. With entropion, the eyelid margin is always rotated toward the globe. Trichiasis and epiblepharon will be discussed in a separate section.

Three forms of entropion are seen. The involutional form is the most common in the USA, but a transient spastic form is also recognized, and cicatricial changes of the conjunctiva and tarsus may cause a cicatricial entropion.

Involutional Entropion

Involutional changes of the eyelid are the most common cause of entropion in the USA. The specific etiologies of involutional entropion are:

Lid laxity
Disinsertion or stretching of the lower lid retractors
Spasm of the preseptal orbicularis causing overriding onto the pretarsal orbicularis
Age-related enophthalmos

Involutional changes leading to horizontal lid laxity cause the eyelid to become unstable. This instability may be exacerbated by age-related enophthalmos, because the globe no longer supports the eyelids in the normal position. Accompanying changes in the lower lid retractors allow the eyelid to rotate inward.

DeRoetth[27] pointed out that involutional entropion can be temporarily cured by an adrenergic drop that stimulates the smooth muscles of the lower lid retractors. Jones[28,29,30] demonstrated the anatomy of the lower eyelid retractors and suggested that aging causes laxity of the retractors. The normal pull of the retractors is toward their attachments at the inferior rectus muscle, so that the inferior border of tarsus is pulled down and posteriorly, holding the eyelid in normal position. As the retractors thin, become lax, or disinsert because of aging, this normal inferoposterior pull is lost. The instability of the lid because of the horizontal lid laxity and loss of retractor tension allows the eyelid margin to rotate toward the eye.

Overriding of the preseptal orbicularis muscle onto the pretarsal muscle probably plays a role in involutional entropion. Using radiopaque markers in the orbicularis muscle, Dalgleish and Smith[29] demonstrated that the preseptal muscle moves up and forward over the lower edge of tarsus in cases of involutional entropion. Sisler[31] reported histological hypertrophy of the preseptal muscles in cases of entropion.

More than 100 procedures and modifications have been devised to correct involutional entropion and prevent its recurrence. Most of these procedures address only one or possibly two etiologic factors associated with entropion. Vertical anterior lamellar shortening was attempted by Ziegler using cautery,[32] and by Hotz using excision of a horizontal ellipse of skin.[33] Horizontal lid tightening has been suggested by Butler,[34] Fox,[35] and Bick.[5] Fibrosis or tightening of the orbicularis muscle was described by Wies[36] and Wheeler.[37] Jones was the first to suggest tightening of the inferior lid retractors.[30] All of these procedures work initially, but often lead to recurrence when used alone.

Collin and Rathbun reported a combination of horizontal lid shortening, orbicularis fibrosis, and retractor reattachment using the "4-snip procedure"[38] originally devised by Quickert. The concept of combining a horizontal lid shortening operation with a retractor reinsertion operation, as conceived by Jones, is used by many surgeons today and remains our choice. A subciliary skin incision is marked, and the lid is infiltrated with local anesthesia. A 4-0 silk traction suture is placed in the lid margin. A scalpel is used to incise the skin. The muscle layer is opened with Westcott scissors. A myocutaneous flap is dissected inferiorly until the preaponeurotic fat is seen. The septum is opened and the fat is retracted to expose the lower lid retractors as a white fibrous sheet. A strip of orbicularis is resected from the lower margin of tarsus and the retractors are separated from the underlying conjunctiva (Fig. 4-12). The free edge of retractors is sutured to the inferior edge of tarsus with four 5-0 Vicryl sutures. Generally the lid is mildly ectropic at this point. If gross ectropion is seen, the retractors are slightly recessed. A tarsal strip operation is performed to further stabilize the lid. The skin is closed with a running suture of 7-0 Vicryl

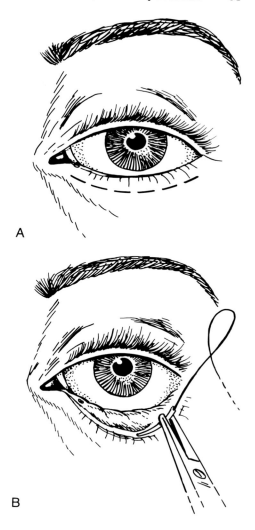

Fig. 4-12 Retractor reinsertion operation for involutional entropion. **(A)** A subciliary incision is marked 2 mm below the lashes. **(B)** Following injection of local anesthetic, a 4-0 black suture is passed into the lid margin for retraction. (*Figure continues.*)

A

B

or 6-0 fast absorbing gut. Three of the four etiologic factors related to entropion are corrected with this procedure. Theoretically the subciliary scar blocks the preseptal orbicularis muscle from overriding the pretarsal muscle.

Spastic Entropion

Acute ocular inflammation or lid swelling accompanied by lid spasm may cause entropion. This is often seen after retinal or anterior segment surgery. Lid laxity probably predisposes patients to this condition, although spastic entropion may occur in young adults. Spastic entropion may be seen as an early sign of involutional entropion. It is not uncommon during surgery for

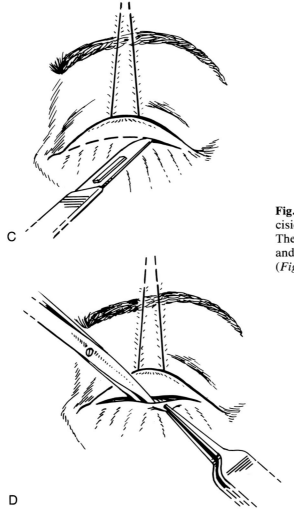

Fig. 4-12 (*Continued*). (**C**) A skin incision is made using a #15 blade. (**D**) The orbicularis muscle is incised and opened medially and laterally. (*Figure continues.*)

unilateral entropion to observe that the sting of topical anesthetic in the contralateral "normal" eye causes a spastic entropion.

In cases where a reversible etiology of the entropion is recognized, Quickert sutures[39] are a good temporizing measure. A double-armed 4-0 chromic suture is passed from deep in the inferior conjunctival fornix anteriorly through the lid, to exit 2 mm below the eyelashes. Medial, central, and lateral double-armed sutures are passed. Sutures are tied tight enough to produce a mild overcorrection of the entropion. The technique is simple and works well as the ocular irritation resolves. Although generally the result is temporary, the technique may be useful in bedridden or ill patients unable to withstand a more

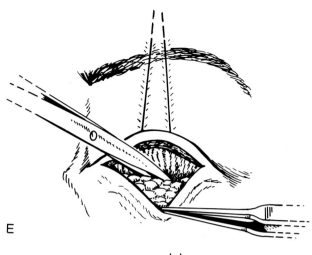

E

Fig. 4-12 (*Continued*). (**E**) The lower lid retractors are identified posterior to the preaponeurotic fat. (**F**) The retractors are dissected free from the underlying conjunctiva and advanced. (**G**) The retractors are sutured to the inferior tarsal margin using 5-0 Vicryl sutures. (*Figure continues.*)

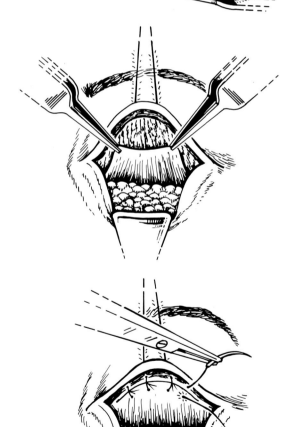

F

G

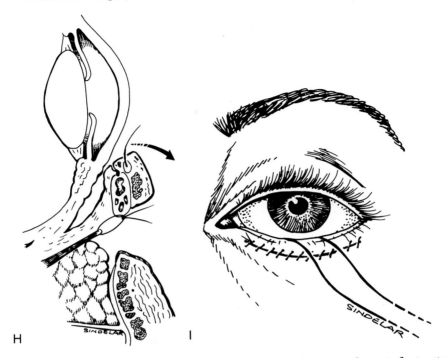

H   I

Fig. 4-12 (*Continued.*) (**H**) Cross section of lower lid showing reattachment of retractors and resultant rotation of lid margin. (**I**) The skin is closed with a running suture.

involved entropion repair. In cases of spastic entropion where no reversible cause can be identified, a retractor reinsertion and lid tightening operation is performed.

Cicatricial Entropion

Shortening of the posterior lamella may cause cicatricial entropion, forcing the lashes against the eyeball. Inflammatory processes, including chronic blepharitis, acne rosacea, chronic allergy, ocular pemphigoid, and Stevens-Johnson syndrome, are common causes. Trauma or chemical injuries may be associated. Trachoma is the leading cause of entropion outside the Western world.

Antimetabolites or steroids may be useful in Stevens-Johnson disease and ocular pemphigoid. In most cases surgical redirection or replacement of damaged tissue is necessary. Procedures that redirect the eyelid are Wies procedure or transverse tarsotomy,[36] and the anterior tarsal wedge resection and anterior lamellar advancement for upper lid entropion.[40] Posterior lamella scarring may be incised and successfully lengthened using buccal mucosa, hard palate mucosa, or nasochondral mucosa. Autogenous ear cartilage and sclera can be used; however, they cause ocular irritation until epithelialization occurs. Sclera exhibits variable degrees of resorption.[17]

Sporadic cases of true congenital entropion and ectropion are rare, and a discussion of these conditions is not included.

TRICHIASIS

Trichiasis is a condition in which misdirected lashes arise from the lid margin and rub against the cornea and conjunctiva. Reflex tearing is stimulated by conjunctival and corneal irritation. Three separate processes can be categorized under trichiasis: distichiasis, aberrant lashes, and metaplastic lashes. Each category has a distinct etiology and suggests a specific treatment.

Distichiasis is an uncommon congenital abnormality in which the multipotential meibomian gland cells of the tarsus develop into hair follicles and form a second row of eyelashes along the posterior margin of the eyelid. The extra row may be complete or incomplete. Often the lashes grow upward and cause exposure keratitis. Anderson et al.[41] described lid splitting and posterior lamellar cryotherapy for surgical treatment of distichiasis. The procedure is tedious, but is successful in destroying the abnormal lashes and preserving the normal lashes.

Aberrant lashes may arise following trauma, eyelid reconstruction after tumor excision, or chronic blepharitis with lid margin scarring. In many cases no cause can be identified. Often the aberrant lashes may be localized and removed by a wedge resection with primary closure of the involved eyelid. More diffuse areas of aberrant lashes should be treated with cryotherapy.

Metaplastic lashes arise following chronic eyelid inflammation. Metaplasia of the meibomian glands produces hair follicles. In most cases, eyelid margin irregularities due to scarring are present. An associated marginal entropion or mild inturning of the lid margin may coexist. A cycle of increasing irritation and metaplastic lashes may ensue. Lid hygiene and topical antibiotics, with or without mild steroids, should be used in an attempt to interrupt the cycle. Misdirected lashes causing corneal or conjunctival changes should be treated.

Epiblepharon and entropion may be confused with trichiasis. Epiblepharon (Fig. 4-13) is a condition in children in which an extra roll of lower lid skin pushes the lashes against the cornea. The eyelid margin is in the normal position. The problem is most common in oriental children. Surprisingly, symptoms and signs of corneal irritation are often minimal despite numerous lashes against the cornea. Generally children outgrow the disease by age 10, as the face assumes more adult features. If symptomatic, the condition can be corrected by a horizontal excision of the extra roll of skin.[33] Entropion is characterized by an inward turning of the eyelid margin, which is generally not seen in association with trichiasis.

The treatment of trichiasis depends on the patient's symptoms, signs of corneal exposure, and the extent of trichiasis. In mild cases where only a few lashes are involved, ocular lubricants or mechanical epilation is possible. Un-

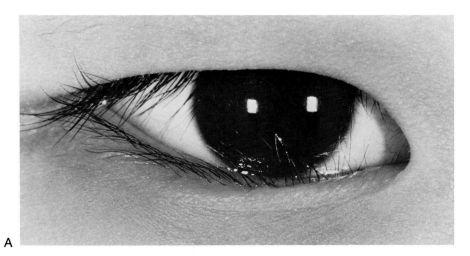

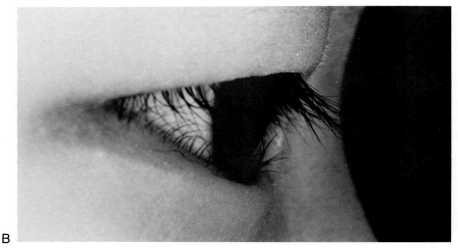

Fig. 4-13 Epiblepharon. (**A**) Normal position of lid margin. (**B**) Note roll of skin turning lashes against cornea.

fortunately, most lashes regrow after epilation in 4 to 6 weeks. In some cases the symptoms are worse as the lashes regrow because the returning lashes act as short, stiff bristles. Electrolysis is possible as a permanent cure; however, 50 to 70 percent of the lashes recur, and multiple treatments are necessary to reduce symptoms. Surgical resection of areas of trichiasis is an excellent option when the misdirected lashes are localized. In cases with more diffuse involvement, cryotherapy is recommended.

Cryotherapy allows destruction of lashes over a large area, with little or no effect on normal eyelid tissue. Hair follicles die at $-20°C$.[42,43] Eyelid and lacrimal tissue can withstand temperatures to $-40°C$ or colder. The exact mechanism of cryonecrosis is poorly understood. Rapid tissue freezing causes formation of intracellular ice crystals. Cells are destroyed as the ice crystals grow and rupture the cellular membrane. Intracellular pH changes cause denaturation of cellular proteins and lipoproteins.[44] A slow thaw period allows recrystallization to form larger ice crystals that are highly destructive to the cell. Cryotherapy also causes vascular thrombosis. A double freeze-thaw cycle increases success.[43]

Cryosurgery for trichiasis is performed as an outpatient procedure under local anesthesia. Patients are asked not to epilate their lashes for two weeks prior to treatment. Lidocaine 2 percent (Xylocaine) with 1:100,000 mg/ml epinephrine mixed with equal parts of bupivacaine 0.75 percent (Marcaine) is injected into the planned treatment area. The epinephrine causes vasoconstriction and therefore results in a faster freeze cycle. The bupivacaine dimishes postoperative pain. A nitrous oxide probe (Cryomedics) is applied to the lid margin, freezing the eyelid for thirty seconds or until 2 to 3 mm ice-ball forms around the probe tip. A thermocouple (temperature probe) can be used to monitor tissue temperature. In theory this is highly desirable; however, exact positioning of the probe at the lash root is necessary and difficult to obtain. We no longer use a thermocouple. Care is taken to protect the globe with a plastic, not metal, corneal protector. As the probe starts to freeze, the lid is retracted off the globe. After a slow thaw, the cryotherapy cycle is repeated. The lashes are then epilated. Effective treatment usually allows the damaged lash to "slide" out with little resistance. Topical antibiotic ointment is applied to minimize air contact with the burn. A narcotic prescription is given to be used as needed for pain. Patients are warned that significant postoperative swelling is normal.

Complications of cryotherapy are infrequent. Approximately 90 percent of lashes are permanently destroyed. Epidermal or full-thickness lid necrosis can occur if the area is overtreated. Cryotherapy causes depigmentation in darkly pigmented individuals because dermal melanocytes die at -10 to $-15°C$, and is rarely used in darkly pigmented individuals. Caution should be exercised in treating ocular pemphigoid patients as exacerbations are alleged to occur. Often, however, these patients are entering an active stage of their disease, which would progress even without cryotreatment.

CONCLUSION

Eyelid malpositions and related conditions are frequent causes of epiphora. Lacrimal pump failure due to lid laxity, or orbicularis muscle paresis may be improved by horizontal lid shortening. Punctal eversion, medial ectropion, or more advanced cases of ectropion may be relieved by lid shortening, often in combination with the medial spindle operation. Entropion can be treated with anatomic reinsertion of the lower lid retractors and the tarsal strip operation. Reflex tearing due to trichiasis is managed by excision or cryodestruction of the lash follicles. Recognition and appropriate treatment of these conditions will relieve and patient's symptoms of epiphora.

REFERENCES

1. Silverstone P: Surgery for involutional ectropion. p. 97. In Bosniak SL, Smith BC (eds): History and Tradition. Vol 5. Advances in Ophthalmic Plastic and Reconstructive Surgery. Pergamon Press, Elmsford, New York, 1986
2. Jones LT: Epiphora II: Its relation to the anatomical structures and surgery of the medial canthal region. Am J Ophthalmol 43:209, 1957
3. Hill JC: Analysis of senile changes of the palpebral fissure. Trans Ophthalmol Soc UK 95:49, 1975
4. Schaefer AJ: Lateral canthal tendon tuck. Ophthalmology 86:1879, 1979
5. Bick MW: Surgical management of orbital tarsal disparity. Arch Ophthalmol 75:386, 1966
6. Kuhnt H: Beitrage zur Operationen. Augenhilkunder. Jean, G. Fischer, 1883, p 45
7. Szymanowski J: Handbuch der Operationen chirugie. Braunschweig, Berlin, 1870, p 243
8. Smith B, Bosniak S, Sachs M: The management of involutional lower lid ectropion. Adv Ophth Plast Reconstr Surg 2:287, 1983
9. Tse DT: Surgical correction of punctal malposition. Am J Ophthalmol 100:339, 1985
10. Nowinski TS, Anderson RL: The medial spindle procedure for involutional medial ectropion. Arch Ophthalmol 103:1750, 1985
11. Smith B: The "lazy-T" correction of ectropion of the lower punctum. Arch Ophthalmol 94:1149, 1976
12. Tenzel RR: Treatment of lagophthalmos of the lower lid. Arch Ophthalmol 81:366, 1969
13. Tenzel RR, Buffam FV, Miller GR: The use of the "lateral canthal sling" in ectropion repair. Can J Ophthalmol 12:199, 1977
14. Anderson RL, Gordy DD: The tarsal strip procedure. Arch Ophthalmol 97:2192, 1969
15. Fox SA: Marginal (tarsal) ectropion. Arch Ophthalmol 63:660, 1960
16. Wesley RE: Tarsal ectropion from detachment of the lower lid retractors. Am J Ophthalmol 93:491, 1982
17. McCord CD, Tanenbaum M, Dryden RM, Doxanas MT: Eyelid malpositions: entropion, eyelid margin deformity and trichiasis, ectropion, and facial nerve palsy. p. 279. In McCord CD, Tanenbaum M (eds.): Oculoplastic Surgery. 2nd ed. Ch. 12. Raven Press, New York, 1987
18. Anderson RL, Hatt MU, Dixon R: Medial ectropion—a new technique. Arch Ophthalmol 97:521, 1979
19. Dryden RM, Wulc AE: The preauricular skin graft in eyelid reconstruction. Arch Ophthalmol 103:1579, 1985
20. Dryden RM, Adams JL: Temporary non-incisional tarsorrhaphy. Adv Ophth Plast Reconstr Surg 1:119, 1985
21. Smellie GD: Restoration of the blinking reflex in facial nerve palsy by a simple load operation. Br J Plast Surg 19:279, 1966
22. Barclay TL, Roberts AC: Restoration of movement to the upper eyelid in facial palsy. Br J Plast Surg 22:257, 1969

23. Muhlbauer WD: Palpebral magnets for paretic lagophthalmos. In Fredericks S, Brady GS (eds): Symposium on the Neurologic Aspects of Plastic Surgery. CV Mosby, St. Louis, 1978
24. Arion HG: Dynamic closure of the lids in paralysis of the orbicularis muscle. Int Surg 57:48, 1972
25. Morel J, Fatio D, LeLardie JP: Palliative surgical treatment of facial paralysis: The palpebral spring. Plast Reconstr Surg 33:447, 1964
26. Baker DC: Facial paralysis. p. 580. In Della Rocca RC, Nesi FA, Lisman, RD (eds): Ophthalmic Plastic and Reconstructive Surgery. Vol. 1. Ch. 23. CV Mosby, St. Louis, 1987
27. DeRoetth A: Mechanism of the senile entropion. Trans Pac Coast Oto Ophthalmol Soc 44:173, 1963
28. Jones LT: The anatomy of the lower eyelid and its relationship to the cause and cure of entropion. Am J Ophthalmol 49:29, 1960
29. Dalgleish R, Smith JLS: Mechanics and histology of senile entropion. Br J Ophthalmol 50:79, 1966
30. Jones LT, Reeh MV, Wobig JL: Senile entropion: A new concept for correction. Am J Ophthalmol 72:327, 1972
31. Sisler, HA, Lebay GR, Finlay JR: Senile ectropion and entropion: A compared and histopathologic study. Ann Ophthalmol 8:319, 1976
32. Ziegler SL: Galvano cautery puncture in ectropion and entropion. JAMA 53:183, 1909
33. Hotz FC: Eine neue operation fur entropium and trichiasis. Arch fur Aufenhix, 1879–1880, pp 68–80
34. Butler JBV: Simple operation for entropion. Arch Ophthalmol 40:665, 1948
35. Fox SA: Correction of senile entropion. Arch Ophthalmol 48:624, 1952
36. Wies FA: Surgical treatment of entropion. J Int Coll Surg 21:758, 1954
37. Wheeler JM: Spastic entropion correction by orbicularis transplantation. Am J Ophthalmol 22:477, 1939
38. Collins JR, Rathbun JE: Involutional entropion: A review with evaluation of a procedure. Arch Ophthalmol 96:1056, 1978
39. Quickert MH, Rathbun E: Suture repair of entropion. Arch Ophthalmol 85:304, 1971
40. Tenzel RR, Miller GR, Rubnzik R: Cicatricial upper lid entropion treated with bank scleral graft. Arch Ophthalmol 93:999, 1975
41. Anderson RL, Harvey JT: Lid splitting and posterior lamella cryosurgery for congenital and acquired distichiasis. Arch Ophthalmol 99:631, 1981
42. Sullivan JH: The use of cryotherapy for trichiasis. Trans Am Acad Ophthalmol Otolaryng 83:708, 1977
43. Sullivan JH, Beard C, Bullock JD: Cryosurgery for treatment of trichiasis. Am J Ophthalmol 82:117, 1976
44. Bedrossian EH, Simonton JT: Management of trichiasis. In Della Rocca RC, Nesi FA, Lisman RD (eds): Ophthalmic Plastic and Reconstructive Surgery. Vol. 1. CV Mosby, St. Louis, 1987

5 | Congenital Lacrimal Disorders and Management

J. Justin Older

Congenital obstruction of the lacrimal drainage system is present in up to 6 percent of newborns.[1] In some cases the problem resolves spontaneously, but in others intervention by the physician is indicated. Symptoms vary from intermittent epiphora to conjunctivitis and dacryocystitis. Proper management of congenital dacryostenosis depends on knowledge of the development of the lacrimal drainage system as well as on the natural course of the condition.

EMBRYOLOGY

Most of the causes of congenital obstruction of the excretory system are related to improper formation of certain structures in the lacrimal drainage system. The lacrimal drainage system develops along the line of the cleft between the lateral nasal and the maxillary processes (Fig. 5-1). A fold of ectoderm extends downward into the underlying mesenchyme and forms a sulcus (the naso-optic fissure) which soon becomes detached from the surface and forms a solid rod of cells between the future medial canthus and the nasal cavity.[2] This rod of cells begins to elongate, and a second rod of epithelial cells emerges from the primitive nasal cavity. These two rods of epithelial cells grow toward each other but may remain separate for some time (Fig. 5-2). Cells from the uppermost rod bifurcate and form the rudiments of the canaliculi. The epithelium of the lid margin plays no part in the formation of the canaliculi.

During the third month, the central cells of the solid rod begin to disin-

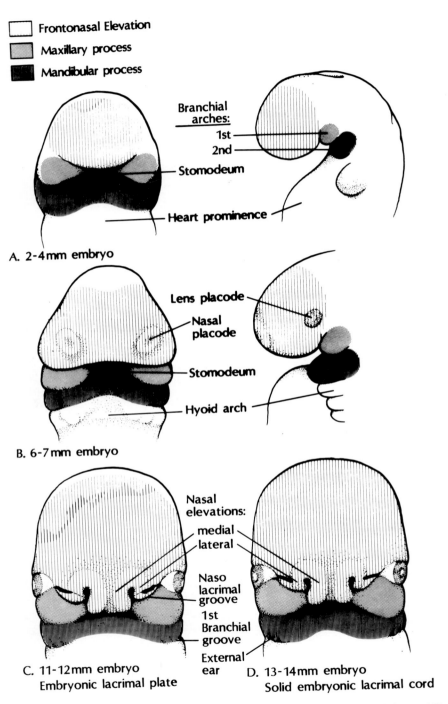

Fig. 5-1 Development of lacrimal drainage system in the embryo and fetus. (*Figure continues.*)

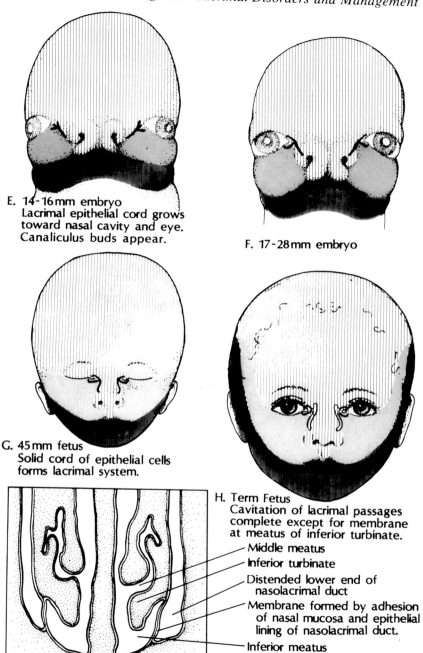

E. 14-16 mm embryo
Lacrimal epithelial cord grows
toward nasal cavity and eye.
Canaliculus buds appear.

F. 17-28 mm embryo

G. 45 mm fetus
Solid cord of epithelial cells
forms lacrimal system.

H. Term Fetus
Cavitation of lacrimal passages
complete except for membrane
at meatus of inferior turbinate.
Middle meatus
Inferior turbinate
Distended lower end of
nasolacrimal duct
Membrane formed by adhesion
of nasal mucosa and epithelial
lining of nasolacrimal duct.
Inferior meatus

Fig. 5-1 (*Continued*).

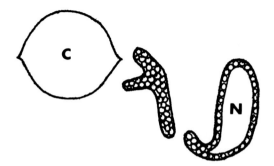

Fig. 5-2 Formation of nasolacrimal system in the 6-week-old embryo. Solid rods of cells beginning to form the nasolacrimal drainage system. C, conjunctival sac; N, nasal cavity. (After Duke-Elder S, Cook C: Normal and abnormal development. Part 1. Embryology. p. 242. In Duke-Elder S (ed): System of Ophthalmology. Vol. 3. CV Mosby, St. Louis, 1963.)

tegrate in a segmental fashion (Fig. 5-3). The canalization of the upper rod begins at the ocular end of the rod and progresses toward the nasal area (Fig. 5-4). Similarly, the rod of cells near the nasal cavity begins to form a canal that opens into the inferior meatus. The lysis of cells at the junction of the two epithelial rods that finally establishes the communication between the lacrimal drainage canal and the nose usually takes place at the end of the sixth month. However, this may be delayed for several weeks or months after birth. At birth, a membrane consisting of the apposed mucosal linings of the cavity of the inferior meatus and the lower end of the lacrimal duct is often still present.[2]

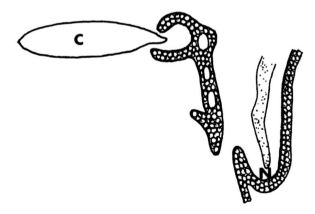

Fig. 5-3 The solid rod begins to disintegrate in a segmental fashion in the 12-week-old fetus. C, conjunctival sac; N, nasal cavity. (After Duke-Elder S, Cook C: Normal and abnormal development. Part 1. Embryology. p. 242. In Duke-Elder S (ed): System of Ophthalmology. Vol. 3. CV Mosby, St. Louis, 1963.)

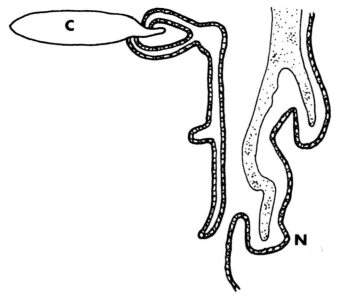

Fig. 5-4   Canalization begins to take place at 3.5 months. C, conjunctival sac; N, nasal cavity. (After Duke-Elder S, Cook C: Normal and abnormal development. Part 1. Embryology. p. 242. In Duke-Elder S (ed): System of Ophthalmology. Vol. 3. CV Mosby, St. Louis, 1963.)

The lacrimal puncta open onto the lid margins just before the lids separate at the seventh month.

CONGENITAL ANOMALIES

Atresia of the Nasolacrimal Duct

Atresia of the nasolacrimal duct is usually due to failure of canalization of the lower end of the nasolacrimal duct, but it may be caused by debris within the duct.[3] Although the blockage may occur at the upper or middle portions of the duct, the most common site is the lower end.

Jones and Wobig described eight types of lower nasolacrimal duct obstruction:

1.   The duct ends at or near the vault of the anterior end of the inferior nasal meatus and fails to perforate the nasal mucosa. This is probably the most common type.
2.   The duct extends to the floor of the nose lateral to the nasal mucosa.
3.   The duct extends several millimeters down, lateral to the nasal mucosa, without an opening.

4. The duct is almost completely absent because of failure of the osseous nasolacrimal canal to form.

5. The lower end of the duct is blocked by an impacted anterior end of the inferior turbinate.

6. The duct ends blindly in the medial wall of the maxillary sinus.

7. The duct ends blindly in the anterior end of the inferior turbinate.

8. A bony nasolacrimal canal extends to the floor of the nose without an opening.[4]

Congenital Lacrimal Amniotocele (Congenital Lacrimal Sac Mucocele)

This condition described by Jones and Wobig[4] consists of a swelling of the tear sac at birth. It is believed to be due to a nasolacrimal obstruction below the tear sac combined with a blockage at the opening of the canaliculi in the tear sac. In some cases the canaliculi enter the tear sac via a sinus of Maier, which may enter the sac at an acute angle. The posterior margin of the sinus is referred to as the valve of Rosenmüller. When the nasolacrimal duct is blocked and fluid builds up in the lacrimal sac, this valve may close off the egress of fluid from the sac into the eye via the canaliculi. If this occurs, a tear sac filled with fluid will be noticed as a swelling in the medial canthal area in the newborn (Fig. 5-5).

Congenital Absence of Valves

If the valve of Hasner at the nasal end of the nasolacrimal duct is absent, pneumatoceles of the sac may occur and nose blowing may cause a retrograde passage of air. If both the valve of Hasner and the valve of Rosenmüller are missing, air can be blown from the nose to the eye.[5]

Absence or Atresia of the Canaliculi

This rare condition is due to a failure of the budding out of the anlage of the lacrimal passage or a failure of the canalization of the solid rod of epithelial cells that form the lacrimal drainage system.[3]

Atresia of the Lacrimal Puncta

Punctal atresia, which is not rare, may be caused by a failure of the conjunctiva, which overlies the canaliculus, to dehisce. A fine membrane persists over the punctal openings. While the punctal area can usually be seen just

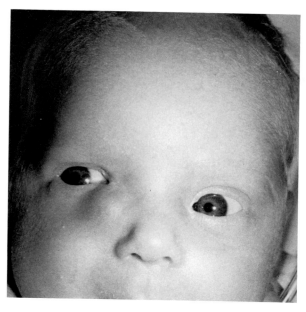

Fig. 5-5 Newborn with congenital lacrimal sac mucocele (amniocele) on the right side. There are no signs of infection and the cystic mass has a bluish color.

below this membrane, it sometimes cannot be identified. Punctal atresia and absence of the canaliculi often have a hereditary component.[3]

Supernumerary Puncta and Canaliculi

Various combinations of extra canaliculi and puncta have been reported. There is often a hereditary component to this type of congenital deformity. Most of these deformities actually represent side openings in the canaliculi.[3] However, Jones and Wobig described true supernumerary canaliculus and punctum. In their cases the rest of the lacrimal drainage system was usually normal and patients often complained of epiphora. These authors suggested the name *lacrimal anlage duct,* believing it was due to the canalization of a rod of epithelial cells extending from the lacrimal sac area. The lacrimal anlage duct usually forms below the inferior canaliculus and may open onto the skin several millimeters below the caruncle (Fig. 5-6).[4]

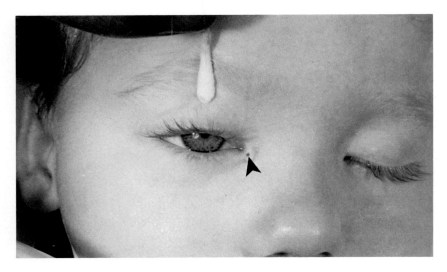

Fig. 5-6   Infant with lacrimal anlage duct at the medial canthus of the right eye. Opening is indicated by an arrow.

Facial Anomalies

The overall incidence of nasolacrimal apparatus problems in children with various facial anomalies is not great, but there is a statistical relationship between children with facial clefts and nasolacrimal abnormalities. About 12 percent of these children have absent puncta, canalicular problems, or nasolacrimal duct obstructions.[6]

DIAGNOSIS

The symptoms of children with congenital nasolacrimal obstruction usually include epiphora (Fig. 5-7), chronic or recurrent conjunctivitis, and dacryocystitis (Fig. 5-8). Physical examination can usually reveal such anomalies as absent puncta or accessory canaliculi (Fig. 5-6). Congenital amniotocele can also be appreciated visually (Fig. 5-5), but massage of the lacrimal sac might be necessary to diagnose a nasolacrimal obstruction with a sac filled with mucus. In many cases there will be a history of chronic epiphora or recurrent infection without physical signs of nasolacrimal abnormality.

Although most methods of evaluating the lacrimal outflow system are not practical with infants, the dye disappearance test can be most helpful. A strip of moistened fluorescein filter paper is touched to the inner aspect of the lower lid. In children with normal lacrimal outflow systems the dye will be gone from the tear meniscus in 5 minutes. Examination with a blue light will aid this

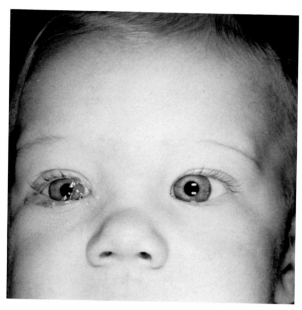

Fig. 5-7   Infant with typical signs of congenital nasolacrimal duct obstruction of the right eye. Epiphora, increased tear lake, mucoid debris, and mattering of lashes are present.

evaluation, especially if the child is uncooperative. If the dye disappearance test is not conclusive, the presumptive diagnosis of congenital nasolacrimal duct obstruction must be based on history alone. A more definitive way to diagnose obstructions of the lacrimal passages is dacryocystography. In a series reported by Hurwitz and Welham,[7] 80 children between the ages of six months and seven years underwent dacryocystography under general anesthesia. Findings included obstruction of the lower sac, the lower duct, and the mid-duct as well as stenosis of the lower sac and of the common canaliculus. Many of these children had had one or more probings before the dacryocystography was done, and this prior treatment may have contributed to some of the obstructions. The study did not correlate each site of obstruction with the number or lack of previous probings.

Dacryoscintigraphy, the use of radioactive tracer to evaluate nasolacrimal drainage, has been found helpful in evaluating lacrimal drainage in children. In the cases reported, general anesthetic was not used but sedation was given to infants and small children who were unable to cooperate.[8]

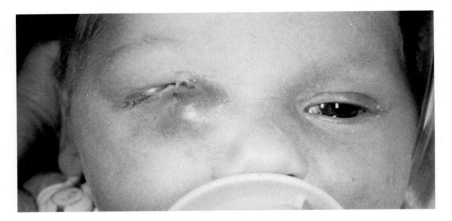

Fig. 5-8 Acute dacryocystitis complicating a congenital lacrimal sac mucocele (amniocele) in a newborn. This *Staphylococcus aureus* infection responded to systemic antibiotics, and the lacrimal obstruction was cured by simple probing.

TREATMENT

Obstruction of the Nasolacrimal Duct

Treatment of a patient with congenital nasolacrimal duct obstruction depends upon the child's age but continues to remain controversial. If the child has had a history of chronic conjunctivitis and epiphora within the first 3 months of life (Fig. 5-7), most ophthalmologists will treat with local antibiotics and

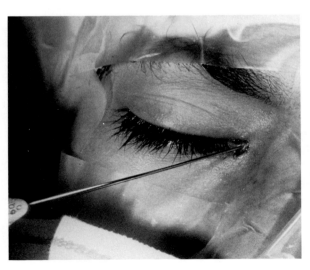

Fig. 5-9 Excision of extra canaliculus (lacrimal anlage duct). Probe has been placed with the extra canaliculus, which is then dissected free from underlying tissue with a collar of skin at the opening. After resection, skin and soft tissues are closed in layers.

massage of the lacrimal sac. However, these therapies may already have been prescribed by the family pediatrician.

When there is a history of epiphora without a mucopurulent discharge, the parents are instructed to massage the child's nasolacrimal duct 2 to 4 times a day. A finger is used to massage the lacrimal sac in an inferior direction for 3 to 4 strokes. The effect of the hydrostatic pressure may force the membrane at the end of the nasolacrimal duct to open, thereby relieving the obstruction.

If there is mucopurulent discharge associated with the epiphora, a drop of antibiotic solution can be instilled in the eye before each massage treatment. If an associated dacryocystitis exists, systemic antibiotics must be used to clear the infection. In both of these cases of associated infection, cultures should be taken before antimicrobial treatment is begun.

If the problem persists for more than a few weeks and is a source of consternation to the family, many ophthalmologists will recommend gentle probing in the office.[4,9] Those physicians who recommend early probing reason that the risk is minimal and the chance of cure is greatest at this stage because chronic inflammation will not have had a chance to worsen the obstruction. They also believe that chronic epiphora and possibly chronic conjunctivitis or recurrent dacryocystitis is a significant problem for both the child and the family. The physicians who recommend early probing perform the procedure in the office without general anesthesia to reduce the anesthetic risk.

Baker reported a series in which 860 eyes were probed in children between 3 and 14 months of age. A second probing was required in 6 percent of the cases, and a third probing was required in only 0.5 percent. Two children required intubation, but they were first seen by the author after the age of 12 months.[9]

A significant number of ophthalmologists[10,11,12] as well as many pediatricians, recommend medical management of epiphora during the first year of life. They reason that about 90 percent of the obstructions will resolve by 13 months of age without the need for surgical intervention.

In a study performed by Paul, 55 infants with nasolacrimal duct obstruction were followed prospectively with medical management. By 1 year of age, 90 percent of these children were without epiphora. Of those infants who were still obstructed at 3 months, 80 percent were clear by one year of age. Seventy percent of the children who were still obstructed at 6 months were without epiphora at 12 months, and of those children who remained obstructed at 9 months, 52 percent were without epiphora at one year of age.[12]

Timing of Initial Probing—The Controversy

The data seem to indicate that the vast majority of congenital nasolacrimal duct obstructions will resolve spontaneously by 1 year of age. However, during that time, the child may have chronic or recurrent conjunctivitis or dacryocystitis. The ophthalmologists who recommend early probing believe that it is a safe procedure with minimal risk and a high cure rate, and that the child and family therefore should not be subjected to many months of the symptoms and medical treatments associated with nasolacrimal duct obstruction. The physicians who recommend medical treatment for the first year cite evidence that most obstructions will resolve with medical treatment and hold that it is unnecessary to submit the child to the risks of surgery.

Both groups involve the family in the decision of probing versus continued medical management. The surgeons who probe early indicate that the families find the problems of chronic infection unacceptable. On the other hand, the ophthalmologists who prefer late probing emphasize that the families participate in the decision and prefer to give medical treatment the maximum trial. As with so many areas of medicine, the decision made by the family usually reflects the opinion of the treating physician.

If the decision to probe is made, best results are obtained if probing is performed within the first 13 months of life. In a retrospective study of 572 eyes with nasolacrimal duct obstruction, Katowitz and Welsh found that the success rate of initial probing was 97 percent in children under 13 months of age. Between 13 and 18 months, the rate dropped to 76.4 percent and fell in a stepwise progression to 33.3 percent for children probed after 24 months.[1]

Probing Techniques

The goal of probing is to open the membrane that is thought to be present at the lower end of the nasolacrimal duct. Since this membrane is usually very thin and tight, gentle pressure will usually be sufficient to "pop" it and cure the obstruction.

The type of anesthesia is usually chosen by the anesthesiologist, but the anesthesiologist may ask the surgeon how long the procedure will take. Whether or not intubation is used may determine the expected length of the operation. Since probing is not always a rapid procedure, intubation may be preferable in order for the surgeon not to feel hurried during the operation. If the child is an infant, the surgeon may elect to use a papoose board to immobilize the child, thereby eliminating the risk of a general anesthetic.

The punctum is gently dilated (Fig. 5-10), and fluorescein solution is irrigated through the upper canaliculus. This maneuver is performed because the diagnosis of a blocked nasolacrimal duct has usually been presumptive until this point. A suction catheter is placed in the corresponding nostril. If dye is recovered in the nostril, it is clear that fluid can pass through the drainage system under pressure. If dye reflexes out of the lower punctum, there is probably a nasolacrimal duct obstruction, especially if there is mucus mixed with the irrigating solution.

A 00 or 000 lacrimal probe is gently introduced into the upper or lower punctum (Fig. 5-11) and advanced in the direction of the medial canthal tendon (Fig. 5-12). When the end is felt to be pressing against the bone, the probe is rotated so that the tip points toward the lateral side of the nostril. Further rotation directs the probe posteriorly since the nasolacrimal canal ends under

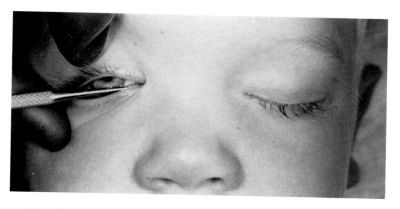

Fig. 5-10 The punctum is gently dilated with a tapered probe.

the inferior turbinate. The surgeon should feel the probe slip into the canal. Significant pressure should not be needed to enter the nasolacrimal canal.

Once in the canal, the probe should be pushed toward the floor of the nose (Fig. 5-13). A "pop" may be felt when the obstruction is penetrated, but this is not always the case. The surgeon may then look into the nose to visualize the probe under the inferior turbinate. Alternatively, another probe may be introduced into the nose to touch the first one, giving a metal-on-metal sensation (Fig. 5-14). In order to check the success of the probing, the fluorescein solution

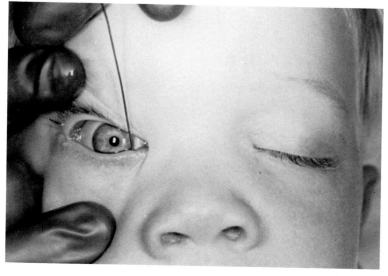

Fig. 5-11 The Bowman probe is inserted through the punctum, perpendicular to the lid margin, until it reaches the ampulla.

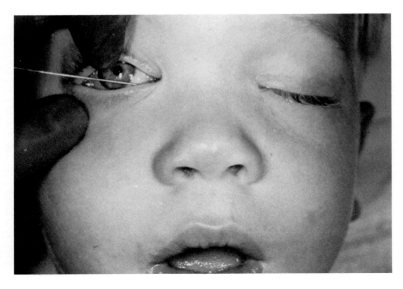

Fig. 5-12   The Bowman probe is advanced through the canaliculus, parallel to the eyelid margin. After passing through the common canaliculus, the tip of the probe rests against the medial wall of the lacrimal sac fossa.

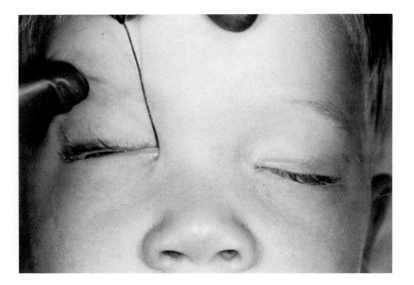

Fig. 5-13   The probe is rotated upward, until the tip falls down into the nasolacrimal duct. The probe is gently advanced toward the nose, until it penetrates the distal obstruction.

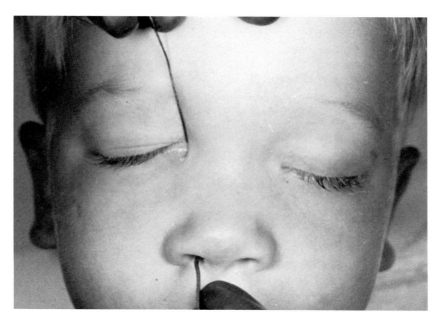

Fig. 5-14 A second probe may be inserted into the nose, under the middle turbinate, in order to verify that the first probe has entered the nasal cavity. The examiner will be able to feel "metal against metal" contact.

can be irrigated through the upper punctum and recovered in the nose via a transparent suction catheter.

Antibiotic drops are instilled in the operated eye after surgery and three or four times a day for the next 5 days. The degree of success will usually be apparent within several days.

Probing Failures

Although most lacrimal probings solve the problem of nasolacrimal obstruction, 5 to 10 percent of these procedures are not successful. If the patient was not cured with the initial probing, but the probe was passed into the nose or irrigation fluid was recovered in the nose, a second probing might succeed. If the surgeon was unable to pass the probe into the nose on the first operation, a dacryocystogram could be performed to determine the site of the obstruction.

In cases of congenital obstruction without multiple previous probings or severe chronic infection, intubation with silicone tubes is often successful when two probings fail (see Chap. 6). In a series of 25 intubations for nasolacrimal obstruction, 84 percent were considered successful. The average number of previous probings in the group was 1.6.[13]

Dacryocystorhinostomy is an appropriate treatment in those patients who do not respond to probing or silicone tube placement. It may also be indicated if there is an obstruction in the common canaliculus or a deformity in the nasolacrimal canal that cannot be penetrated by a lacrimal probe. Surgery is usually delayed until the child is at least 18 months old (see Chap. 9). Welham and Hughes reported the results of dacryocystorhinostomy in 49 patients with congenital nasolacrimal duct obstruction and a history of unsuccessful probings (average 3). The children ranged in age from 17 months to 16 years. A success rate of 93 percent was reported, with a follow-up time of 33 months.[14]

Congenital Amniotocele

As with the treatment of the more common types of nasolacrimal duct obstruction, treatment of congenital amniotocele is also controversial. Scott et al. write that "congenital mucocele is one of the few indications for immediate lacrimal system probing in the neonatal period."[15] Conversely, Levy states that "probing of the nasolacrimal system may not be necessary in the treatment of uncomplicated congenital amniotocele of the lacrimal sac."[16]

In a retrospective study of seven infants born with tense, blue-gray swellings (Fig. 5-6) inferior to the medial canthal tendon, Weinstein et al. reported that four had uncomplicated mucoceles. One of the children was treated successfully with massage, but the other three had infections of the lacrimal sac (Fig. 5-9) that required immediate probings. All three probings were successful, and cultures from these lacrimal sacs yielded *Staphylococcus* organisms. Two of these infants developed recurrent lacrimal sac swellings which responded to repeat probings at 3 months of age.[17]

Although medical treatment may be attempted if there is no evidence of infection, I believe early probing is probably indicated in cases of congenital amniotocele.

Atresia of the Lacrimal Puncta

If a punctum is absent, it is often because a membrane covers the area over the canaliculus. A dimple may be present, indicating the top of the canaliculus. In these cases, a sharp probe or a needle may be sufficient to pierce the membrane and create the punctum. The system can then be irrigated to see if it is patent. If it is patent, no further surgery is needed, but if other areas of obstruction exist, probing or more extensive surgery may be indicated.

An alternative approach is to make an incision, as one would do to begin a dacryocystorhinostomy, and try to find the lacrimal sac. If the sac can be found, the next step is to try to pass a probe in a retrograde fashion from the common canaliculus toward the appropriate punctum. Methylene blue injected into the lacrimal sac area can be helpful in locating the canaliculus. The surgeon can then cut down to the tip of the probe to create a punctum. After this procedure the entire lacrimal drainage system can be intubated with silicone tubing. If there is blockage in the lacrimal duct or the lacrimal sac, a dacryocystorhinostomy with silicone intubation may be required.

Atresia of the Canaliculi

When there is a true absence of the canaliculi, a conjunctivodacryocystorhinostomy with implantation of Jones Pyrex tubes is the treatment of choice (see Chapter 15).

Supernumerary Canaliculi (Lacrimal Anlage Duct)

These extra canaliculi are best treated by excision if the rest of the drainage system is patent. A dye such as methylene blue can be injected into the duct to outline its length. A probe is then passed into the duct and a skin incision is made over the probe (Fig. 5-9). Blunt dissection is then continued to outline the duct. After this procedure the duct is removed, with care being taken not to injure the lacrimal sac or normal canaliculi.[4]

EDITOR'S COMMENTS

As stated by Dr. Older, dacryocystorhinostomy (DCR) is usually deferred in infants until the age of 18 months. Unfortunately, some infants with congenital obstruction will develop bacterial dacryocystitis. These infections can be serious, requiring intravenous antibiotics and hospitalization, especially if a virulent organism is identified. If dacryocystitis is recurrent, there is a serious threat of septicemia, and definitive treatment is required.

If routine probing of silicone intubation fails, these infants may require DCR at an age earlier than 18 months. The editor has had occasion to perform DCRs under these circumstances on 6 infants ranging in age from 2 weeks to 1 year.

Although the anatomy was small in size, the surgery was not technically difficult. The DCR has been successful in each case, with no unexpected complications. To date, there has been no evidence of nasal deformity resulting from this surgery at an early age.

Thus, when serious bacterial infections are recurrent, and routine probing fails, it is possible to perform DCR on infants.

REFERENCES

1. Katowitz JA, Welsh MG: Timing of initial probing and irrigation in congenital nasolacrimal duct obstruction. Ophthalmology 94:698–705, 1987
2. Duke-Elder S, Cook C: Normal and abnormal development. Part 1. Embryology.

In Duke-Elder S (ed): System of Ophthalmology. Vol. 3. CV Mosby, St. Louis, 1963

3. Duke-Elder S: Normal and abnormal development. Part 2. Congenital deformities. In Duke-Elder S (ed): System of Ophthalmology. Vol. 3. CV Mosby, St. Louis, 1963

4. Jones LT, Wobig JL: Surgery of the Eyelids and Lacrimal System. Aesculapius, Birmingham, 1976, p. 160

5. Schaefer AJ, Campbell CB, Flanagan JC: Congenital lacrimal disorders In Smith BC et al. (eds): Ophthalmic Plastic and Reconstructive Surgery. Vol. 1. CV Mosby, St. Louis, 1987

6. Whitaker LA, Katowitz JA, Randall P: The nasolacrimal apparatus in congenital facial anomalies. J Maxillofac Surg 2:59, 1974

7. Hurwitz JJ, Welham RAN: The role of dacryocystography in the management of congenital nasolacrimal duct obstruction. Can J Ophthalmol 10:346, 1975

8. Heyman S, Katowitz JA: Dacryoscintigraphy. In Treves ST (ed): Pediatric Nuclear Medicine. Springer-Verlag, New York, 1985

9. Baker JD: Treatment of congenital nasolacrimal system obstruction. J Pediatr Ophthalmol Strabismus 22:34, 1985

10. Petersen RA, Robb RM: The natural course of congenital obstruction of the nasolacrimal duct. J Pediatr Ophthalmol Strabismus 15:246, 1978

11. Nelson LB, Calhoun JH, Menduke H: Medical management of congenital nasolacrimal duct obstruction. Pediatrics 76:172, 1985

12. Paul TO: Medical management of congenital nasolacrimal duct obstruction. J Pediatr Ophthalmol Strabismus 22:68, 1985

13. Durso F, Hand JR. SI, Ellis FD, Helveston EM: Silicone intubation in children with nasolacrimal obstruction. J Pediatr Ophthalmol Strabismus 17:389, 1980

14. Welham RAN, Hughes SM: Lacrimal surgery in children. Am J Ophthalmol 99:27, 1985

15. Scott WE, Fabre JA, Ossoinig KC: Congenital mucocele of the lacrimal sac. Arch Ophthalmol 97:1656, 1979

16. Levy NS: Conservative management of congenital amniotocele of the nasolacrimal sac. J Pediatr Ophthalmol Strabismus 16:254, 1979

17. Weinstein GS, Biglan AW, Patterson JH: Congenital lacrimal sac mucoceles. Am J Ophthalmol 94:106–110, 1982

6 | Silicone Intubation of the Nasolacrimal Drainage System*

James A. Katowitz
Donald A. Hollsten

The use of silicone tubing to facilitate repair of the nasolacrimal system was first described by Gibbs, who reported its use in the repair of damaged canaliculi in 1967.[1] Before that time, polyethylene and nylon had been used for intubation of the nasolacrimal system.[2-5] Since then, a number of authors have described the use of silicone intubation in the treatment of both congenital and acquired lacrimal drainage disorders.[6-9] Silicone has proven to be nonirritating and flexible, and to give generally favorable results for intubation of the nasolacrimal duct. It can be used as an intermediate between lacrimal probing with turbinate infracture and dacryocystorhinostomy (DCR) in the management of dacryostenosis.[10] (See Chapter 5.)

As with any surgical procedure, knowledge of the anatomy is essential if silicone intubation of the nasolacrimal system is to be performed safely and effectively.

---

* The opinions or assertions contained herein are the private views of the authors and are not to be construed as official or as reflecting the views of the Department of the Army or the Department of Defense.

ANATOMY

The nasolacrimal drainage system in humans consists of tubes lined with respiratory epithelium which extend from the medial aspect of both lids to the inferior meatus of the nostril (Fig. 6-1). The nasolacrimal duct and lacrimal sac are said to be partially lined by ciliated epithelium, whereas the canaliculi are free of cilia.[11] Tears enter the lacrimal drainage system through a punctum located in the medial aspect of each lid. The lower lid puncta are believed to be responsible for most tear drainage, but it is possible to have atresia of the lower lid puncta without epiphora, so the upper canaliculus can often provide adequate lacrimal drainage. The puncta open into an ampulla approximately 1.5 to 2.0 mm in diameter. This dilation of the canaliculus extends into the lid, perpendicular to the margin, for approximately 2 mm before turning 90 degrees to course nasally. The canaliculi roughly parallel the lid margin, passing slightly posterior between the anterior and posterior crus of the medial canthal tendon. The horizontal portions of the canaliculi are approximately 8 mm long. In 90 percent of individuals, the upper and lower lid canaliculi join to form a common canaliculus before entering the lacrimal sac. In some instances the two canaliculi do not join, and enter the sac separately. A fold of mucosa, the valve of Rosenmüller, is usually present at the junction of the common canaliculus and the lacrimal sac.

The lacrimal sac is oriented vertically. The fundus of the sac extends superiorly from the valve of Rosenmüller for about 5 mm before ending blindly. The inferior aspect of the sac extends from the valve of Rosenmüller to the nasolacrimal duct, a distance of approximately 10 mm. The duct, coursing inferiorly and slightly posteriorly, travels through bone for 12 mm and through mucosa for approximately 5 mm before opening into the inferior meatus. The nasolacrimal ostium is about 30 to 35 mm from the external nares.

The functional portion of the nasolacrimal drainage system in the adult measures approximately 37 mm from the punctum to the end of the nasolacrimal duct at the valve of Hasner. These dimensions are smaller in children, depending on the age of the child.

The lacrimal drainage system can be divided into two functional portions. The upper system consists of the puncta and canaliculi, and the lower system consists of the lacrimal sac and nasolacrimal duct (Fig. 6-1).

INDICATIONS FOR INTUBATION

Intubation of the nasolacrimal system has been advocated for a variety of indications. A number of authors have discussed the efficacy of silicone intubation in congenital dacryostenosis not responsive to probing and irrigation.[10,12–14] Other problems for which silicone intubation has been used include acquired dacryostenosis in adults, canalicular obstruction, canalicular laceration, and as a DCR stent.[9,10,12–14]

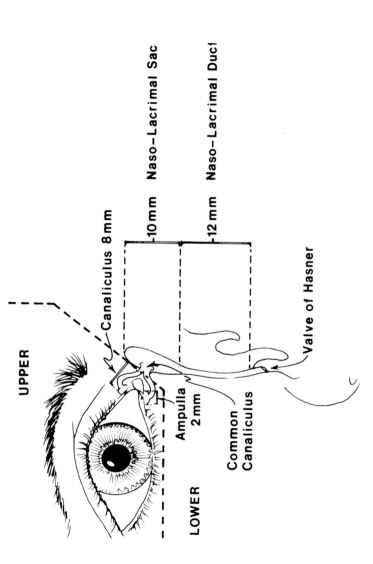

Fig. 6-1 Normal anatomy of the lacrimal drainage system. Dotted lines show upper and lower portions of the system.

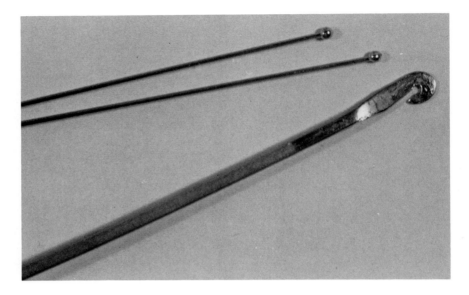

Fig. 6-2   Crawford hook and probes.

INTUBATION MATERIALS

Silastic tubing of 0.25 mm external diameter is preferred for pediatric and adult use. Although the tubing can be glued in place over a #0 tapered probe with silicone bonding glue prior to autoclaving, we prefer to use prepackaged intubation sets with the Silastic already attached to two probes.[7,12] While this is slightly more expensive, it greatly facilitates use of the Silastic tubing by avoiding the sometimes troublesome step of attaching the tubing to the probe during intubation.

Several types of probes are available, which vary in malleability and design. It is important to use a probe that is malleable enough not to traumatize the lacrimal drainage system. Also, the bonding method should prevent tube slippage while the lacrimal drainage system is intubated. We prefer the Crawford intubation set because of the malleability of the probes and the ease of retrieval from the nose. The probe is designed with a bulbous tip that can be caught with a specially designed hook[7,12] (Fig. 6-2).

ANESTHESIA FOR SILASTIC INTUBATION

In children, general anesthesia via an endotracheal tube is indicated, not only to protect the airway from any bronchospasm induced by irrigation or hemorrhage but because the length of the procedure cannot be predicted. While nasolacrimal probing with Silastic tubing intubation is usually a short operative procedure, it can, on occasion, require 45 minutes or longer even in the hands of the most experienced practitioner. For these reasons, endotracheal intubation is indicated.

In adults, on the other hand, Silastic intubation is performed under either local or general anesthesia. If additional surgical procedures are planned, the patient may select general anesthesia. However, local anesthesia can be used if the patient chooses or if the patient's health makes general anesthesia dangerous. To perform the procedure under local anesthesia, a topical anesthetic agent is placed on the eye three or four times over a 5-minute interval. In addition, a cotton swab moistened with 4 percent cocaine solution is placed in the inferior meatus at the opening of the nasolacrimal duct. A local anesthetic agent is irrigated through the lacrimal drainage system by placing an irrigating cannula into one of the canaliculi. The intubation can be attempted at this time. If the patient is still uncomfortable, the anesthesia can be augmented with local infiltration of 1 percent or 2 percent lidocaine. These techniques will usually allow the intubation to be performed with little or no discomfort.

TECHNIQUES OF INSERTION

Although the accomplished ophthalmic surgeon may frequently perform a rapid and atraumatic intubation of the lacrimal drainage system, problems will sometimes arise. The probe must negotiate several right-angle turns before exiting the nostril. The probe can also be very difficult to retrieve from the floor of the inferior meatus. In children the inferior meatus is narrow, with little space between the nasal floor, lateral wall, and inferior turbinate.[10] These factors combine to make an apparently simple procedure often quite challenging.

Intubation begins at the lower lid. The punctum should first be dilated with a punctal dilator to insure an adequate opening. Care should be taken to avoid creating a false passage with the dilator. On rare occasions it may be necessary to perform a one-snip punctoplasty to ensure an adequate opening without creating a false passage.

After the lower punctum is dilated, the probe tip is introduced into the punctum at a right angle to the lid margin. Insertion to a depth of 1 to 2 mm will place the tip at the base of the ampulla. At this time, the lateral aspect of the upper lid should be anchored with the surgeon's finger in order to avoid an accordion-like folding of the nasal lid when the probe is passed through the horizontal canaliculus. Such folding will impede passage of the probe and will also increase the likelihood of a false passage.

The probe is passed nasally parallel to the lid margin until the lacrimal sac is entered and the firm nasal wall of the lacrimal sac encountered. The valve of Rosenmüller at the entrance of the canaliculus is called a "soft stop" and differs in quality from the "hard stop" encountered when the probe hits the nasal wall of the lacrimal fossa. If the practitioner is unsure whether a soft stop has been encountered, it is helpful to release the lateral tension on the lid and gently advance the probe nasally. If the probe has encountered a soft stop, nasal movement of the probe will usually be accompanied by nasal movement of the eyelid, most visible in the medial canthal area. On the other hand, if the probe has encountered a hard stop, nasal movement of the probe is not accompanied by a corresponding movement in the lid. A soft stop can be safely passed with little difficulty if the surgeon maintains gentle nasal pressure on the probe while maintaining lateral tension on the eyelid, and directs the probe along the anatomic pathway of the canaliculus (parallel to the lid margin and slightly posterior).

Once the soft stop of the valve of Rosenmüller has been passed and the practitioner is sure that the hard stop of the nasolacrimal wall has been encountered, it is necessary to direct the probe down the lacrimal sac and nasolacrimal duct. To accomplish this, the lateral tension on the eyelid is released and the probe redirected. The probe is rotated 90 degrees until it is directed inferior and slightly posterior. It is sometimes necessary to rotate the probe past the sagittal plane, directing it slightly temporal in order to place the tip in the superior opening of the duct. It is important to recognize when the probe tip has reached the inferior meatus. Continued pressure once the nasal floor has been encountered can curl the probe posteriorly, making retrieval more difficult.

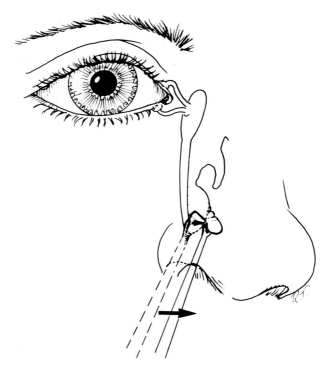

Fig. 6-3 Infracture of the inferior turbinate with the blunt edge of the periosteal elevator.

After the probe has been passed through the lacrimal drainage system, it is necessary to retrieve the tip from the inferior meatus. This can be the most difficult step of the procedure, especially in the child whose inferior meatus is more of a potential space, and smaller than that of the adult.[10] Malleable probes will greatly facilitate this portion of the procedure. It is useful to shrink the nasal mucosa of the inferior meatus with 4 percent cocaine solution or oxymetazoline (Afrin). The inferior turbinate can also be infractured to enlarge the meatus (Fig. 6-3). Infracture is usually a valuable step in the pediatric patient but not always required in adults, where the space for probe retrieval is often adequate. Depending on the type of intubation system used, actual retrieval of the probe can be accomplished by several different methods. For the Quickert-Dryden system, a grooved director can be inserted into the nostril and an attempt made to "capture" the probe tip in the groove.[4] This can be difficult, however, and the tip may curve posteriorly rather than anteriorly. The tip may also be grasped with a small hemostat. One commercially marketed probe system is illuminated by fiberoptics to facilitate the retrieval. As described earlier, the newer, malleable Crawford-type probes with the bulbous tip offer a significant advantage; they can be retrieved with a special hook[12] (Fig. 6-4). This system facilitates probe retrieval in the infant as well as the adult.

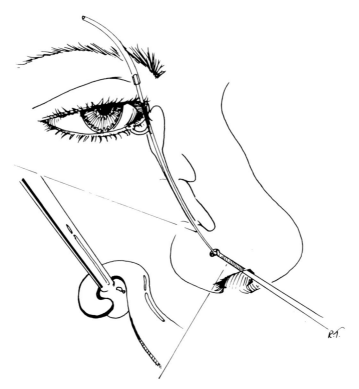

Fig. 6-4   Retrieval of the probe from inferior meatus with the Crawford hook.

Once the probe tip is captured and ready for extraction from the nostril, it is helpful to lubricate the distal probe and tubing with an antibiotic ointment. Lubrication will allow the Silastic tubing to slide through the lacrimal drainage system with mimimum resistance. The probe must be pulled from the nose with a smooth, quick motion. These two techniques will minimize the possibility of the tubing separating from the probe as it is pulled through the system. Bending the probe into a curve will minimize trauma to the lacrimal system and protect the cornea.

The upper canaliculus makes a shallower angle at its entrance into the lacrimal sac, and is therefore both easier to intubate and less likely to be traumatized by the second probe.

When the lower lid has been intubated, the second probe (attached to the other end of the Silastic tubing) is then inserted through the upper canaliculus and retrieved from the nose in a similar fashion.

FIXATION OF THE TUBING

Fixation of the tubing is necessary after the system has been successfully intubated. The ends of the tubing must be tied and secured with the proper amount of tension. A Silastic tube that is too loose can protrude from the canaliculus and rub the cornea. Likewise, a tube that is too tight can cause erosion and slitting of the punctum, particularly in the young child who will grow rapidly during a 6-month period of intubation.

In children, the use of multiple square knots alone to fix the tubing in the inferior meatus can lead to problems. The child may catch the loop of tubing in the medial canthal area while rubbing the eye, and pull the knot up into the nasolacrimal duct or even the lacrimal sac. The excess tubing will then protrude from the puncta. This usually results in an urgent phone call from the parents.

Several methods of fixation have been proposed.[15] These include use of multiple knots in the inferior meatus, fixation of the tubing to the nasal mucosa with a nonabsorbable suture, and attachment of a retinal sponge to prevent migration of the Silastic knots up the nasolacrimal duct. We prefer a cuff of larger bore tubing. A small piece of neurosurgical shunt tubing makes a useful cuff that is also radiopaque (Silastic Peritoneal Catheter, Dow Corning Medical Products, Midland, MI). The cuff should be cut to a length of about 4 mm (Fig. 6-5). Both ends of the Silastic tubing are placed through the cuff before they are detached from the probes. The ends of the tubes are then tied with multiple square knots, creating a knot larger than the bore of the cuff (Fig. 6-6). Fixation of the cuff can be reinforced with a nonabsorbable suture placed through the cuff and between the knots as they are tied. The cuff creates a mass that is too large to pass up the nasolacrimal duct even if the tube is grasped by a child.

The proper amount of tension on the Silastic tubing can be estimated by tying a temporary knot and then pulling the slack tubing from the puncta to see how far over the surface of the eye it will extend. When properly tightened,

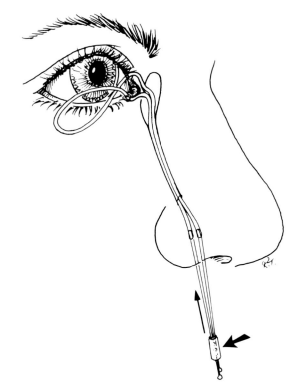

Fig. 6-5 The probes are passed through a cuff of neurosurgical shunt tubing.

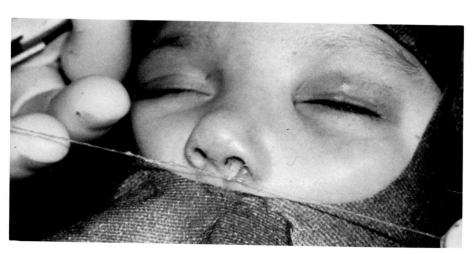

Fig. 6-6 Multiple surgical knots are tied below the cuff.

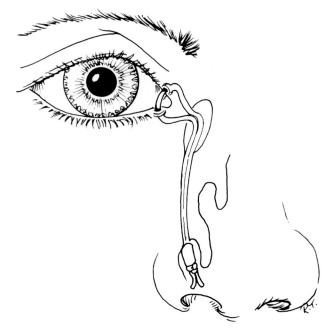

Fig. 6-7   The cuff is positioned below the inferior turbinate after excess length tubing below knots is cut off.

the slack tubing should extend 2 mm to 3 mm from the puncta without tension. A handy landmark is the nasal limbus with the eye in primary position. The slack tubing should extend from the puncta no further than the nasal limbus in a young child or halfway to the limbus in an adult. After the appropriate tension has been determined, multiple knots are placed in the Silastic tubing and the excess ends cut. The cuff and knots are then placed at the inferior meatus of the nostril (Fig. 6-7).

POSTOPERATIVE MANAGEMENT AND COMPLICATIONS

Immediate postoperative care consists of twice daily application of antibiotic ointment. This can be tapered after several days to bedtime use only. Patients should be seen one week postoperatively and then 3 to 4 weeks later. If no complications are discovered, followup every 2 to 3 months is routine.

Careful and frequent followup is necessary after successful intubation of the lacrimal drainage system to allow early diagnosis of complications. Frank rejection of the Silastic tubing by the host is, fortunately, extremely rare. Dacryocystitis is more common but still unusual. The tubing in the nasolacrimal duct occupies a significant cross-sectional area, and can itself obstruct the outflow, which can lead to dacryocystitis. Unless systemic antibiotics result in complete remission, the tubing should be removed. Dacryocystitis is an ominous sign and usually indicates that a dacryocystorhinostomy will be required to cure the patient's nasolacrimal obstruction.

A more common complication is cheesewiring of the canaliculi. This complication is usually caused by tying the tubing too tightly. In children, rapid growth of the face in the presence of a Silastic loop of fixed length loop can be responsible for canalicular slitting. Careful clinical judgment is required when tying the tubing. As described earlier, some slack should be left to allow for growth, but not so much as to allow corneal irritation. A small amount of canalicular cheesewiring can be tolerated and is not an absolute indication for removal. Close follow-up with determination of the amount and progression of cheesewiring is essential. A slit of up to one-half of the canaliculi does not seem to cause problems after tube removal. Cheesewiring beyond one-half of the canalicular length needs to be weighed against the benefit to be obtained by allowing the tube to remain in place. If the potential benefits are not great, the tube should be removed.

A common but usually minor complication of Silastic intubation is the formation of a pyogenic granuloma at the punctum. An unpleasant odor may accompany this type of growth. In most cases the granuloma can be effectively treated with excision and careful bipolar cautery. Formation of a granuloma is not by itself an indication for removal of the tube.

Nasal hemorrhage is a complication of Silastic intubation often seen in the immediate postoperative period. Bleeding may result from penetration of an obstruction in the lacrimal duct or at the valve of Hasner, but most often it results from trauma to the nasal mucosa during infracture of the inferior turbinate or retrieval of the probes from the inferior meatus. The hemorrhage is usually mild and easily managed with vasoconstrictor spray, cold compresses, and head elevation. More severe cases may require placement of a nasal pack. Severe nosebleeds can require cautery, hospitalization, and assistance from a rhinologist. Nasal bleeding in children needs to be observed closely because of their smaller total blood volume.

A complication seen more commonly in children is retrograde migration of the knots through the nasolacrimal duct into the lacrimal sac. This usually occurs when the child applies traction to the exposed tubing in the medial canthal area, either by rubbing the eye or by actually grasping the tubing. The child will present with a long loop of tubing protruding from the puncta, usually in a fashion that irritates the eye (Fig. 6-8). It would appear that this complication could be addressed by cutting the loop in the medial canthal area and pulling the knots through the common canaliculus and out one of the puncta. Unfortunately, such a maneuver could damage the upper drainage system by causing a stricture, and should only be considered if the knot is known to be very small, on the order of a single square knot. Our preferred method is to cut the loop in the medial canthal angle and place a small probe into the lumen of the tubing emerging from the upper lid canaliculus (Fig. 6-9). The probe, with tubing attached, can then be passed down the lacrimal drainage system.

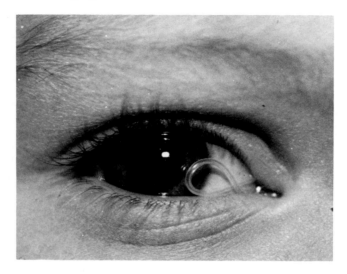

Fig. 6-8   Silastic tubing pulled from the inner canthus.

The probe tip is then identified in the inferior meatus and the tubing extracted from the nostril (Fig. 6-10). If further intubation treatment is necessary, the system can then be intubated with fresh Silastic tubing. This technique avoids trauma to the common canaliculus and its opening into the lacrimal sac. The upper lid is chosen for passage of the probe with its swaged-on tubing in order to avoid damage to the more important lower lid drainage system. Retrograde knot migration can also occur in the adult, usually when the tubing has been tied incorrectly, with too much slack in the Silastic loop. Correction in the adult is simple. The loose ends of tubing can usually be visualized in the inferior meatus. A head lamp or indirect ophthalmoscope can be used to assist visu-

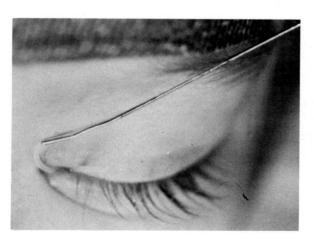

Fig. 6-9   The tube loop is cut and a triple 0 Bowman probe threaded into the lumen of the tubing from the upper canaliculus.

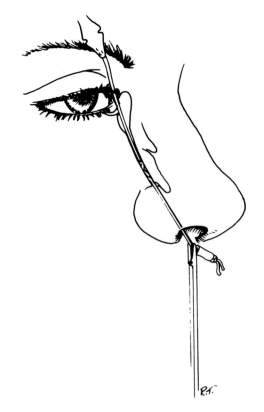

Fig. 6-10 The triple 0 Bowman probe is passed down the system into the nose and the tubing is retrieved with alligator forceps. (If needed, an intubation of the system can now be performed with a new intubation set.)

alization. The tube ends can be grasped with a small forceps and gently pulled out the nostril. With the tube thus stretched, a 5-0 or 6-0 silk suture can be tied around both arms of tubing proximal to the knot. This suture effectively shortens the loop and prevents the complication from recurring. The tube ends are then returned to the inferior meatus.

REMOVAL OF TUBING

The timing of tube removal is determined by balancing the benefits of leaving the Silastic material in place against any complications that may have developed. The original 6-week concept has evolved over the years to a more extended period. Six months of intubation is now considered appropriate in most clinical situations.[7–10, 12, 13] One reason for this change in philosophy has been the application of the increased understanding of wound healing. Wound healing is known to include four phases: inflammatory, fibroblastic, maturation, and contraction.[16] The maturation phase begins about 1 month after trauma and continues for years. The scar reaches its maximum strength at about 12 weeks. It is desirable to leave the Silastic tubing in place at least until wound healing is well into the maturation phase. If it is removed earlier, wound contracture may occur in any strictures that have been penetrated, which could lead to recurrence of epiphora.

A conceptual distinction needs to be made between what may occur in the nasolacrimal duct of a child with Silastic intubation and in that of an adult. In the very young child, the presence of a stent in the duct may stimulate expansion as well as prevent wound contracture. This is similar to the use of a prosthesis to expand the microphthalmic orbit—skeletal and soft tissue growth is increased by the pressure of foreign material used to stretch and stimulate growth. In the adult, the effect of such expansion in the orbit is very limited, and this is probably the case in the nasolacrimal duct as well. The potential for reducing wound contracture by the presence of a stent is, however, probably a more critical factor.

In the adult, 6 months of treatment with Silastic tubing is indicated for most situations unless a complication necessitates earlier removal. Indications for early removal include dacryocystitis, rejection, and cheesewiring of more than one-half of the canalicular length. Removal in adults is usually simple. The tube is cut in the medial canthal area and the patient asked to blow his or her nose into a tissue. This often results in passage of the cut tube through the lacrimal drainage system and capture in tissue. If this maneuver is not successful, the nostril can be opened with a nasal speculum and the tube ends visualized directly. Again, illumination from the indirect ophthalmoscope or other headlight is very helpful. After it has been visualized, the tubing can usually be grasped with a small forceps or hook.

Timing of tube removal is more critical in children. Facial growth can result in cheesewiring. It is desirable to leave the tube in place as close to 6 months as possible. Treatment can be longer than 6 months if clinical observation reveals good tube placement with no complications. Removal of the tube in children usually requires endotracheal intubation with general anesthesia. However, removal in the office can be performed on cooperative children as young as 5 or 6 years of age. The technique differs from removal in adults in that children are not asked to blow their nose. The tube is first grasped with direct visualization using a hemostat by the practitioner. The loop in the inner canthus is then cut and the ends withdrawn from the nostril.

SUMMARY

Silastic intubation of the nasolacrimal duct has proven an effective alternative to dacryocystorhinostomy in selected pediatric and adult cases of nasolacrimal duct stenosis. When properly inserted and monitored, it may avoid further surgery. Although Silastic tubing could, perhaps, be left in the nasolacrimal duct for a more extended period, the current recommended period before removal is approximately 6 months.

REFERENCES

1. Gibbs DC: New probe for the intubation of lacrimal canaliculi with silicone rubber tubing. Br J Ophthalmol 51:198, 1967
2. Shannon GM, Hamdi TN: Repair of injuries of the lacrimal canaliculus. Am J Ophthalmol 62:974, 1966
3. Griffith TP: Polythene tubes in canaliculus surgery. Br J Ophthalmol 47:203, 1963
4. Quickert MH, Dryden RM: Probes for intubation in lacrimal drainage. Trans Am Acad Ophthalmol Otolaryngol 74:431, 1970
5. Werb A: Surgery of epiphora. Int Ophthalmol Clin 4:377, 1964
6. Keith CG: Intubation of the lacrimal passages. Am J Ophthalmol 65:70, 1968
7. Crawford JS: Intubation of obstruction in the lacrimal system. Can J Ophthalmol 12:289, 1977
8. Soll DB: Silicone intubation: An alternative to dacryocystorhinostomy. Ophthalmology 85:1259, 1978
9. Pashby RD, Rathbun JE: Silicone tube intubation of the lacrimal drainage system. Arch Ophthalmol 97:1318, 1979
10. Katowitz JA: Lacrimal drainage surgery. In Duane TD (ed): Clinical Ophthalmology. Vol. 5. Harper & Row, Philadelphia, 1983
11. Duke-Elder S: The Anatomy of The Visual System. Vol. II. System of Ophthalmology. CV Mosby, St. Louis, MO, 1961
12. Kraft SP, Crawford JS: Silicone tube intubation in disorders of the lacrimal system in children. Am J Ophthalmol 94:290, 1982
13. Dortzbach RK, France TD, Kushner BJ, et al: Silicone intubation for obstruction of the nasolacrimal duct in children. Am J Ophthalmol 94:585, 1982
14. Katowitz JA, Welsh MG: The timing of initial probing and irrigation in congenital nasolacrimal duct obstruction. Ophthalmology 94:698,
15. Lauring L: Silicone intubation of the lacrimal system: pitfalls, problems, and complications. Ann Ophthalmol 8:489, 1976
16. Wilkins RB, Kulwin DR: Skin and tissue techniques in oculoplastic surgery. pp. 1–14. In McCord CD (ed): Oculoplastic Surgery. Raven Press, New York, 1981

7 | Intranasal Procedures

Ralph E. Wesley

The lacrimal drainage system transports tears from the conjunctival cul de sac to the intranasal cavity. Therefore successful lacrimal surgery requires knowledge of both the ocular and nasal anatomy, including knowledge of intranasal structures not required for traditional cosmetic rhinoplasty or for procedures to improve airway obstruction.[1,2] This chapter describes three intranasal procedures that facilitate lacrimal surgery: infracture of the inferior turbinate in congenital lacrimal obstruction, silicone intubation of the lacrimal system for canalicular lacerations, and removal of the middle turbinate to facilitate dacryocystorhinostomy (DCR) and conjunctivodacryocystorhinostomy (CDCR) surgery.

INTRANASAL ANATOMY AND EXAMINATION

The clearance of the lower nasolacrimal duct relative to the inferior turbinate and the relationship of DCR and CDCR sites to the upper nasal septum and anterior middle turbinate are anatomic characteristics that the lacrimal surgeon must frequently consider. The Jones tube and CDCR are likely to function better in a large nose with a wide bridge than in a small nose or one that has had fractures with callus telescoping inward from the medial canthus and lacrimal sac. In the placement of a Jones tube, a large intranasal space near the medial canthus means that the length of the tube will be less critical and the positioning less tedious. Callus near the medial canthus means that intranasal scarring will be more likely. Such scarring can close a DCR tract performed to alleviate dacryocystitis following a nasal fracture.

A fiberoptic headlight, nasal speculum, and topical decongestant provide the best opportunity for evaluation of the nose prior to surgery. The nasal speculum should be placed into the nose with the handle held horizontally so that the blades separate vertically. Spreading the blades horizontally presses against the patient's nasal septum, causing significant pain and discomfort.

Examination of the nose without a topical decongestant usually provides only a view of the inferior turbinate and some of the lower septum. The inferior turbinate can be seen lying just inside the nose along the lateral wall; it is frequently mistaken for a polyp by ophthalmologists. The middle turbinate, situated at the level of the medial canthus, usually cannot be seen without decongestion.

Topical 0.25 percent phenylephrine drops sprayed into the nose or applied with a cotton applicator will produce the vasoconstriction required for a good intranasal examination. A nasal tetracaine solution can be applied if anesthesia is required. Cocaine 4 percent solution works well as a vasoconstrictor and anesthetic agent, but we have stopped using cocaine because of the potential for systemic toxicity and the risk of theft.

Once the nasal mucosa has been decongested, the anterior nasal cavity can be examined. The position of the septum affects CDCR surgery. The septum may enlarge or be deviated as it extends upward toward the medial canthus. The space between the septum and the lateral wall of the nose may determine the success of a DCR or CDCR. The position and size of the middle turbinate will also provide information as to whether the middle turbinate should be removed to provide adequate space for the DCR to function. (In my experience, the anterior portion of the middle turbinate must always be removed for a CDCR to function.)

Examination of the inferior turbinate will sometimes reveal a cast coming from the inferior portion of the nasolacrimal duct that may be removed to restore flow of the lacrimal drainage system. Identification of the inferior turbinate is required to retrieve silicone tubes used in lacrimal intubation or to infracture the turbinate in congenital nasolacrimal duct obstruction.

A few relationships need emphasis. The nasolacrimal duct drains tears from the lacrimal sac of the medial canthus into the nose. The lower end of the nasolacrimal duct empties under the inferior turbinate. Figure 7-1 shows that the lacrimal sac and medial canthus correspond to the anterior tip of the middle turbinate. The rhinostomy from the lacrimal sac in DCR surgery enters the nose above the inferior turbinate and anterior to or at the middle turbinate.

The middle turbinate is part of the ethmoid bone attached to the roof of the nose. Just above the nasal roof lies the intracranial cavity separated by the thin cribriform plate. Pulling on the middle turbinate can cause a cerebrospinal fluid leak. The septum is cartilaginous inferiorly but consists of bone superiorly near the area where the DCR or CDCR drains into the nose, which makes septoplasty in the area near a rhinostomy more difficult.

The frontal sinus drains under the middle turbinate, as do the maxillary sinus and most of the ethmoid sinuses. Surgery on the middle turbinate or intranasal packing material can thus block the drainage of the frontal sinus. The superior turbinate can rarely be identified during surgery.

Intranasal relationships can be best appreciated during surgery when the

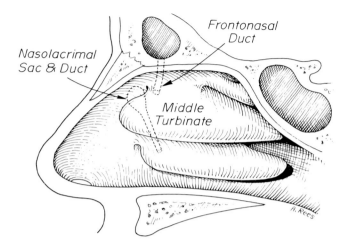

Fig. 7-1 The nasolacrimal duct drains beneath the inferior turbinate. The lacrimal sac fossa, the site of the opening of a DCR into the nose, lies near the middle turbinate. The anterior middle turbinate may need removal (e.g., Fig. 7-6) to provide adequate drainage for a DCR or CDCR. Note that the frontal sinus drainage can be affected by removal of the anterior middle turbinate.

surgeon examines the anatomy both through the nose and through a rhinostomy. Placing a cotton-tipped applicator or suction tip through the rhinostomy while viewing through the nare allows immediate appreciation of the relationship of intranasal structure to lacrimal drainage function. Placing a probe up through the nose while viewing through the rhinostomy will give added perspective as to the position of the septum. Constant comparison using both techniques will provide the needed visual orientation, which is extremely important in smaller noses or in those with anatomic variations.

For hemostasis during surgery, phenylephrine drops can be applied with cotton balls or cotton applicators using bayonet forceps. With friable mucosa or a highly vascular mucosa that needs stronger vasoconstriction, local anesthetic with 1:100,000 epinephrine can be injected for further vasoconstriction. If the patient has severe hypertension or arrhythmias, the epinephrine can be diluted for greater safety.

Polyps, previous surgery, or anatomic variation makes the examination of intranasal anatomy a constant challenge as well as a rewarding learning experience. The assistance of an otorhinolaryngologist can be helpful when performing a procedure under difficult or unfamiliar circumstances. I recommend that the lacrimal surgeon freely call upon the valued experience of colleagues when performing new procedures. The cooperation of specialties can provide a learning experience for each surgeon and a gratifying result for the patient.

INFRACTURE OF THE INFERIOR TURBINATE FOR CONGENITAL NASOLACRIMAL DUCT OBSTRUCTION

Most newborns with congenital nasolacrimal duct obstruction have only brief episodes of tearing and mattering, which resolve spontaneously in the first several weeks or months of life as the nasolacrimal duct epithelium opens into the nose.[4] If the obstruction fails to resolve with massage and topical medications, a simple probe and irrigation usually alleviate the nasolacrimal duct obstruction.

In some children, congenital nasolacrimal duct obstruction persists despite probing and irrigation. In the past, children who did not respond to probing were treated with silicone intubation of the nasolacrimal duct.[5-7] Silicone intubation of the nasolacrimal duct usually solves the problem, but even this procedure sometimes fails and the child may need a DCR.

A study at Vanderbilt University Medical Center of patients with congenital nasolacrimal duct obstruction that failed to respond to one or two probings[8] showed that simple infracture of the turbinate with a straight hemostat had an extremely high rate of success. This procedure requires simple equipment and far less skill than does silicone intubation. It may have a higher rate of success than silicone intubation in problem patients with congenital nasolacrimal duct obstruction, but no comparison study has been performed.

The infracture of the inferior turbinate[9] moves the body of the inferior turbinate away from the lower end of the nasolacrimal duct and stretches open the obstruction of the inferior nasolacrimal duct. In a study of 50 problem patients[8] (either older children or children for whom nasolacrimal duct obstruction had failed to resolve despite one to four previous probings), all but four responded to infracture. Three of these failures were found to have no nasolacrimal duct, and required a DCR.

The infracture of the turbinate is performed after a routine probing with the overhead operating lights and visualization with a pediatric speculum of the inferior turbinate (just inside the nares along the lateral wall of the nose). Many surgeons unfamiliar with intranasal anatomy mistake the inferior turbinate for a polyp. The middle turbinate usually cannot be seen well without vasoconstriction since it lies up near the medial canthus.

Phenylephrine $\frac{1}{8}$ percent on cotton packing should be placed inside the nose beside the inferior turbinate. After 3 minutes the cotton can be removed and a small, straight hemostat placed into the nose so that one blade slips under the inferior turbinate (Fig. 7-2).

The inferior turbinate on the involved side frequently appears both smaller and plastered against the lateral wall of the nose compared with the more normal side. The blades of the hemostat should be opened and placed around the inferior turbinate (Fig. 7-3). The hemostat should be firmly closed to avoid abrading the mucosa when the hemostat is twisted. The turbinate should be rotated a full 90 degrees toward the midline nasal septum in an aggressive infracture (Fig. 7-4). The turbinate will be felt to "give" when the infracture is properly performed.

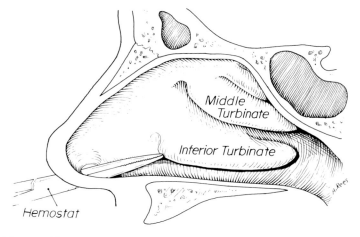

Fig. 7-2 Most problem cases of congenital nasolacrimal duct obstruction can be cured by simply infracturing the inferior turbinate with a straight hemostat. The hemostat is advanced to the tip of the inferior turbinate which lies along the lower, lateral nasal wall.

The firm grip of the hemostat on the turbinate prevents slipping and abrasion of the nasal mucosa, reducing the chance of nosebleed. The hemostat will leave a crushed mark on the turbinate, which helps prevent bleeding from the mucosa. Follow-up of these patients has shown that the turbinate later returns to nearly the original position. Airway obstruction has not been created.

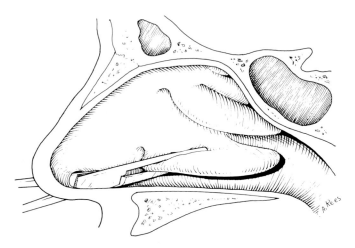

Fig. 7-3 The blades of the hemostat should be opened and the hemostat slipped onto the inferior turbinate. If the turbinate is plastered against the lateral wall of the nose, the lateral blade must be forced between the turbinate and the lateral wall of the nose.

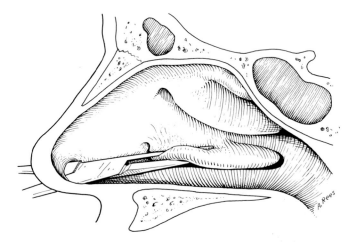

Fig. 7-4   With the blades of the hemostat firmly clamped, the inferior turbinate should be twisted a full 90 degrees toward the midline. This moves the inferior turbinate toward the nasal septum and away from the opening of the nasolacrimal duct.

Following infracture of the turbinate, irrigation should be attempted. If the irrigation is successful, a small piece of Gelfoam can be placed under the inferior turbinate for additional hemostasis. The parents are told that the child may tear for a week or so while the Gelfoam at the base of the nasolacrimal duct dissolves and the edema of the lacrimal system from the probing subsides. No medication is given and the patient is re-examined one month after the infracture procedure.

Just after infracturing the turbinate, it may not be possible to irrigate into the nose. The duct will slowly stretch open during the subsequent weeks and the tearing or purulence will subside. However, the surgeon will be reassured if he can irrigate into the nose while the child is on the operating table. This can be accomplished by using a muscle hook from below to pop open any residual obstruction.

The muscle hook test is performed by inserting a small tenotomy muscle hook into the nose with the tip pointed upward as it passes under the inferior turbinate. The tip will fall upward into the lower end of the nasolacrimal duct (Fig. 7-5). This gives a very definite feel—in fact, the child's head can frequently be lifted off the table with the tip of the muscle hook in the nasolacrimal duct. The surgeon can then irrigate into the nose immediately, rather than waiting for the duct to stretch open.

The muscle hook maneuver also provides important diagnostic and prognostic information. If no nasolacrimal duct can be found with the muscle hook from below, the child most likely has an abnormal nasolacrimal duct (congenital nasolacrimal anomaly), which probably will require a DCR for relief.

While performing this maneuver in over 90 children, I have encountered three who had anomalous development of the nasolacrimal duct, rather than

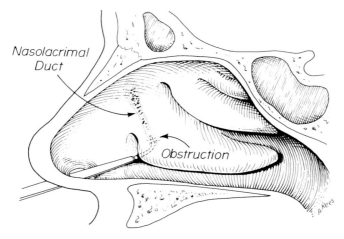

Fig. 7-5   A small tenotomy muscle hook inserted with the tip pointed upward can be used to verify the presence of the nasolacrimal duct. The tip of the hook will fall up into the nasolacrimal duct and pop open any residual obstruction so that the surgeon can irrigate into the nose.

membranous obstruction of the distal duct. They had been probed multiple times. In each case, the muscle hook test revealed no nasolacrimal duct opening under the inferior turbinate. This finding suggested that a DCR was required. All three patients responded well to this procedure. In all three, a lacrimal sac was identified during DCR, but no nasolacrimal duct.

Most surgeons still use silicone intubation in problem cases of congenital nasolacrimal duct obstruction. Insertion of silicone tubes requires considerable skill, and once inserted, the tubes must be left in place for up to six months. They frequently extrude, and sometimes fail to alleviate the problem. Infracture of the turbinate avoids use of the silicone tubes and can be accomplished with simple equipment. I suspect that some of the success associated with silicone intubation is related to the fact that infracture of the turbinate is often required for placement of the silicone tubes.

I avoid cocaine drops in children because of the potential for toxicity.[10] Phenylephrine drops provide adequate vasoconstriction and carry much less risk of cardiac arrhythmia than epinephrine or cocaine. A small piece of Gelfoam beneath the inferior turbinate and a few drops of thrombin in the nose help to prevent nosebleed. Children often have some bloody drainage from the nose after infracture. An active nosebleed in a child requires examination, since the amount of blood loss is critical and cannot be adequately assessed by telephone. In case of active nosebleed, I instruct the parents to remain calm, occlude the external nose, and report to their nearest emergency room. To date, there have been no late nosebleeds following infracture of the turbinate.

Infracture of the turbinate is a powerful tool for the treatment of congenital nasolacrimal duct obstruction, whether or not the muscle hook maneuver is used. The unusual patients who require a DCR may be identified at the time of probing by the muscle hook technique, thus avoiding repeated, unnecessary probings or what might be considered "the anesthesia tolerance test."

REMOVAL OF THE MIDDLE TURBINATE IN DCR AND CDCR

With a DCR, the tears are rerouted by opening a hole into the lacrimal sac fossa medial to the lacrimal sac to permit drainage of the tears directly into the nose, bypassing a blocked nasolacrimal duct. The CDCR[3,11] is used to bypass the entire lacrimal drainage system in patients with blockage of the canaliculi. A Pyrex Jones tube is placed from the conjunctiva into the nasal cavity through a rhinostomy.

The rhinostomy in either of these procedures should be placed anterior and inferior to the lacrimal sac. The inferior position aids gravity drainage, and the anterior position helps to avoid the anterior portion of the middle turbinate, just inside the nose (Fig. 7-1). A large, anteriorly developed middle turbinate can compromise either a DCR or a CDCR. In a CDCR, the anterior portion of the middle turbinate must nearly always be removed for the glass Jones tube to function (Fig. 7-6). If the middle turbinate is allowed to remain in place, contact of nasal mucosa with the tube can cause bleeding, discharge, and pain. The tube may change position, irritating the eye and ceasing to function.

I have consulted on several DCR failures in which reoperation revealed that the rhinostomy site was adequate, but that blockage resulted from an

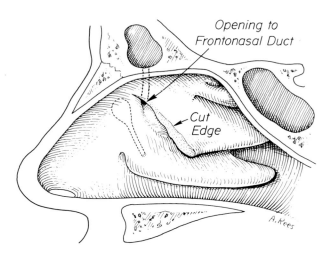

Fig. 7-6 The lateral wall of nose after the tip of middle turbinate has been removed. Cautery of the turbinate or packing can block the frontal sinus because of proximity of the frontonasal duct to the middle turbinate.

enlarged, anteriorly developed middle turbinate. During surgery, the effect of leaving the middle turbinate in place will frequently be misjudged, since the turbinate is shrunken by topical or injected vasoconstrictor agents. When the turbinate returns to normal size it can change the position of the Jones tube or obstruct the DCR site. After the middle turbinate is removed, a larger space is available for placing a Jones tube or performing a DCR.

When the nasal septum is significantly deviated toward the rhinostomy site, I find removal of the turbinate more effective than submucous resection of the nasal septum. In many instances septoplasty results in a midline position for the lower septum, but not for the upper bony septum so critical to lacrimal drainage. Furthermore, because of the risk of cerebrospinal fluid leakage, resection of the superior septum for lacrimal surgery is much more hazardous than the lower airway septoplasty typically performed by general plastic surgeons and otorhinolaryngologists. The most effective superior nasal septoplasty is performed under direct visualization through the rhinostomy at the time of Jones tube placement. If the septoplasty is performed via an incision made externally through the nose, visualization through the rhinostomy will direct the surgeon's instruments to the exact level at which bony septum needs to be removed, yet provide the greatest margin of safety against intracranial penetration.

To remove the anterior portion of the middle turbinate, local anesthetic containing epinephrine should be injected into the turbinate for hemostasis. I prefer to cut the turbinate cleanly, using nasal scissors through the nose or rongeur through the medial canthal rhinostomy. Frequently, I score the middle turbinate with a 15 Bard Parker blade to facilitate the turbinectomy. Leaving the bone of the turbinate exposed can produce prolonged nasal discharge and late nasal bleeding. Twisting the turbinate can rip the superior attachment from the roof, causing cerebrospinal fluid leakage and possible meningitis.

After removing the turbinate, I pack Gelfoam soaked in thrombin onto the bare turbinectomy site for hemostasis. The Gelfoam should not be packed superiorly, as it can block the frontonasal duct (Fig. 7-6), causing a postoperative frontal sinusitis. The Gelfoam slowly dissolves during the first 1 to 2 postoperative weeks.

I used to use unipolar electrocautery to remove the middle turbinate. This method provided excellent hemostasis, but I encountered four patients who developed frontal sinusitis postoperatively.[12] These patients had redness and swelling near the incision, suggestive of cellulitis. Percussion of the frontal sinus and subsequent radiographs documented frontal sinusitis (Fig. 7-7). I have also encountered frontal sinusitis when Gelfoam was packed up against the roof of the nose. None of the cases required surgical decompression of the frontal sinus, as they resolved with steroids and antibiotics. Since the frontonasal duct drains into the nose just beneath the middle turbinate[13,14] (Figs. 7-1 and 7-6), electrocautery near the frontonasal duct may lead to a transient blockage of the frontal sinus. Because the size and shape of the middle turbinate varies with each patient, a large, anteriorly developed middle turbinate may be mistaken for the nasal septum when viewed through the rhinostomy during

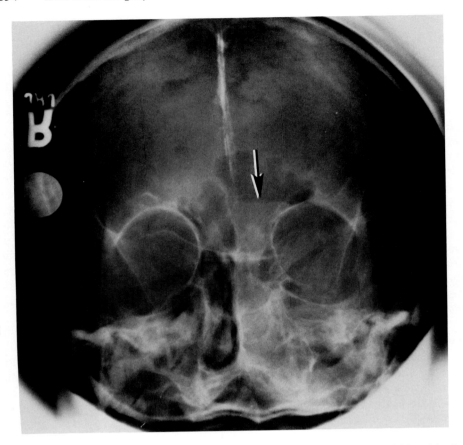

Fig. 7-7   Radiographic verification of frontal sinusitis after DCR. Air-fluid level in the left frontal sinus (arrow) and tenderness to percussion confirm the diagnosis. Patients with pain after DCR should have frontal sinus percussion to check for inflammation of the frontal sinus.

surgery. The middle turbinate should be assessed in each DCR or CDCR by examination both through the nose and through the rhinostomy.

Some patients have a large, anteriorly placed middle turbinate that is pneumatized by a large ethmoid air cell. When the rhinostomy is performed the opening appears to communicate with the nasal cavity, but actually ends blindly in the air cell within the middle turbinate. Unless the middle turbinate is removed, the lacrimal procedure is doomed. This error can be avoided by examining the turbinate both intranasally and through the DCR incision.

When the superior septum deviates toward the rhinostomy placement of a Jones tube during CDCR is extremely difficult. The traditional septoplasty will not provide as much chance for success as will removal of the middle turbinate. After trabeculectomy the tube can be angled posteriorly into the space created by the resection.

Placing Gelfoam soaked in thrombin onto the cut edge of the middle turbinate or using it to stent open a DCR has eliminated the need for gauze or catheter stents inside the nose. Gauze packing requires an uncomfortable removal procedure a day or so after surgery and may cause a nosebleed when pulled away from the bare surface of the nose. The Gelfoam slowly dissolves as the mucosal epithelium heals spontaneously, thus allowing the patients to be discharged from the hospital without waiting for the packing to be removed.

SILICONE INTUBATION OF THE LACRIMAL SYSTEM

Silicone intubation of the lacrimal system is performed most often during repair of canalicular lacerations, and to treat common canalicular obstruction and congenital nasolacrimal duct obstruction. In my experience, placement of silicone tubes during repair of canalicular lacerations not only provides a stent for the lacrimal system, but helps pull the lid posteriorly along the posterior medial canthal tendon.

An avulsed medial eyelid must be attached to the posterior head of the medial canthal tendon for successful eyelid and lacrimal reconstruction. I frequently see a medial canthus that is flattened with a space between the lid, caruncle, and globe since the reconstructive force is greater along the lines of the anterior canthal tendon than along the posterior canthal tendon. Silicone tubes direct this force posteriorly and allow the surgeon to identify the proper position for the lid repair.

Though I do not personally use silicone tubes for congenital lacrimal duct obstruction, they have a success rate of over 90 percent.[5-7] Silicone tubes are probably the most frequently used modality in children who have failed to respond to probings of the nasolacrimal duct.

Several types of silicone tubes that are various modifications of the original method described by Quickert and Dryden[5] are available. I use the prefabricated Guibour tubes (Concept, Inc.)[1] or the Crawford tubes (Jed Med, Inc.).[2] The Crawford tubes have a knob on the end with a fairly flexible probe. In some instances, the extreme flexibility of the Crawford probe makes it difficult to pass down the nasolacrimal duct, requiring the use of the stiffer Guibour tubes. The Crawford tubes offer to novices the advantage of a knob on the end that makes for ease of retrieval with a hook under the inferior turbinate.

The following techniques help in retrieving either type of tube.

First, good vasoconstriction in the intranasal cavity is important. Using a nasal speculum, phenylephrine-soaked cotton balls are placed near the inferior turbinate. Inexperienced surgeons often place the packing too high. The vasoconstrictor needs to be down beside the inferior turbinate and, if possible, underneath the inferior turbinate. Maximum vasoconstriction is then obtained by injecting the inferior turbinate with a mixture of lidocaine with epinephrine

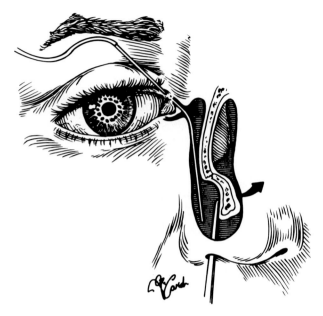

Fig. 7-8 Retrieval of silicone tubes becomes much easier if the inferior turbinate has been fractured away from the lateral wall.

and allowing this mixture to further decongest the nose and reduce the chances of bleeding.

Next, the inferior turbinate should be infractured with a large, straight hemostat in adults, or with a small, straight hemostat in infants. This will give better visualization or, at least, access to the area underneath the inferior turbinate from which the probe must be retrieved (Fig. 7-8).

Next, retrieval will be greatly expedited if the hemostat or Crawford hook is placed underneath the inferior turbinate as soon as the probe starts down the nasolacrimal duct. If the surgeon passes the probe down the nasolacrimal duct and then tries to retrieve it, he or she will find the probe has turned back toward the nasopharynx and lies in an anteroposterior direction. The ideal retrieval is easiest if the probe and the instrument for retrieval, such as the hemostat, are at right angles; therefore, the hemostat or Crawford hook should be underneath the inferior turbinate when the probe starts down. The surgeon can frequently feel the probe and retrieve it. If not, it can be seen with good decongestion and a headlight.

One frequent mistake is passing the hook or hemostat into the nose at too high an angle so that it goes above the inferior turbinate rather than under the middle turbinate (Fig. 7-9). It is impossible to retrieve the tube once this mistake has been made. With the patient lying on the operating table, the retrieval instrument usually needs to be angled inferiorly rather than perpendicular to the operating table. By hugging the floor of the nose, the proper positioning will be accomplished (Fig. 7-10).

Once the tubes have been retrieved from the nose there are many methods of securing them, but I prefer a simple square knot. The tubes are stretched

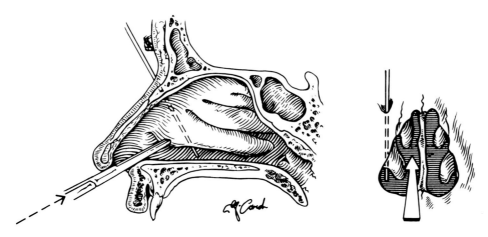

Fig. 7-9 Incorrect technique for retrieval of silicone tubes from the nasal cavity. The hemostat has been inserted above the lower border of the inferior turbinate. The surgeon must identify by sight or by feel the lower edge of the inferior turbinate and pass the instrument beneath the inferior turbinate to retrieve the tubes.

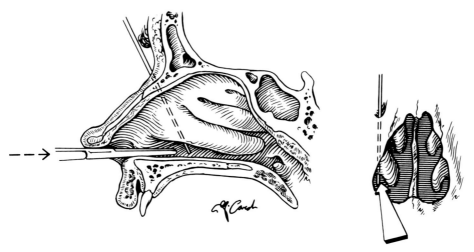

Fig. 7-10 The hook or hemostat to retrieve silicone tubes from the nose must be passed under the inferior turbinate as illustrated. If bleeding obscures visualization, proper placement can be accomplished by hugging the floor of the nose during attempted insertion of the tube retriever under the inferior turbinate.

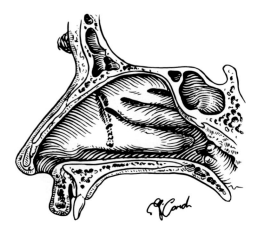

Fig. 7-11 The silicone tubes are secured with a single square knot and allowed to retract under inferior turbinate. Removal is by the eyelid approach.

and tied over the tip of a muscle hook. Once the square knot is secured the muscle hook is removed and the tubes retract under the inferior turbinate (Fig. 7-11).

When the tubes are to be removed, perhaps 6 months later, the easiest path is via the eyelids. Even with uncooperative children, removal from the eyelids can be accomplished in the office so that general anesthesia can be avoided.

The loop of tubing (Fig. 7-12) between the eyelids can be pulled out until

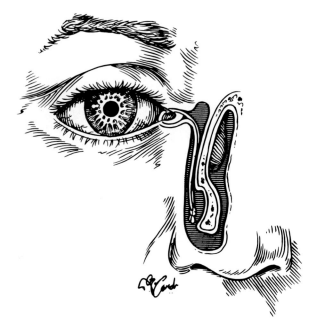

Fig. 7-12 Silicone intubation of the lacrimal system with a square knot under the inferior turbinate. Removal can be accomplished by pulling the eyelid portion until the square knot reaches the common cannaliculus. The square knot is pulled out of the canaliculus; then the tubing can be cut and easily removed.

it is stopped by the square knot reaching the common canaliculus. The square knot is then pulled out of the canaliculus in a hand-over-hand fashion. A single square knot will pass through a canaliculus, whereas multiple knots and tie-downs may not. Once the knot is worked out of the eyelid, the tubing can be cut and the rest of the silicone slides out easily.

NOSEBLEED AFTER INTRANASAL PROCEDURES

The seriousness of nosebleed from lacrimal procedures can vary from nuisance to life-threatening complication. Noses with friable mucosa will bleed profusely when touched with a cotton applicator but usually clot spontaneously in a few minutes if the surgeon is patient. The most serious nosebleeds occur in patients who had little bleeding at the time of surgery because of temporary hemostasis from the vasoconstrictor rather than from active clotting of vessels. Later in the day, as the vasoconstriction subsides, the nose starts to bleed slowly, with the pace increasing gradually because no clots had really formed over the constricted vessels. The other type of serious nosebleed occurs in the patient who starts to bleed approximately 4 days after surgery. In this case, the clot on a larger vessel dissolves before healing has taken place, and the bleed may be persistent.

Almost all nosebleeds will subside spontaneously if the patient's head is elevated and cold or pressure placed on the external nose. The blood pressure should be checked to make sure the patient is not hypertensive. If the nosebleed is chronic, hypotension must be ruled out. If the nosebleed occurs after the patient has left the hospital, the hematocrit must be checked. One cannot tell the seriousness of blood loss from the patient's history. With acute bleeds, the hematocrit will not drop for several hours.

The most important factor in prevention of a serious nosebleed is to assure that patients do not use platelet inhibitors. The most potent common drug is aspirin. Other nonsteroidal antiinflammatory drugs can cause bleeding, but none so severe as those I have encountered in patients taking aspirin.

When the bleeding persists, I inject lidocaine with epinephrine around the bleeding site, using good suction and a headlight, and try to apply cautery directly to the bleeding site. The cautery itself is rarely successful, but good visualization and the opportunity for direct injection with a vasoconstrictor improves hemostasis. Packing the area with cotton balls moistened by cocaine solution will usually provide temporary relief.

If blood loss cannot be controlled or recurs, the patient is taken to the operating room. The rhinostomy site is opened under sterile conditions, the periosteum is reflected from the medial wall of the orbit, and the anterior ethmoidal artery is ligated. In my experience, once the anterior ethmoidal supply has been interrupted, nasal bleeding from lacrimal surgery will cease. Fortunately, few patients require this procedure; however, the lacrimal surgeon should know of this maneuver for use in the proper instance. Most bleeding stops without treatment, but the surgeon should consider that most patients today would prefer to have anterior ethmoidal artery ligation rather than risk exposure to acquired immunodeficiency syndrome (AIDS) by transfusion.

ACKNOWLEDGMENT

Supported in part by a grant from Research to Prevent Blindness, Inc., New York, New York.

EDITOR'S COMMENTS

There is a real need in lacrimal surgery for experience and instruction in intranasal techniques. Dr. Wesley's present chapter and past publications are a valuable resource in this regard.

Dr. Wesley's intranasal approach to congenital lacrimal obstruction is innovative and promising. Although this approach has not been widely accepted, every lacrimal surgeon will find these techniques important in selected cases.

The description of turbinectomy is especially valuable, since few ophthalmologists receive training in this technique. I have not found it necessary to routinely perform turbinectomy with DCR or Jones tube insertion, but in patients with a hypertrophied anterior turbinate, the procedure is mandatory. Although the need for these techniques in routine cases is controversial, the important point is that every ophthalmologist will encounter occasional patients who require turbinectomy for successful lacrimal surgery. As has been emphasized, collaboration with an otorhinolaryngologist is appropriate when the ophthalmologist first uses new intranasal procedures.

REFERENCES

1. Jones LT: An anatomical approach to problems of the eyelids and lacrimal apparatus. Arch Ophthalmol 66:111, 1961
2. Dortzbach RK: Dacryocystorhinostomy. Ophthalmology 85:1267, 1978
3. Jones LT: Conjunctivodacryocystorhinostomy. Am J Ophthalmol 59:773, 1965
4. Peterson RA, Robb RM: The natural course of congenital obstruction of the nasolacrimal duct. J Pediatr Ophthalmol Strabismus 15:246, 1978
5. Quickert MH, Dryden RM: Probes for intubation in lacrimal drainage. Trans Am Acad Ophthalmol Otolaryngol 74:431, 1970
6. Anderson RL, Edwards JJ: Indications, complications and results with silicone stents. Ophthalmology 86:1474, 1979
7. Lauring L: Silicone intubation of the lacrimal system: Pitfalls, problems and complications. Ann Ophthalmol 24:489, 1976
8. Wesley RE: Inferior turbinate fracture in the treatment of congenital nasolacrimal duct obstruction and congenital nasolacrimal duct anomaly. Ophthalmic Surg 16:368, 1985

9. Havins WE, Wilkins RB: A useful alternative to silicone intubation in congenital nasolacrimal duct obstructions. Ophthalmic Surg 14:666, 1983
10. Meyers EF: Cocaine toxicity during dacryocystorhinostomy. Arch Ophthalmol 98:842, 1980
11. Campbell CB III, Flanagan JD: Mucous membrane graft and conjunctivodacryocystorhinostomy (Jones tube placement). p. 216. In Wesley RE (ed): Techniques in Ophthalmic Plastic Surgery. John Wiley & Sons, New York, 1986
12. Wesley RE, Bond JB: Intranasal procedures for successful lacrimal surgery. Ophthalmic Plast Reconstr Surg 2:153, 1986
13. Templer JW: Inflammatory disease of paranasal sinuses & nose. p. 280. In English EM (ed): Otolaryngology: A Textbook. Harper & Row, Hagerstown, NJ, 1976
14. Davies J: Embryology & anatomy of the head, neck, face, palate, nose & paranasal sinuses. In Paparella MM, Shumrick DA (eds): Otolaryngology. WB Saunders, Philadelphia, 1980

8 | Outpatient Dacryocystorhinostomy and Anesthesia Techniques

Steven C. Dresner

Surgeons have traditionally performed dacryocystorhinostomy (DCR) as an inpatient procedure; however, outpatient DCR has recently been more commonly performed. With proper patient selection, either local or general anesthesia may be employed on an outpatient basis with safety and a high degree of patient acceptance.

Patient selection for outpatient DCR is very similar to patient selection for outpatient cataract surgery. Generally, most patients with dacryostenosis are suitable candidates for outpatient surgery. Patients with unstable cardiovascular status and diabetic patients who are difficult to manage may be better served with inpatient observation. Other considerations for inpatient monitoring include bleeding diatheses or severe psychiatric conditions.

LOCAL ANESTHESIA

Local anesthesia for DCR has several advantages over general anesthesia. The risks of general anesthesia are avoided as well as many of the side effects, such as nausea, vomiting, laryngeal discomfort and musculoskeletal pains. The recovery period is appreciably reduced, which may expedite outpatient treatment. Most important, bleeding is a smaller problem under local anesthesia because inhaled anesthetics are all potent vasodilators.[5]

Since the risks of general anesthesia can be avoided, DCR may be offered to elderly patients with cardiovascular or other disorders for whom general anesthesia is contraindicated. The offer of local anesthesia makes patients more willing to accept the procedure. Most surgeons will also find that they prefer local anesthesia because it minimizes intraoperative hemorrhage and therefore expedites completion of the procedure.

Proper selection of patients suitable for local anesthesia is important. Children, adolescents, and overly anxious patients should not be considered for local anesthesia. It is helpful to discuss the sequence of events that the patient will experience during surgery when the patient is in the office for consultation. A general description of the proposed anesthetic and the surgical technique will usually help allay fears. The patient should be advised that after the anesthetic is delivered no pain will be felt; however, the patient will be able to hear the bone being removed. When patients are instructed in this way, acceptance is high, and neither patient nor surgeon should experience any unpleasant surprises intraoperatively.

The surgeon may use local anesthesia alone or monitored anesthesia care. If monitored anesthesia care is used, it is helpful to consult with the anesthesiologist or nurse anesthetist just before surgery; the surgeon then can discuss the type of blocks and agents intended for use and communicate any special requirements to the anesthetist.

Anesthetic Agents

Lidocaine with epinephrine is the agent recommended for local anesthesia in DCR. Lidocaine is an aminoethylamide with a low percentage of hypersensitivity reactions.[1] Preparations of lidocaine with epinephrine 1:100,000 or 1:200,000 allow for more prolonged anesthesia and less toxicity per dose because vasoconstriction induced by the epinephrine inhibits systemic absorption. The duration of action for peripheral nerve blocks of lidocaine 2 percent with 1:200,000 epinephrine solution ranges up to 3 hours.[2] The normal dosage of lidocaine should not exceed 7 mg per kg, and it is recommended that the maximum dose not exceed 500 mg.

Bupivacaine hydrochloride (Marcaine) is an amide-type local anesthetic that produces a more prolonged anesthesia than lidocaine and enables the surgeon to obtain nerve blocks of up to 6 hours. It is available in 0.25, 0.5, and 0.75 percent solutions, with or without epinephrine 1:200,000. A mixture of lidocaine 1 percent with epinephrine 1:100,000 and bupivacaine 0.5 percent plain is a useful preparation for DCR, yielding an intermediate and long-acting anesthesia with adequate epinephrine for hemostasis.

Cocaine is the topical anesthetic generally used on the nasal mucosa in DCR. It not only provides good local anesthesia, but also vasoconstricts and shrinks the nasal mucosa. It is prepared in a solution ranging between 4 and 10 percent. The duration of anesthesia is 90 minutes. The maximum recommended dosage of cocaine is 3 mg/kg. Cocaine inhibits catecholamine uptake and has a sympathetic potentiating effect. Cocaine combined with topical epinephrine or phenylephrine hydrochloride (Neo-Synephrine) may lead to toxic cardiovascular effects; therefore, the use of these two potentiating agents together on the mucosal surface is not recommended.[3] The judicious use of 4 percent cocaine solutions and limitation of the total dose should prevent most toxic reactions.

Topical anesthesia of the conjunctival surface is obtained by repeated drops of tetracaine hydrochloride (Pontocaine). This is provided as a 0.5 percent solution. Toxicity is not a consideration in topical anesthesia of the eye. Hypersensitivity, however, is a consideration since tetracaine is an ester derivative, and most reported true allergic reactions are caused by this type of agent.[4]

Technique

After preoperative sedation, the patient is placed in a supine position, and the nasal cavity is packed. (Fig. 8-1) Half- or quarter-inch gauze packing moistened with 4 percent cocaine is placed in the middle meatus, between the middle

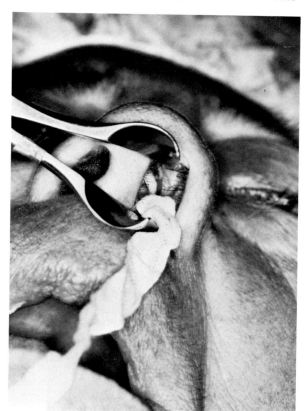

Fig. 8-1 The middle meatus is packed with a cocaine-moistened gauze packing strip under direct visualization using a headlight, nasal speculum, and bayonet forceps.

and inferior turbinates. Alternatively, cocaine-moistened 3-inch cottonoids may be used. A headlight, nasal speculum, and bayonet forceps are used so that the pack may be placed under direct visualization. A 4 percent cocaine or 0.5 percent tetracaine spray can be used prior to packing to minimize discomfort. The pack is left in place until it is removed intraoperatively.

After the nose has been packed, the surgeon marks the incision at the preferred site. Regional anesthesia is obtained by blocking the infratrochlear and anterior ethmoidal nerves, which are branches of the nasociliary nerve. The anterior ethmoidal nerve branches from the nasociliary nerve and exits the orbit through the anterior ethmoidal foramen about 25 mm posterior to the medial orbital rim. It supplies sensation to the anterior ethmoidal sinuses, which are often encountered in DCR. After giving off the anterior ethmoidal nerve, the nasociliary nerve extends anteriorly as the infratrochlear nerve. The infratrochlear nerve runs along the superior border of the medial rectus muscle and penetrates the orbital septum. The infratrochlear nerve supplies the medial skin of the eyelids, side of the nose, medial conjunctiva, and lacrimal sac and caruncle.[6]

A 25-gauge 1½ inch needle is used with a 5 ml syringe. With the patient in the supine position, the needle is placed approximately 1 cm above the medial canthus and directed posteriorly 2 cm along the medial orbital wall. (Fig. 8-2) Two to three millileters of the anesthetic solution is injected. An additional

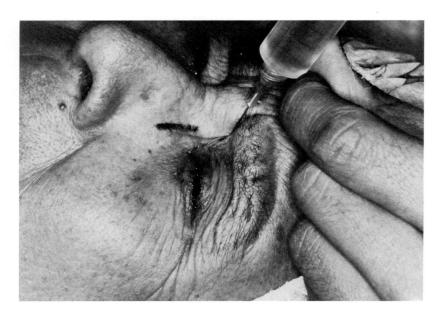

Fig. 8-2 The infratrochlear and anterior ethmoidal block is performed using a 25-gauge 1½-inch needle, placing the needle approximately 1 cm above the medial canthus and directed posteriorly 2 cm along the medial orbital wall. Two to 3 ml of the solution is injected.

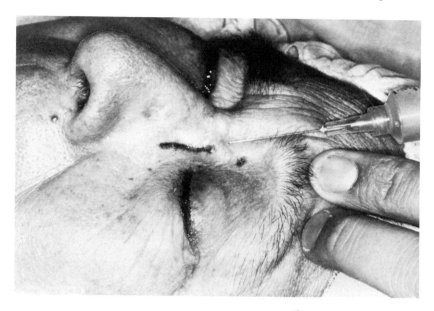

Fig. 8-3 Local anesthesia is obtained by subcutaneous infiltration.

milliliter is then injected subcutaneously beneath the previously marked incision (Fig. 8-3).

Topical tetracaine is dropped on the conjunctival surface and used repetitively when needed during the surgery. After local infiltration, the patient is prepared and draped while the surgeon scrubs; thus when the surgeon returns to the operating room, adequate vasoconstriction will have been obtained prior to incision.

Complications

The complications of local anesthesia include severe hypertension, cardiovascular instability, and cocaine toxicity.[3,7] Judicious use of local anesthetics and avoidance of improper combinations of topical adrenergic compounds with cocaine should help prevent these occurrences. Retrobulbar hemorrhage, globe perforation, and extraocular motility imbalance are possible complications of the anterior ethmoidal nerve block. Vision-threatening hemorrhage or globe perforation would preclude proceeding with DCR until the condition had been properly treated.

GENERAL ANESTHESIA

General anesthesia can be used for DCR on an inpatient or outpatient basis. If outpatient surgery is planned, recovery may be made easier by using shorter-acting narcotics such as fentanyl, sufentanyl, and alfentanyl, rather than morphine or meperidine (Demerol). Among inhaled anesthetics, enflurane has become extremely popular in the outpatient setting for maintenance of anesthesia because it has a more rapid recovery than halothane and may produce fewer postoperative side effects than isoflurane.[8]

After general anesthesia is induced, the nose is packed with cocaine-moistened gauze or cottonoids to provide hemostasis and shrinkage of the nasal mucosa. A local anesthetic with epinephrine is then injected subcutaneously underneath the incision for the hemostatic effect alone. No infratrochlear or anterior ethmoidal block is necessary.

COMPLICATIONS OF OUTPATIENT DCR

The most common immediate complication of DCR is postoperative hemorrhage. A petrolatum- or antibiotic-impregnated nasal pack placed at the completion of surgery will ensure that this does not occur. The pack, if carefully placed under direct visualization after the anterior flaps have been fashioned and prior to skin closure, will not affect flap viability. The pack is removed 24 to 48 hours later in the office. If bleeding persists, the pack can be replaced if necessary. Alternatively, a Gelfoam-thrombin stent may be placed intraoperatively between the flaps and left in place until it liquefies.[9]

EDITOR'S COMMENTS

Medicare and private insurance carriers have placed increasing pressure on ophthalmologists to perform outpatient surgery. In a few areas of the United States, justification is required if DCR is performed on an inpatient basis. In discussions with oculoplastic specialists across the United States, I have discovered that perhaps one third are performing outpatient DCRs under local anesthesia. Some authorities on lacrimal surgery are strongly opposed to outpatient DCR, fearing serious hemorrhage during the first 24 hours. My experience with outpatient DCR over the past 2 years has been very positive, and patient acceptance has been high.

The need for routine anterior ethmoidal nerve block in local anesthesia for DCR is controversial. I have used local anesthesia for nearly all DCR surgery over the past 8 years, without routine anterior ethmoidal nerve block. My technique includes a nasal packing moistened with cocaine, and local infiltration of 2 percent lidocaine with epinephrine 1/200,000 under the incision, over the infraorbital foramen, and over the supraorbital notch. With this combination, at least 90 percent of patients are free of pain. For the occasional patient who experiences deep pain, the anterior ethmoidal nerve block can be placed during surgery.

The disadvantage of routine anterior ethmoidal nerve injection is the potential for serious complication. As Dr. Dresner has explained, orbital hemorrhage, globe perforation, diplopia, and transient visual loss are all possible.

Individual techniques for DCR vary, and surgeons who often resect the tip of the middle turbinate or ethmoid air cells may routinely require the medial orbital injection for adequate anesthesia.

REFERENCES

1. Ruzicka T, Gerstmeier M, Przybilla B, Ring J: Allergy to local anesthetics: Comparison of patch test with prick and intradermal test results. J Am Acad Dermatol 16:1202, 1987
2. Savarese JJ, Covino BG: Basic and clinical pharmacology of local anesthetic drugs. p. 985. In Miller RD: Anesthesia. 2nd Ed. Vol. 2. Churchill Livingstone, New York, 1986
3. Meyers EF: Cocaine toxicity during dacryocystorhinostomy. Arch Ophthalmol 98:842, 1980
4. Aldrete JA, Johnson DA: Allergy to local anesthetics. JAMA 207:356, 1969
5. Mailer CM, Webster AC: Controlled sedation, sphenopalatine and nasociliary blocks, and bloodless flap suturing in dacryocystorhinostomy. Can J Ophthalmol 17:189, 1982
6. Doxanas MT, Anderson RL: Clinical Orbital Anatomy. Williams & Wilkins, Baltimore, 1984
7. El-Din, A, Mostafa SM: Severe hypertension during anesthesia for dacryocystorhinostomy. Anesthesia 40:787, 1985
8. White PF: Outpatient anesthesia. p. 1985. In Miller RD: Anesthesia. 2nd Ed. Vol. 3. Churchill Livingstone, New York, 1986
9. Leone CR: Gelfoam-thrombin dacryocystorhinostomy stent. Am J Ophthalmol 94:412, 1982

9 Dacryocystorhinostomy

James R. Patrinely
James W. Gigantelli

Disorders of the lacrimal drainage system are, at the least, very annoying to the patient, and when serious infection is present may threaten vision and life. The definitive treatment for most lacrimal drainage system disorders is surgical.

Surgery of the lacrimal drainage system is one area of ocular adnexal surgery that has not been actively encroached on by other specialists. This may be because the diagnosis, indications, and satisfaction with results are all related to the eye.

Dacryocystorhinostomy (DCR), a procedure that fistulizes the lacrimal sac and nasal cavity, is the most frequent lacrimal drainage procedure. With the exception of the occasional otorhinolaryngologist or plastic surgeon, ophthalmologists are responsible for the vast majority of DCRs performed. However, many eye physicians are uncomfortable with bone surgery, lacrimal and nasal anatomy, potential bleeding problems, and nasal examination.

HISTORICAL BACKGROUND

An early account of a procedure analogous to DCR was recorded in the first century by Celcus, who described pushing a hot iron probe through the lacrimal bone into the nasal cavity.[1] However, before the early 20th century, surgical treatment of lacrimal outflow disorders mainly consisted of removal of the lacrimal sac (dacryocystectomy). Toti's description, in 1904, of a fistulization procedure heralded the modern era of DCR. In his operation, the lacrimal sac was exposed through an external skin incision, a lacrimal fossa rhinostomy performed, the nasal mucosa and medial portion of the lacrimal sac excised, and the wound closed with skin sutures alone.[2]

Toti's procedure had a high failure rate (85 to 90 percent) secondary to cicatrization of the rhinostomy site. These failures encouraged the experimentation and modification that has led to development of the modern procedure.[3] Kuhnt (1914) and Ohm (1920) were able to improve the surgical success rate by suturing the lacrimal sac mucosa to the periosteum or nasal mucosa.[4,5]

In 1921, Dupuy-Dutemps described a very successful procedure (94.8 percent success in over 1,000 cases) that became the forerunner of contemporary DCR.[6,7] In this procedure, rather than excising a portion of the sac, the lacrimal sac was incised, forming both anterior and posterior flaps, and then carefully anastomosed to the nasal mucosa.[6]

Numerous modifications of this surgical procedure have since been proposed; however, modern improvements have mainly resulted from advances in surgical technique and instrumentation.

INDICATIONS

Indications for DCR include acquired nasolacrimal duct obstruction with patent canaliculi, or this condition combined with a distal common canalicular obstruction, persistent congenital nasolacrimal duct obstruction following probing and intubation, chronic dacryocystitis, and lacrimal sac foreign bodies.

The only absolute contraindication to DCR is malignancy of the lacrimal sac, which is treated by dacryocystectomy. Acute dacryocystitis has been cited as a contraindication to immediate DCR; however, some authors have reported good success in these cases without an increase in complications when parenteral antibiotics are started 24 hours preoperatively.[8]

ANESTHESIA

DCR can be performed under either local or general anesthesia. When combined with mild sedation, local anesthesia is favored for most patients except children. Even when using general anesthesia, nasal packing with vasoconstrictors should be performed and external injections of local anesthetics given to facilitate hemostasis and improve visualization.

The nasal cavity should be packed with $\frac{1}{4}$-inch-wide cotton strips, umbilical tape, or neurosurgical cottonoids lightly moistened with 4 percent cocaine solution to constrict the vascular mucosa. Nasal packing should be performed under direct visualization using a headlight, nasal speculum, and bayonet forceps. Visualization is facilitated by decongesting the mucosa with cocaine spray before packing. The use of a premixed 4 percent (40 mg/ml) cocaine solution provides excellent intranasal anesthesia, and its intrinsic vasoconstrictive properties obviate the need for an additional vasoactive agent such as 0.25 percent phenylephrine. This cocaine solution also appears to cause less burning and discomfort than cocaine crystals. Unlike pharmacy-compounded solutions of cocaine, which can lose up to 59 percent of their potency in one week, premixed topical cocaine hydrochloride solution remains chemically stable for up to 9 months from manufacture.[9] The fatal dose of cocaine has been reported as 1.2 g, although severe toxic effects have been reported from doses as low as 20 mg. Generally, up to 50 mg can be safely used, although dosages should be reduced for children and for elderly or debilitated patients.[10] The maximum dose should not exceed 3 mg/kg.

It is important to place the superior nasal packing near the head of the middle turbinate, at the planned rhinostomy site. Excessive upward force with the bayonet packing forceps should be avoided to prevent damage to the lamina cribrosa with resultant cerebrospinal fluid leakage.

External anesthesia is achieved with topical anesthetic drops and local infiltration. Hemostasis is maximized with a subcutaneous injection of 1 to 2 percent lidocaine containing 1:200,000 mg/ml epinephrine at the incision site and into the lacrimal fossa. The injection should be given 5 to 10 minutes before surgery. These measures will provide adequate operative anesthesia, allowing the entire procedure to be performed under local anesthesia with sedation.[11]

In addition to local infiltration, some authors suggest regional nerve blocks of the nasociliary and infraorbital nerves.[3,12] The anterior ethmoidal branches of the nasociliary nerve may be anesthetized by injecting 1 ml of anesthetic along the medial orbital wall, inferonasal to the trochlea and immediately above the medial canthal tendon. This technique anesthetizes a portion of the intranasal cavity, the tip of the nose, and the medial canthal region. The infraorbital nerve block is performed by injecting 0.5 ml of anesthetic at the external ostium of the infraorbital canal, approximately 1 cm inferior to the mid-portion of the infraorbital rim. This technique anesthetizes the lower eyelid and malar region.

TECHNIQUE

Proper preparation and instrumentation will greatly facilitate the surgery. Because the surgeon will be working in a small, deep incision, a fiberoptic headlight and magnifying loupes are indispensible. Traditionally, there have been two separate schools of thought regarding skin incisions for DCR; they differ essentially in their relation to the angular vessels and medial canthal tendon (Fig. 9-1). Fasanella suggests placing the incision 3 to 4 mm nasal to the medial canthus (medial to the angular vessels) and carrying the incision inferiorly over the anterior lacrimal crest.[13] We favor the more medially placed incision described by Werb, Callahan and others.[3,14,15] Placed 10 to 12 mm nasal to the medial canthus, the incision begins at the level of the inferior edge of the medial canthal tendon and continues inferolaterally, tangent to the inferonasal rim of the orbit, in a straight line for 15 to 20 mm along the side of the nose. This incision is parallel and medial to the large angular vessels and leaves an inconspicuous scar in the thicker nasal skin. The position of this incision tends to avoid the postoperative cicatricial web that can occur if the incision is curved or crosses into the thinner skin of the eyelid. Modification

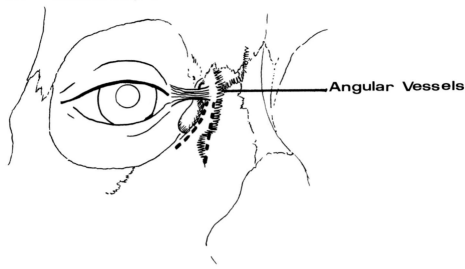

Angular Vessels

Fig. 9-1   Popular incision sites (dotted lines) for DCR. The lateral incision is temporal to the angular vessels and follows the curvature of the anterior lacrimal crest. The more medial incision is linear and 10 to 12 mm nasal to the medial canthus beginning at the lower border of the medial canthal tendon. This incision (our preference) is parallel to the angular vessels and lies within the thicker nasal skin.

of the skin incision placement is necessary in Orientals who have a flat nasal bridge and in patients with prior midfacial trauma or DCR. A more lateral, and thus posterior, incision may be preferred in patients with epicanthal folds or with lateral displacement of the lacrimal system, as can be found following naso-orbital fractures. Incisions for reoperation of DCR should be hidden within the scar of the first procedure.

Following the skin incision, the orbicularis is bluntly dissected down to the periosteum of the frontal process of the maxilla. Some authors prefer to dissect sharply through both skin and orbicularis with one pass of the scalpel.[8] Theoretically, this insures that once deeper structures have been localized by external palpation, there is less chance of misguided dissection. However, we have not had difficulty guiding our deep dissection and believe that hemostasis is improved by bluntly dissecting the vascular orbicularis muscle with spreading motions parallel to the angular vessels. It is important to incise the subcutaneous tissues for the full extent of the skin incision in order to maximize deep exposure. Care must be taken to cauterize the subcutaneous vessels meticulously. The use of small, blunt rake retractors aids both visualization and hemostasis.

The periosteum is next incised 3 to 4 mm anterior and parallel to the anterior lacrimal crest and reflected posteriorly with a Freer or Cottle periosteal elevator. The surgeon will find that the periosteum is most firmly adherent to the underlying bone at the anterior lacrimal crest. Sometimes bone bleeding comes from the sutura notha, a small vascular groove just medial to the anterior lacrimal crest that carries a branch of the infraorbital artery.[16] When rounding the anterior lacrimal crest, the surgeon must take care to avoid lacerating the lacrimal sac. The periosteum posterior to the anterior lacrimal crest is loosely adherent. The lacrimal sac and proximal nasolacrimal duct are reflected laterally with their periosteal covering (Fig. 9-2).

Next, an osteotomy in the lacrimal fossa is created and the nasal mucosa exposed. A variety of instruments, including a trephine attached to a Stryker saw, an air drill with a burr attachment, and an osteotome and mallet, have been advocated for this purpose. We have found that with care, a curved hemostat may be used to rupture the thin, incompletely ossified bone at the junction of the lacrimal bone and maxillary bone in the middle of the lacrimal sac fossa (Fig. 9-3). The bony opening can then be enlarged by spreading the hemostat blades. The nasal mucosa is rarely disturbed. By using this anatomic bone window, we find that bulky and time-consuming power instruments are unnecessary.

The osteotomy is then enlarged using Kerrison rongeurs, Citelli bone punches, or Hardy-Sella punches. The bone removed includes the lacrimal bone, the superior nasal wall of the nasolacrimal canal, the anterior lacrimal crest region, the bone beneath the medial canthal tendon, and occasionally anterior ethmoidal bone (Fig. 9-4). Care is taken not to penetrate or engage the nasal mucosa with bites of the instrument. Preservation of nasal mucosa may be facilitated by removing the nasal pack prior to enlarging the osteotomy and hugging the inner bone surface with the rongeurs. An oval osteotomy, 14 mm deep and 17 mm long, will usually suffice. The osteotomy is about the size of a dime or the surgeon's thumbnail. Postoperative nasal endoscopy has shown that in most cases the fistula shrinks to about 2 mm, regardless of the original osteotomy size (see Ch. 16).[17]

A thorough knowledge of the surrounding anatomy can prevent many undesirable complications of osteotomy. The anterior ethmoidal artery, 25 mm posterior to the medial canthal tendon, is a potential source of hemorrhage during posterior dissection.[16,18] The average distance from the superior edge of the osteotomy to the anterior cranial fossa floor is 5.0 mm.[19] The thinnest area of the cribriform plate overlies the posterior portion of the nasal window.[19] Ethmoidal air cells may enlarge superiorly with age, altering the anterior cranial fossa floor lateral to the cribriform plate. Therefore, rotational forces with rongeurs in the superoposterior portion of the osteotomy, and inadvertent superior dissection, could fracture the cranial floor and/or cribriform plate, resulting in a cerebrospinal fluid leak.[19] Conversely, inadequate bone removal and failure to recognize and remove anterior ethmoidal tissue, which may compromise the rhinostomy, are common errors that can lead to obstruction. Lempert straight rongeurs or Takahashi ethmoidectomy forceps are helpful in performing an anterior ethmoidectomy.

Most surgeons agree that anastomosis of lacrimal sac mucosa and nasal mucosa improves the success rate of DCR. Controversy exists regarding the use of a single anterior or posterior flap, or combined anterior and posterior

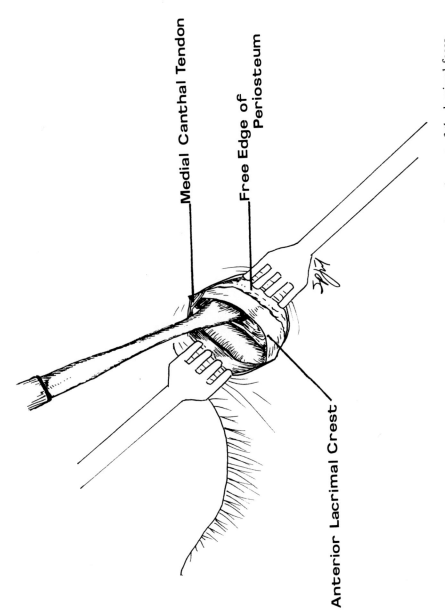

Fig. 9-2 Lateral displacement of the lacrimal sac and its periosteal covering out of the lacrimal fossa with a Freer elevator.

Medial Canthal Tendon

Free Edge of Periosteum

Anterior Lacrimal Crest

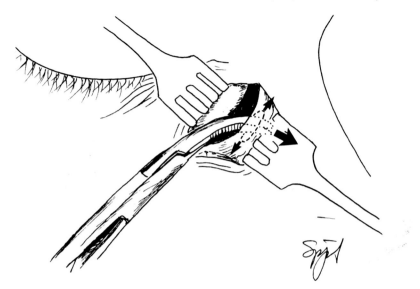

Fig. 9-3 Careful directed inward force (large arrow) with a curved hemostat into the middle of the lacrimal fossa will easily rupture the thin bone. The osteotomy can then be enlarged by spreading the hemostat blades (small arrows).

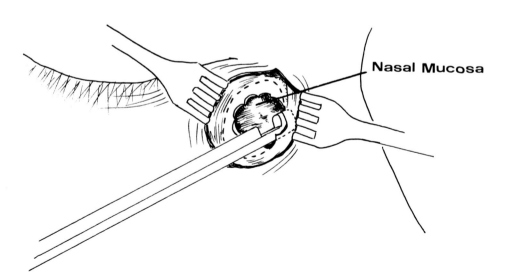

Fig. 9-4 Narrow Kerrison rongeurs are used to remove the lacrimal fossa bone, the anterior lacrimal crest, and the superonasal wall of the nasolacrimal duct. The blunt end of the rongeur is used to push back and preserve the nasal mucosa when biting the bone.

flaps. A review of the literature suggests that all three alternatives can produce similar results.[6,7,20-27] We usually remove the posterior nasal and lacrimal sac flaps and suture together the anterior nasal and lacrimal sac flaps. We believe that the anterior flaps help prevent scar tissue from growing into the ostium and that a wide open posterior region into the nose is as good as posterior flaps and better than poorly created or sutured posterior flaps, which may actually block the nasal opening. Postoperative nasal endoscopic studies have shown that the ostium cicatrized to the same small size (approximately 1.8 mm), regardless of whether anterior flaps alone, or both anterior and posterior flaps were used.[17]

In the creation of mucosal flaps, the lacrimal sac is incised first, because it causes less hemorrhage and facilitates planning of the nasal mucosal incision. A 000 or 00 Bowman lacrimal probe is passed through the lower canalicular system into the lacrimal sac, tenting the wall of the medial sac (Fig. 9-5). This technique positions the lacrimal sac incision opposite the internal ostium of the common canaliculus. Some authors suggest irrigating 1 percent methylene blue solution into the lacrimal sac in order to facilitate identification of the mucosal surface and verify full-thickness incision of the sac.[15,21] This modification, however, does not provide localization of the sac incision site over the internal common canalicular ostium, and offers no advantage over visualization of the Bowman probe in the assurance of a full-thickness incision. The methylene blue often spills into the surgical field and interferes with subsequent tissue identification following incision into the sac.

When incising the lacrimal sac, the surgeon must consider the type of flaps and anastomosis planned. Advocates of a single anterior or posterior flap usually make either a straight vertical incision or a U-shaped incision. The base of a U-shaped incision is placed anterior or posterior (Fig. 9-5). Proponents of combined anterior and posterior flaps make a horizontal H-shaped incision.

It is important to remember that the lacrimal sac mucosa is being incised through a periosteal layer, and therefore direct visualization of the probe placed within the sac is necessary to verify a full-thickness opening into the sac. A curved #12 or straight #11 Bard-Parker blade can be used to incise the sac from the upper fundus down to the proximal nasolacrimal duct. Because these blades have long cutting edges and are used in a deep incision, inadvertent skin incisions can occur. They can be prevented by wrapping the blade with a Steristrip, leaving only the distal 4 mm exposed.

Following sac incision, a complete inspection of the mucosal surface and contents is mandatory with particular attention to the possibility of neoplasms, polyps, masses, dacryoliths, and scarring of the common canalicular ostium. If common canalicular stenosis or scarring prevents passage of the Bowman probe, then a common canalicular opening can be created by resecting the scarred internal ostium with a Westcott scissors or #11 blade. The patent canaliculi are then intubated with silicone stents. This reconstruction is successful in up to 73 percent of patients.[27]

Incision of the nasal mucosa should also be planned in accordance with the preferred type of flap and anastomosis. The pattern of the incision usually

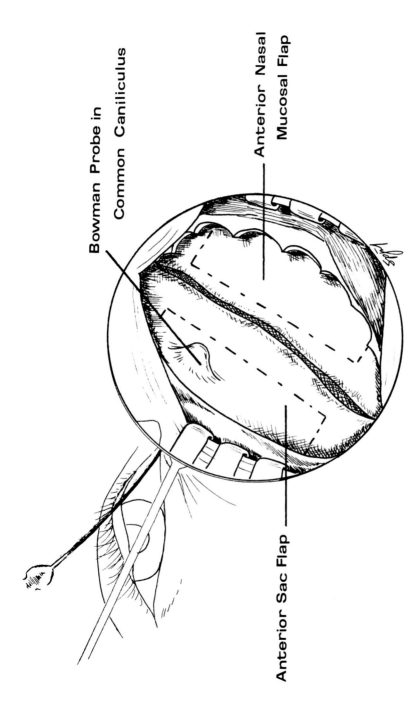

Bowman Probe in Common Caniliculus

Anterior Nasal Mucosal Flap

Anterior Sac Flap

Fig. 9-5 Magnified view of operative field, showing Bowman probe in lower canaliculus tenting the medial wall of the lacrimal sac. The planned anterior lacrimal sac and nasal mucosal flaps are outlined (dashed lines). The posterior mucosal flaps may be excised or anastomosed.

mirrors the shape of the lacrimal sac incision. Hyperemia of the nasal mucosa suggests the possibility of significant hemorrhage following incision. Topical vasoconstrictive agents or mucosal infiltration with anesthetic solution containing epinephrine can decrease mucosal bleeding. Also, the increased tissue turgidity following injection of local anesthetic facilitates cutting the normally floppy nasal mucosa. The nasal packing may be removed from the nostril prior to incising the nasal mucosa, or removed through the wound after the mucosa is opened. At this time, further inspection of nasal anatomy is possible. It is not uncommon to find an association of nasal pathology with lacrimal drainage system disorders, especially in males and following trauma.[28] Certain pathologic conditions should be managed by an otorhinolaryngologist before lacrimal system surgery, including such conditions as nasal and sinus malignancy, nasal polyps, and impacted inferior turbinate. Appropriate management of these conditions may obviate the need for lacrimal system surgery. A deviated septum may narrow the intranasal cavity, leading to postoperative synechiae and fibrous overgrowth. Most DCRs will be successful when the septum is moderately deviated, but a septoplasty should be performed if the deviation threatens to obstruct the fistula site.

Sometimes intranasal pathology is discovered intraoperatively and must be managed by the ophthalmologist (Fig. 9-6). The ethmoidal air cells are usually located posterior to the lacrimal sac, and the head of the middle turbinate is normally recessed away from the lacrimal fossa (Fig. 9-6A). Malposition or enlargement of these structures is common, and failure to recognize and treat the abnormality can lead to postoperative failure. In approximately one third of adults with nasolacrimal duct obstruction, the anterior position of the ethmoidal air cells can block the posterior portion of the osteotomy site (Fig. 9-6B).[29] These cells increase the distance between the intranasal cavity and the lacrimal sac and can obstruct the osteotomy site. The encroaching ethmoidal air cells can be removed piecemeal with a hemostat or front-biting rongeurs (ethmoidectomy forceps) in order to enlarge the rhinostomy. Some surgeons believe that placing posterior flaps over the exposed ethmoidal air cells helps prevent subsequent fibrous overgrowth, but several reports suggest this step is unnecessary.[30]

The head of the middle turbinate may be greatly enlarged and, located anteriorly, may block the rhinostomy site (Fig. 9-6B). Even if the turbinate appears to be minimally occluding the rhinostomy, the surgeon must remember that when vasoconstricted it is smaller than normal and the postoperative size may obstruct or create adhesion to the rhinostomy site. If necessary, the head of the middle turbinate is resected with front-biting or up-biting rongeurs after the mucosa has been injected with lidocaine containing 1:200,000 mg/ml epinephrine. Trimming the head of the turbinate with a unipolar electrocautery may cause inflammation of the frontonasal duct with secondary frontal sinusitis.[31] After removal of the turbinate head, the cut surface is packed with Gelfoam soaked in liquid thrombin.

A variety of stents have been recommended to maintain the surgical fistula. These materials include lubricated nasal packing, silicone sponge, or Gel-

the nose gently and lowering the head for 20 minutes. If these measures fail, then a nasal pack consisting of cotton gauze impregnated with antibiotic ointment, phenylephrine, or thrombin may be required. The authors prefer packing with absorbable thrombin-soaked Gelfoam rather than risk dislodging a stable thrombus when removing a gauze packing. Refractory cases are usually caused by hemorrhage from anterior ethmoidal vessels, and surgery may become necessary in order to place a vascular clip. Although most postoperative hemorrhages are manifested by epistaxis, orbital hemorrhage has also been reported.[18]

Despite the routine use of prophylactic antibiotic drops and ointment, postoperative infections do occur. Acute infections necessitate the use of systemic antibiotics, warm compresses, and surgical drainage of any abscess. The presence of a chronic postoperative infection often signifies recurrent lacrimal obstruction and may require surgical exploration. Dacryoliths not removed during DCR may also cause a chronic infection resistant to antibiotics.

Other reported intraoperative complications include hypertension and CSF rhinorrhea. Late postoperative complications include hypertrophic and cosmetically disfiguring (tented or bowstring) scars. Scarring is usually minimal, but often the incision will be transiently indurated and elevated. As the scar matures, this induration regresses and is usually inconspicuous at 3 months.

In skilled hands, DCR is an effective technique in the treatment of lacrimal drainage system disorders. In reported series, both with and without silicone stent canalicular intubation, the success rate approaches 95.0 percent.[21,22,25–27] Even in children, where hypertrophic scarring has been implicated as a cause for failure, the success rate is 83 percent.[44] In most series, closure of the rhinostomy or stenosis of the common canaliculus by fibrous tissue account for the great majority of DCR failures.[21,22,24,25] Secondary closure of the ostium and return of epiphora usually occurs within the first three months after surgery. It is sometimes possible to dilate the stenotic ostium in the office under topical cocaine anesthesia. A small muscle hook may be inserted into the intranasal ostium and used to aggressively stretch the ostium in all directions. The intranasal ostium may also be enlarged with front-biting rongeurs.[45] If these maneuvers are unsuccessful, the patient will usually require a secondary DCR with resection of scar tissue and enlargement of the rhinostomy.

Even in cases of failed DCR, with careful surgical technique and appreciation of the surgical anatomy, the success rate of secondary DCR approaches 71 percent.[25]

REFERENCES

1. Chandler PA: Dacryocystorhinostomy. Trans Am Ophthalmol Soc 34:240, 1936
2. Toti A: Nuovo metodo conservatore di cura radicale delle suppurazioni croniche del sacco lacrimale (dacriocistorinostomia). Clin Med 10:385, 1904
3. Demorest BH: Dacryocystorhinostomy. p. 455. In Stewart WB (ed): Ophthalmic Plastic and Reconstructive Surgery. American Academy of Ophthalmology, San Francisco, 1984

4. Kuhnt: Notiz zur Technik der Dacryozystorhinostomie nach Toti. Z Augenheilkd 31:379, 1914
5. Ohm: Sitzungsberichte. 36. Versammlung des Vereins rheinischwestfälischer Augenärtz. 1. Demonstration von Instrumenten. Klin Mbl Augenheilkd 64:847, 1920
6. Depuy-Dutemps B: Procede plastique de dacryocystorhinostomie et ses results. Ann Ocul 158:241, 1921
7. Depuy-Dutemps B: Cure de la dacryocystite chronique et du larmoiement par la dacryorhinostomie plastique. Presse Med 40:833, 1922
8. Iliff LE, Iliff WJ, Iliff NT: Lacrimal tract surgery. p. 171. In Iliff CE, Iliff WJ, Iliff NT (eds): Oculoplastic Surgery. WB Saunders, Philadelphia, 1979
9. Murray JB, Al-Shoura H: Stability of cocaine HCl in aqueous solution. J Pharm Pharmacol 28:24, 1976
10. Ritchie JM, Green NM: Local anesthetics. p. 313. In Goodman LS, Gilman A, et al. (eds): The Pharmacological Basis of Therapeutics. 7th Ed. Macmillan, New York, 1985
11. Kirschner H: Local anesthesia in external dacryocystorhinostomy. p. 267. In Bosniak SL (ed): Advances in Ophthalmic Plastic and Reconstructive Surgery. Vol. 3. Pergamon Press, Elmsford, NY, 1984
12. Moazed KT, Cooper WC: Dacryocystorhinostomy. p. 229. In Blitzer A, Lawson W, Friedman WH (eds): Surgery of the Paranasal Sinuses. WB Saunders, Philadelphia, 1985
13. Fasanella RM: Pitfalls and complications in surgery and trauma of the lacrimal apparatus. p. 110. In Fasanella RM (ed): Complications in Eye Surgery. WB Saunders, Philadelphia, 1965
14. Werb A: Surgery of the lacrimal sac and nasolacrimal duct. p. 156. In Milder B, Weil BA (eds): The Lacrimal System. Appleton-Century-Crofts, Norwalk, CT, 1983
15. Callahan MA, Callahan A: Lacrimal system. p. 103. In Callahan MA, Callahan A (eds): Ophthalmic Plastic and Orbital Surgery, Aesculapius Publishing Company, Birmingham, AL, 1979
16. Doxanas MT, Anderson RL: Clinical Orbital Anatomy. Williams & Wilkins, Baltimore, 1984
17. Linberg JV, Anderson RL, Bumsted RM, et al.: Study of intranasal ostium external dacryocystorhinostomy. Arch Ophthalmol 100:1758, 1982
18. Slonim CB, Older JJ, Jones PL: Orbital hemorrhage with proptosis following dacryocystorhinostomy. Ophthalmic Surg 15:774, 1984
19. Neuhaus RW, Baylis HI: Cerebrospinal fluid leakage after dacryocystorhinostomy. Ophthalmology 90:1091, 1983
20. Iliff CE: A simplified dacryocystorhinostomy. Arch Ophthalmol 85:586, 1971
21. McLachlan DL, Shannon GM, Flanagan JC: Results of dacryocystorhinostomy: Analysis of the reoperations. Ophthalmic Surg 11:427, 1980
22. Older JJ: Routine use of a silicone stent in a dacryocystorhinostomy. Ophthalmic Surg 13:911, 1982
23. Taiara C, Sargent RA, Smith B: Dacryocystorhinostomy: The Kasper operation. Ann Ophthalmol 6:1333, 1974
24. Pica G: A modified technique of external dacryocystorhinostomy. Am J Ophthalmol 72:679, 1971
25. McPherson SD Jr, Egleston D: Dacryocystorhinostomy: A review of 106 operations. Am J Ophthalmol 47:328, 1959
26. Leone CR, VanGemert JV, Underwood L: Dacryocystorhinostomy: A modification of the Dupuy-Dutemps operation. Ophthalmic Surg 10:35, 1979

27. Hurwitz JJ, Rutherford S: Computerized survey of lacrimal surgery patients. Ophthalmology 93:14, 1986
28. Zolli CL, Shannon GM: Dacryocystorhinostomy: A review of 119 cases. Ophthalmic Surg 13:905, 1982
29. Patrinely JR, Anderson RL: A review of lacrimal drainage surgery. Ophthalmic Plast Reconstr Surg 2:97, 1986
30. Hatt M: The excretory lacrimal pathways. p. 74. In Hatt M (ed): Ophthalmic Plastic and Reconstructive Surgery. Thieme, New York, 1986
31. Wesley RE, Ballinger WH: Acute frontal sinusitis after lacrimal surgery. Ann Ophthalmol 18:350, 1986
32. Bosniak SL: Editorial comment: Dacryocystorhinostomy technique. p. 239. In Bosniak SL (ed): Advances in Ophthalmic Plastic and Reconstructive Surgery. Vol 3. Pergamon, Elmsford, NY, 1984
33. Cassady JR: A simplified dacryocystorhinostomy technique. Ophthalmic Surg 11:319, 1980
34. Small RG, Bonham R, Sobol S: The silicone sponge stent dacryocystorhinostomy. p. 253. In Bosniak, SL (ed): Advances in Ophthalmic Plastic and Reconstructive Surgery. Vol. 3. Pergamon, Elmsford, NY, 1984
35. Leone CR Jr: Gelfoam-thrombin dacryocystorhinostomy stent. Am J Ophthalmol 94:412, 1982
36. Anderson RL, Edwards JJ: Indications, complications and results with silicone stents. Ophthalmology 86:1474, 1979
37. Crawford JS: Intubation obstructions in the lacrimal system. Can J Ophthalmol 12:289, 1977
38. Tse DT, Anderson RL: A new modification of the standard lacrimal groove director for nasolacrimal intubation. Arch Ophthalmol 101:1938, 1983
39. Dortzbach RK, France TD, Kushner BJ, et al.: Silicone intubation for obstruction of the nasolacrimal duct in children. Am J Ophthalmol 94:585, 1982
40. Jordan DR, Anderson RL: Prevention of prolapsed silicone stents in dacryocystorhinostomy surgery. Arch Ophthalmol 105:455, 1987
41. Harvey JT, Anderson RL: Transcanalicular removal of prolapsed Silastic tubing after nasolacrimal intubation. J Ocular Ther Surg 2:294, 1982
42. Gonnering RS: Gentle, technically simple repositioning of displaced lacrimal tubing. Ophthalmic Surg 16:307, 1985
43. Cobden RH, Thrasher EL, Harris WH: Topical hemostatic agents to reduce bleeding from cancellous bone: A comparison of microcrystalline collagen, thrombin, and thrombin-soaked gelatin foam. J Bone Joint Surg 58A:70, 1976
44. Nowinski TS, Flanagan JC, Mauriello J: Pediatric dacryocystorhinostomy. Arch Ophthalmol 103:1226, 1985
45. Burns JA, Cahill KV: Management of ostium stenosis of dacryocystorhinostomy. p. 174. In Wesley RE (ed): Techniques in Ophthalmic Plastic Surgery. John Wiley and Sons, New York, 1986

10 Pathology of Nasolacrimal Duct Obstruction

Clinicopathologic Correlates of Lacrimal Excretory System Disease

Steven A. McCormick
John V. Linberg

Nasolacrimal duct obstruction is a common ophthalmic problem, accounting for up to 3 percent of clinic visits in some series.[1,2] It affects patients of every age, from birth through senescence, and results from a wide variety of causes. However, in most cases—those comprising the clinical syndrome of primary acquired nasolacrimal duct obstruction—the pathogenesis is poorly understood. In this group of patients, as well as in patients in whom the etiology of nasolacrimal obstruction is implied from clinical history or operative findings, the opportunity to study the affected tissues from the nasolacrimal canal has rarely been afforded to the ophthalmic pathologist. This situation results from the fact that the most common surgical procedure used to alleviate the clinical obstruction, namely dacryocystorhinostomy (DCR), neither exposes nor requires removal of the offending tissues. Fortunately, DCR remains a most effective surgical treatment in most cases,[3,4] and, therefore, there has been little impetus to study the underlying disease processes leading to obstruction of the nasolacrimal duct.

Understanding of any disease process is aided by pathologic examination of the affected tissues. Indeed, a basic tenet in the practice of surgery is the biopsy, resection, and examination of pathological tissue. Whether pertaining to resection of an obstructed segment of bowel, bypass of coronary arteries narrowed by atherosclerosis, or innumerable other surgical situations, understanding of the pathogenesis of the underlying disease processes has resulted largely from tissue examination. In situations where tissue is not or cannot be removed during surgery, at least postmortem study has been possible. This basic tenet has not been applied to the nonneoplastic disease processes affecting the nasolacrimal excretory system. The anatomy of the nasolacrimal canal essentially precludes routine evaluation at the time of autopsy; therefore, surgical exploration is the only practical way to obtain tissue for pathologic study.

We have previously reported a technique that allows removal of the entire soft tissue contents of the nasolacrimal canal during routine DCR.[5] This technique has been performed successfully in over 40 patients undergoing DCR at our institution since 1983. All operations were performed by one of the authors (JVL). In rare patients, the procedure was not performed, usually because of unrelated medical or anesthetic complications. Postoperative complications have not been encountered in any patient.

OVERVIEW

As a preamble to the discussion of the pathology of the nasolacrimal excretory system, we include a description of the DCR and biopsy techniques used. We also describe the clinical spectrum of conditions affecting the lacrimal excretory pathways as a whole before detailing the pathologic alterations of the nasolacrimal duct. From our study of the ductal tissues obtained by biopsy, we describe cases with obstruction secondary to a variety of specific etiologies, and also our experience with that larger category of idiopathic cases we have designated "primary acquired nasolacrimal duct obstruction" (PANDO). The histology of the tissues of the lacrimal excretory system and the pathologic reaction patterns of the nasolacrimal duct are described. From this analysis, we infer possible pathogenetic mechanisms of PANDO, and we offer a clinicopathologic classification scheme for nasolacrimal duct obstruction.

DCR AND BIOPSY TECHNIQUE

The technique of excisional biopsy of the tissues of the nasolacrimal canal, developed and routinely employed by one of us (JVL), is described below.[5] Because individual DCR techniques vary, the initial steps in this approach are described as a prelude to the actual biopsy technique.

External DCR

Surgery is usually performed under local anesthesia, and preoperative sedation with intramuscular meperidine (50 mg) and promethazine (50 mg) is routine. One hour before surgery, the nasal passages are decongested with 0.05 percent oxymetazoline nasal spray. Immediately before surgery, further decongestion is achieved with 0.5 percent phenylephrine spray. Two cotton pledgets are moistened with 1.5 ml of 4 percent cocaine solution. Surface anesthesia of the nasal mucosa is obtained with 0.5 percent tetracaine nasal spray. Using a headlight, speculum, and bayonet forceps, the first cotton pledget is packed into the superior nasal recess just anterior to the middle turbinate, and the second is placed under the inferior turbinate in the area of the nasolacrimal ostium. Regional anesthesia is completed with the injection of 2 percent lidocaine with epinephrine (1:200,000) in the medial canthus, over the infraorbital foramen, and over the supraorbital notch.

The skin is incised for 2.5 cm inferiorly from a point midway between the medial canthal angle and the bridge of the nose. Dissection is carried down to the periosteum, which is then incised and reflected toward the anterior lacrimal crest. Using Freer elevators, the fascia surrounding the lacrimal sac is gently reflected from the entire lacrimal sac fossa. This usually necessitates cutting the inferior portion of the medial canthal tendon. Inferiorly, the neck of the sac is exposed where it enters the nasolacrimal canal. It may have to be separated from fibers of the inferior oblique muscle that sometimes originate at the lateral margin of the canal.

The thin lacrimal bone is perforated, and rongeurs are used to resect the bone of the lacrimal sac fossa, anterior lacrimal crest, and some bone medial to the crest. An opening of at least 10 × 10 mm is created. The thin bone between the proximal portion of the nasolacrimal duct and the nasal mucosa is grasped with tips of a Hartman rongeur and resected. At this stage of the standard external DCR, the nasolacrimal duct biopsy is performed.

Nasolacrimal Duct Biopsy

The skin incision is retracted inferiorly with blunt rakes or traction sutures. The blunt ends of two Freer elevators are used to expose the entire rim of the entrance of the nasolacrimal canal. Care is taken not to tear or enter the lacrimal sac. The periosteum is readily separated from the bone of the proximal (2 to 3 mm) nasolacrimal canal with the Freer elevators. The junction of the sac and duct is hooked with a small Stevens tenotomy hook, modified by bending the tip into a "J" shape (Fig. 10-1). The hook is held in the surgeon's nondominant hand, and provides gentle upward traction during the remainder of the biopsy.

A Penfield #4 dissector (Fig. 10-1) is used to create a plane of dissection between the soft tissues within the canal and the osseous wall. These tissues readily separate from the bone, in much the same manner as the periorbita readily separates from the orbital walls. No difficulty or bleeding is encoun-

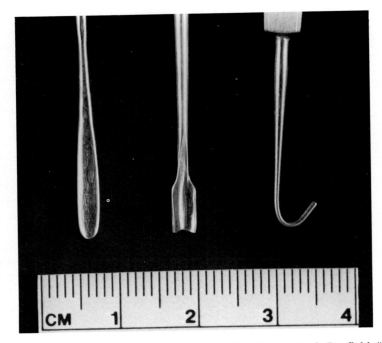

Fig. 10-1   Instruments required for nasolacrimal duct biopsy. *Left,* Penfield #4 dissector. This neurosurgical instrument is used to separate the periosteum from the bone
within the nasolacrimal canal. *Center,* modified 3-mm Freer septum chisel. This custom-
modified otolaryngology instrument is used to cut the distal attachments of the nasolacrimal duct to the nasal mucosa. *Right,* modified Stevens tenotomy hook. It has been
bent from the usual "L" shape into a "J" shape, and is used to hook the proximal end
of the nasolacrimal duct and maintain traction during the dissection.

tered. The soft tissue contents of the canal are mobilized along the entire length
of the nasolacrimal canal. At this point the cylinder of tissue within the canal
remains attached distally to the nasal mucosa. These attachments are now
severed with a modified 3-mm Freer chisel (Fig. 10-1).

The inner surface of the Freer chisel we use is hollow-ground to a 3-mm
radius, and the convex outer surface is ground to a 5-mm radius. These custom
modifications turn the chisel into a gouge with a concave cutting (front) edge
and a point at each corner (Figs. 10-1 and 10-2). The modified chisel is inserted
into the canal with the convex outer surface against bare bone and the inner
surface against the ductal tissue. It is passed inferiorly without engaging the
tissue until it reaches the distal canal (Fig. 10-2). At the end of the canal, the
points engage a portion of the nasal mucosa that is attached to the duct. This
attachment is cut by a sharp forward movement of the instrument. The chisel
is now withdrawn a few millimeters, rotated to a new quadrant, and again
advanced. As this maneuver is repeated, gentle upward traction on the duct is

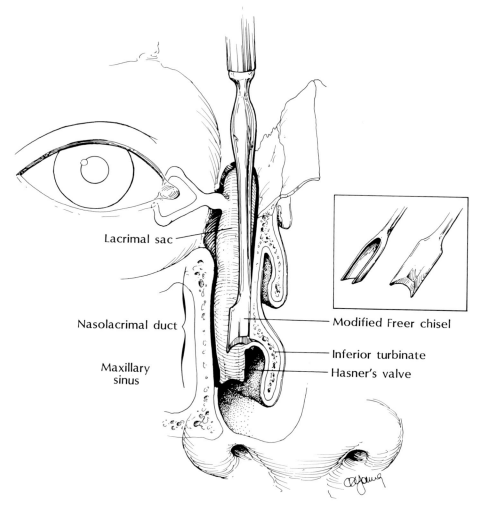

Fig. 10-2   Modified 3-mm Freer chisel is shown cutting the attachments of the distal nasolacrimal duct to nasal mucosa.

maintained with the tenotomy hook. When the final strands of attachment are cut, the entire soft tissue contents of the nasolacrimal canal are withdrawn. The distal end is marked with a suture. The neck of the lacrimal sac is then transected with a Wescott scissors at the point where it entered the canal. This cut releases a specimen that typically includes a margin of lacrimal sac mucosa proximally, fragments of nasal mucosa distally, and all the soft tissue contents of the osseous nasolacrimal canal (Fig. 10-3).

The DCR may now be completed in the usual manner. Once the lacrimal sac is transected inferiorly, the lumen is easily identified in the stump. One

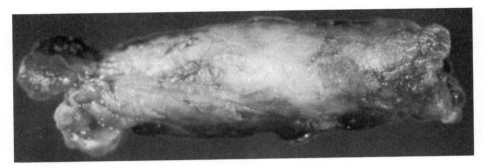

Fig. 10-3 Fresh surgical specimen of soft tissue from within nasolacrimal canal, 4 mm in diameter and 15 mm in length. Fragments of nasal mucosa are attached to distal (left) end.

point of a Wescott scissors is inserted into the sac, which is opened with a single snip. This technique is simple and avoids the difficulties sometimes encountered with the usual scalpel incision into the lacrimal sac.

CLINICAL SPECTRUM OF LACRIMAL EXCRETORY SYSTEM DISEASE

A primary manifestation of lacrimal excretory obstruction is epiphora. This nonspecific symptom can result from complete or partial obstruction, atresia, or absence of any of the structures in the lacrimal pathways, including the puncta, canaliculi, lacrimal sac, or lacrimal duct. The methods of clinical evaluation of the lacrimal system are described in Chapter 2.

Proximal Excretory Pathways

Abnormalities of the proximal excretory pathways are less often the cause of epiphora than abnormalities of the sac and duct. Clinical evaluation usually discloses the source of these deviations. Congenital absence and atresia of one or both puncta or canaliculi are well recognized entities but are relatively uncommon.[6] They generally result from abnormal development or canalization in utero (see Ch. 5 for a discussion of embryogensis of the lacrimal pathways).

Acquired punctal or canalicular stenosis and obstruction can also result from a variety of neoplastic and inflammatory conditions affecting the medial canthal region. Most notably, carcinomas of the canthus or medial eyelid margin can secondarily compromise these structures. Cicatrizing conjunctival or skin processes also can involve the puncta, with either stenosis or secondary punctal eversion leading to epiphora.

Intrinsic neoplasms of the upper lacrimal pathways are extremely rare,[6] but canaliculitis is more common.[7] A celebrated infectious cause of canalicular obstruction is colonization by actinomycetes. Dacryoliths—concretions composed of viable and nonviable organisms with calcification—can often be removed from the canaliculus in this situation. Uncommonly, canalicular obstruction can result from canaliculops—seromucinous cystic dilation of the proximal canaliculus.[8]

In the above situations, with the exception of neoplastic conditions, histopathologic documentation is usually unnecessary or impractical.

Lacrimal Sac

In contrast to disorders of the upper pathways, obstruction at the level of the lacrimal sac is usually an acquired phenomenon. Neoplasms of the sac are uncommon, but their recognition is of paramount importance. Classically, in association with obstruction and tumor of lacrimal fossa, "bloody tears" are said to signal a malignant process.[9] However, in one large series[10] this symptom was lacking in all but one case. Clinical findings and history should be carefully assessed in the evaluation of patients with dacryocystitis, to exclude before surgery the possibility of an underlying neoplasm. Nevertheless, neoplasms are usually not suspected prior to surgery, largely because of their rarity. Routine biopsy of the nasolacrimal tissues can readily rule out the presence of underlying pathologies, including malignancy, responsible for the symptoms of obstruction.

Neoplasms of the sac are usually of epithelial origin, and mimic the neoplasms of the upper aerodigestive tract. The most common histologic types are squamous cell carcinoma, transitional-like carcinoma, and mixtures of the two,[10] although occasional adenocarcinomas have been reported.[11,12] Distinguishing between squamous papillomas, both exophytic and inverted, and well-differentiated carcinoma is often difficult for the pathologist,[6] and careful histologic examination is imperative for choosing the correct therapy. Several case reports of less common carcinomas and sarcomas involving the tissues of the lacrimal fossa have appeared, and many of these are reviewed in Table 10-1.

Dacryocystitis can present as either an acute or chronic inflammatory process. However, acute exacerbations frequently complicate the course of chronic dacryocystitis.

Before the introduction of antibiotics, dacryocystitis was often difficult to manage medically. Dacryocystectomy was frequently necessary to eradicate the chronic infectious and/or inflammatory processes. Series reporting the histopathology of these tissues were published in the first quarter of this century,[13,14,15] but did not address the pathogenesis of lacrimal sac obstruction and revealed only the end stage of a chronic inflammatory process. Since the advent of DCR, dacryocystectomy has rarely been performed. More recent reports have discussed several specific but uncommon infectious etiologies, including trachoma and leprosy (Table 10-1). However, microbiologic studies

Table 10-1. Specific Causes of Secondary Acquired
Nasolacrimal Duct Obstruction

Primary neoplasms
  Papilloma[9,10]
  Squamous cell carcinoma[9,10,41]
  Hemangiopericytoma[42]
  Fibrous histiocytoma[43]
  Oncocytic adenocarcinoma[11]
  Fibroma[46]
  Melanoma[44,45]

Secondary involvement by neoplasms
  Lymphoma[47]
  Leukemia[34,48]
  Lethal midline lymphoma[49]
  Basal cell carcinoma[50]
  Neurofibroma[51]
  Maxillary sinus tumors[52]

Specific inflammatory conditions
  Granulomatous "pseudotumors"[53,54]
  Sarcoidosis[35,55]
  Wegener's granulomatosis[56]

Infectious etiologies
  Trachoma[57,58]
  Leprosy[59]
  Tuberculosis[60]
  Rhinosporidiosis[61]

of the sac suggest that dacryocystitis is polymicrobial in most cases, resulting probably from overgrowth of the normal conjunctival flora.[16-20]

In approximately 15 percent of patients with distal lacrimal obstruction, "dacryoliths" develop within the lacrimal sac. In our experience, these concretions are not truly lithic, because they are rarely significantly mineralized. Rather, they consist of irregular but concentric laminae of dessicated seromucinous material with widely scattered inflammatory cells and apparent lipid material (Fig. 10-4). Occasionally, foreign body giant cells are seen at the periphery, where bacterial colonization is also frequently seen. However, we have never discovered large numbers of organisms in lacrimal sac dacryoliths, as opposed to dacryoliths of the canaliculi.

How dacryoliths develop and how they are temporally related to dacryocyctitis is not entirely clear, but we suggest that low (or no) flow states, such as might be seen in partial, intermittent, or complete distal (ductal) obstruction, predispose to dacryolith formation in the sac. This contention is supported by the fact that we have found minute but histologically identical "liths" in the nasolacrimal duct immediately proximal to focal regions of obstruction (Fig. 10-5). In one of our cases, we removed a large dacryolith from the lacrimal sac during DCR, and the nasolacrimal canal biopsy specimen showed fibrosis of nearly the entire length of the duct. However, it remains unclear why dacryoliths form in relatively few cases of nasolacrimal duct obstruction.

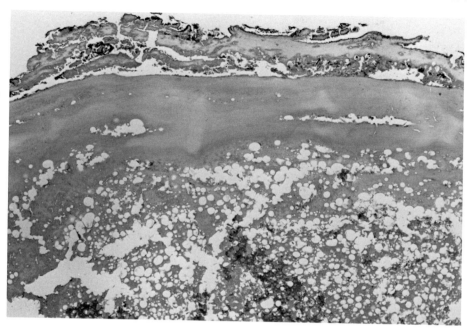

Fig. 10-4 Dacryolith from the lacrimal sac. Dacryoliths from this location generally lack significant calcification, and consist instead of dessicated seromucinous and lipid material with little microbial colonization.

Mucoceles of the lacrimal sac can also complicate distal lacrimal obstruction.[21] We observed complete fibrous obliteration of the nasolacrimal duct in an 83-year-old woman with no history of chronic or acute dacryocystitis who presented with a mucocele of the sac.

Nasolacrimal Duct

Because of the anatomy of the region, obstruction of the excretory pathway originating at the level of the nasolacrimal duct is less likely to produce obvious external signs of inflammation. Because the duct is encased in a bony canal for most of its length, edema and other soft tissue manifestations are generally masked. Usually external signs are present only when obstruction leads to secondary dacryocystitis. In this situation, inflammation over the lacrimal sac inferior to the medial canthal tendon usually becomes clinically evident.

To our knowledge, neoplasms definitely originating in the duct have not been reported. However, secondary invasion of the canal leading to ductal obstruction can occur in advanced neoplasms of the nasal passages or adjacent sinuses. We encountered one patient in whom epiphora associated with nasal obstruction was the presenting sign of a malignant fibrous histiocytoma origi-

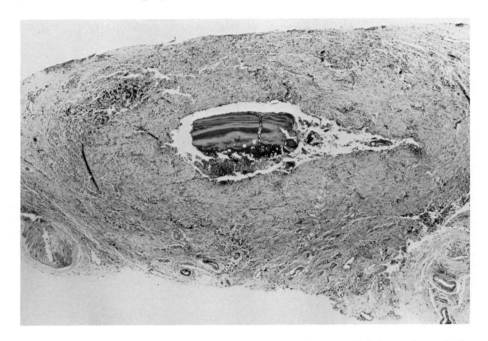

Fig. 10-5   Cross section of the nasolacrimal duct, with a small lith nearly occluding the lumen. Periductal fibrosis with luminal narrowing is present.

nating in the maxillary sinus. Other neoplasms, such as nasopharyngeal carcinoma and esthesioneuroblastoma, more frequently arise in the tissues contiguous to the canal, and are therefore more likely to be associated with secondary ductal obstruction. Obviously, all patients with ductal obstruction should be evaluated to rule out malignancy or other pathologic alterations of the structures adjacent to the canal.

Another important cause of nasolacrimal duct obstruction is mid-facial trauma. Fractures of the maxilla involving the nasolacrimal canal are most notable, and ductal obstruction occurs in about 10 percent of these patients. The duct is compromised by unreduced fractures of the canal, and possibly by soft tissue reactions to the fracture (edema, inflammation, etc.).

The role of the osseous canal in primary acquired nasolacrimal duct obstruction has frequently been discussed.[22,23] The canal is longer and narrower in women than in men and in whites than in nonwhites.[22,24] This evidence has been offered as an explanation of the higher prevalence of duct obstruction in women and in whites.[22,24] Skull measurements of patients with lacrimal obstruction reveal a high prevalence of brachycephaly, which is also associated with narrower canals.[25,26] However, anatomic studies have revealed remarkable variation in the dimensions of the normal canal.[27] In our experience, a 3-mm chisel can easily be inserted and manipulated along the full length of the canal. Thus, the minimum diameter of the canal clearly exceeded 3 mm in all of our patients. Osseous narrowing or obstruction was not encountered. Previous radiologic studies have documented that the inlet of the canal in patients with PANDO is equal in size to that of normal controls.[28] This evidence suggests that stenosis of the osseous canal is not a cause of nasolacrimal duct obstruction except in patients with traumatized or congenitally aberrant canals. If osseous narrowing is documented, we suggest that the patient be evaluated for other osseous pathology (e.g., Paget's disease).[29,30]

Idiopathic or primary acquired nasolacrimal duct obstruction (PANDO)—by far the most common cause of nasolacrimal duct obstruction—is very poorly understood. PANDO is a clinical syndrome defined by complete or functional acquired nasolacrimal duct obstruction without other lacrimal excretory system pathology.

In the past, the inciting factors, pathogenesis, and histologic features of PANDO had not been previously elucidated, owing to a lack of tissue for study. We recently reported our initial clinico-pathologic observations of this syndrome,[5] and the remainder of this chapter is devoted largely to an extension of these histopathologic studies.

PATHOLOGY OF THE NASOLACRIMAL DUCT

By employing routine excisional biopsy of the soft tissue contents of the nasolacrimal canal during DCR, we have had the opportunity to study a large group of patients with PANDO, as well as patients with secondary nasolacrimal duct obstruction of various specific etiologies. We have been impressed that in several patients with PANDO, pathologic examination revealed the specific etiology of the obstruction. These cases will be discussed in detail after a description of the normal histology of the region and our histopathologic observations on idiopathic duct obstruction (PANDO).

Normal Histology of the Excretory Pathways

The normal histology of the lacrimal pathways receives little attention in texts on general histology or ocular anatomy; therefore, we present a review of these structures as a prelude to the histopathologic changes observed in the nasolacrimal duct. See Chapter 1 for a discussion of the macroscopic (surgical) anatomy of the region.

At the punctum, there is a gradual transition from the conjunctival epithelium to the nonkeratinizing stratified squamous epithelium of the canaliculi (Fig. 10-6). This epithelium varies irregularly from three to eight cells in thickness. In some specimens from normal individuals, isolated mucus-containing cells are occasionally seen in the canicular epithelium, and, rarely, acinar collections of secretory goblet cells are associated with areas of mild subepithelial chronic inflammatory infiltration. The canalicular epithelium rests on a delicate basement membrane, subjacent to which is a dense, collagenized connective

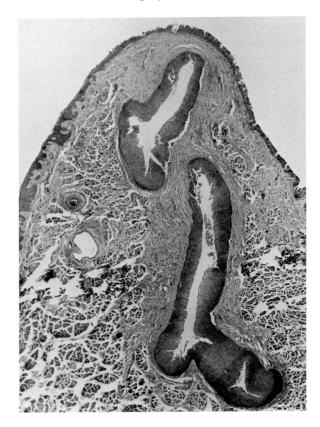

Fig. 10-6 A gradual transition from the skin, *left*, and conjunctival, *right*, epithelium occurs at the normal punctum, giving rise to the nonkeratinizing squamous epithelium of the canaliculus. In this plane of section, the punctal opening is not visualized, and the lumen of the mildly tortuous proximal canaliculus is likewise not completely demonstrated.

tissue forming a tubular structure. It is this dense structure that is recognized as the canaliculus during surgical exploration.

At the junction of the common canaliculus and the lacrimal sac, the epithelium abruptly changes. The squamous epithelium of the canaliculus becomes the stratified columnar epithelium of the sac, which contains many goblet cells and variable numbers of small simple secretory glands. Occasionally, this transition occurs within the common canaliculus (Fig. 10-7).

The mucosae of the lacrimal sac and the lacrimal duct show remarkable variation, even in specimens from individuals with no evidence of disease (Figs. 10-8 and 10-9). In our anatomic studies of midface/orbit specimens obtained from "normal" donor cadavers, we have seen remarkable variation in the degree of chronic inflammatory infiltration of the stroma beneath the stratified columnar epithelium of the sac and duct (Fig. 10-10). Likewise, there is wide variation in the goblet cell components of this epithelium. In some specimens, distinct glandular structures are associated with the epithelium of the sac. Scattered regions with ciliated surface cells are also occasionally encountered.

The subepithelial connective tissues of the lacrimal sac and duct normally

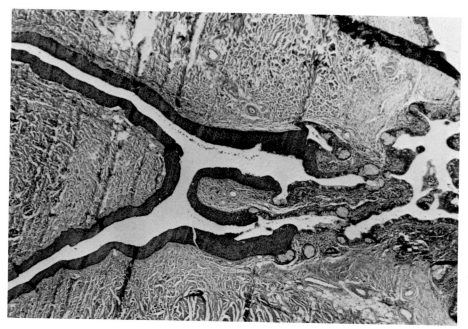

Fig. 10-7 The upper and lower canaliculi join to form the common canaliculus. An abrupt transition from the canalicular epithelium to the secretory stratifield columnar epithelium of the lacrimal sac occurs in this region. In this section a mucosal ridge is seen within the lumen of the common canaliculus.

contain a mild cellular infiltrate composed primarily of mature lymphocytes with occasional plasma cells. The amount of infiltrate varies widely among normal individuals; it is usually heavier in the region of the sac than in the canal. Lymphoid follicles are not normally present. In contrast to the nasal mucosa, eosinophils are very rarely identified.

The caliber of the nasolacrimal duct lumen, as studied in longitudinal histologic sections of normal specimens, also shows some variation (Figs. 10-8 and 10-9), as does the complexity of the mucosal folds along the duct. These variations reflect a difference in the amount of surrounding stromal tissue, rather than a difference in the caliber of the osseous canal, which is a fairly constant 4 to 5 mm. Whether or not a narrow ductal lumen or the presence of redundant mucosal folds predisposes an individual to primary nasolacrimal duct obstruction can only be speculated.

The stromal tissues surrounding the duct uniformly contain an extensive venous plexus reminiscent of the nasal mucosa (Fig. 10-10). Although transient nasolacrimal duct obstruction during acute allergic reactions has been demonstrated radiographically, it is not known if this is secondary to engorgement of the venous plexus or to other reactions. Only a very few of our patients with PANDO give a history of chronic nasal congestion or sinusitis, and we

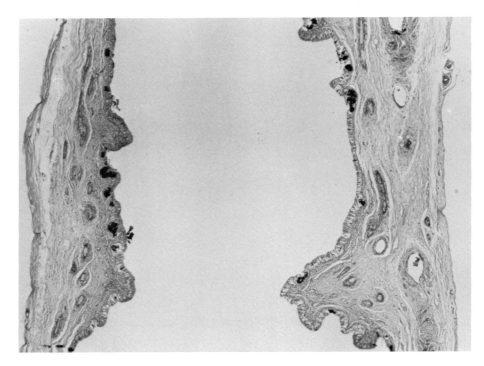

Fig. 10-8   Normal nasolacrimal duct. This normal specimen has a widely patent lumen and numerous mucosal rugae with a few well-developed folds. The mucosa contains numerous collections of goblet cells (darkly stained by PAS technique).

believe that chronic allergic conditions with resultant stromal venous congestion and edema do not play a significant role in the pathogenesis of PANDO. Epiphora associated with nasal stimulation or congestion is well recognized and is usually explained by transient obstruction at the level of the inferior meatus or by reflex tearing. However, it is possible that congestion of the venous plexus of the periductal tissue also contributes to this phenomenon.

The histology of the distal, membranous portion of the duct more closely resembles that of the nasal passages. Near Hasner's valve, mucinous and seromucinous glands are present in the subepithelial stroma (Fig. 10-11). Ciliated respiratory-type epithelium is common in this area.

Histopathologic Reaction Patterns of the Nasolacrimal Duct

Regardless of the specific etiology of nasolacrimal obstruction, the histopathologic reaction patterns of the tissues within the nasolacrimal canal show many similar features. Inflammation, as at any other site, leads to vascular congestion, edema, and inflammatory cellular migration into the connective

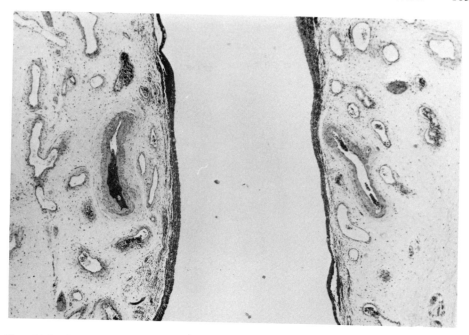

Fig. 10-9 Normal nasolacrimal duct. This normal specimen has a lumen that is narrower than in Figure 10-8 but still widely patent. The mucosa lacks folds and intraepithelial glandular formations, and is more simplified than in Figure 10-8. Stromal tissues are also more abundant.

tissues of the region. As the inflammatory process subsides, fibrosis (cicatrization) ensues.

In complete or partial ductal obstruction, stagnation of tear flow may lead to accumulation of organisms, cellular debris, and other potentially noxious agents normally present in the tear film. Presumably these incite an inflammatory reaction in the ductal tissues, particularly if the barrier function of the epithelium is compromised by erosion or ulceration. Because the nasolacrimal duct lies in the relatively narrow and rigid confines of the osseous canal, edema or inflammatory exudation can result in soft tissue compression of the ductal lumen. Regardless of the inciting cause, it has long been suggested that stasis and secondary infection lead to complete obstruction,[31] and several microbiologic studies have documented colonization of the lacrimal pathways by increased numbers of pathologic organisms.[17–20,32] However, we have not observed significant numbers of organisms or invasive infections in any of the excisional biopsy specimens we have examined, including those with acute inflammation and ulceration. Nonetheless, this cycle of stasis and inflammation with or without infection remains a likely scenario in the pathogenesis of chronic nasolacrimal duct obstruction.

Most of our patients had no history of acute dacryocystitis. Nevertheless,

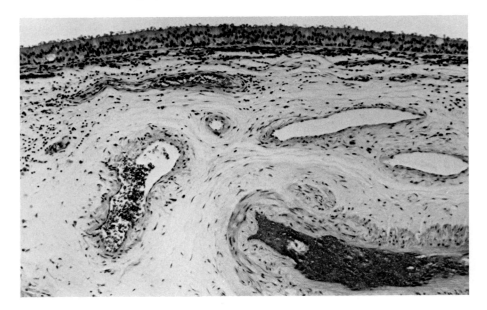

Fig. 10-10 The normal lacrimal duct mucosa displays a partially ciliated stratified columnar epithelium, scattered subepithelial mononuclear inflammatory cells, and a prominent vascular plexus in the surrounding connective tissue.

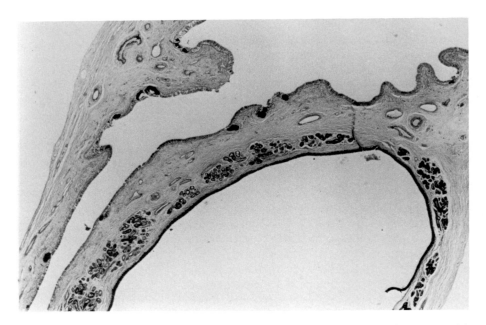

Fig. 10-11 Normal distal nasolacrimal duct and Hasner's valve. Nasal mucosa with numerous secretory glands lines the nasal portion of the valve (bottom).

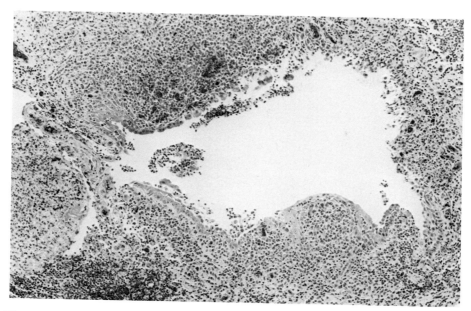

Fig. 10-12 Ulceration with granulation tissue and acute and chronic inflammatory infiltrates are occasionally seen at limited foci in specimens from patients with PANDO. Regenerating epithelium is present in several areas in this specimen.

if acute inflammatory events occurred at localized foci within the canal, it is quite possible that they went unnoticed by the patient. In chronic dacryocystitis with nasolacrimal duct obstruction, we not uncommonly see minute erosions and limited foci of acute inflammation affecting the ductal epithelium (Fig. 10-12). We believe that such episodes of ulceration and acute inflammation within the duct, with the concommitant tissue-altering healing processes (e.g., granulation and fibrosis), are of paramount importance in the progression to complete nasolacrimal duct obstruction.

The epithelium of the duct undergoes a variety of reactive changes in the face of chronic inflammation. We frequently observe squamous metaplasia and reserve cell hyperplasia in areas of severe chronic inflammation and near areas of erosion and ulceration (Fig. 10-13). Goblet cell hyperplasia and, in other areas, goblet cell depletion in the stratified columnar epithelium are also seen. Occasionally, oncocytic metaplasia of the ductal epithelium occurs, particularly in the distal portion of the duct (Fig. 10-14). This finding is sometimes accompanied by hyperplasia and oncocytic change of the nasal seromucinous glands near Hasner's valve.

Despite the chronic inflammatory process, lymphoid follicles are only rarely observed (Fig. 10-15). Rather, the inflammatory infiltrate consists of a lymphoplasmacytic cellular infiltration, heaviest immediately subjacent to the epithelium in the so-called adenoid layer. In more severely and chronically

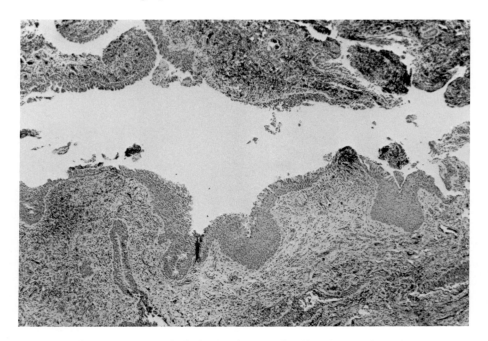

Fig. 10-13   Squamous metaplasia in the ductal epithelium is prominent in some specimens with duct obstruction. This specimen (especially toward the bottom) shows a spectrum of reactive epithelial changes ranging from reserve cell hyperplasia to mature metaplasia.

inflamed areas, marked epithelial basement membrane thickening is seen (Fig. 10-16).

Primary Acquired Nasolacrimal Duct Obstruction

We have studied nasolacrimal ducts removed at various intervals beginning with the onset of symptoms, in our patients with the clinical syndrome of PANDO. Histopathology was correlated with clinical histories. Although some overlap exists, three main categories of histologic change are recognized, which correlate roughly with the duration of clinically recognized obstruction. Obviously it is difficult to obtain tissue very shortly after the onset of epiphora in PANDO, given the usual delay before seeking treatment for this complaint. Our earliest specimen was obtained approximately three months after the onset of epiphora, while many were obtained several years after the onset of obstruction.

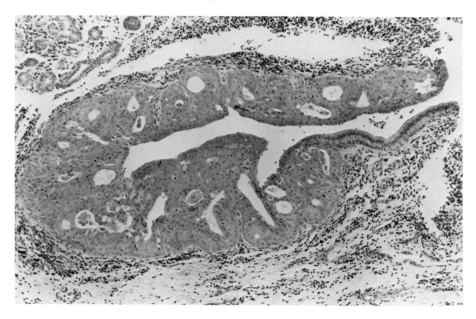

Fig. 10-14 Oncocytic metaplasia, a common reactive change of nasal respiratory mucosa, is shown here in a mucosal invagination. Intraepithelial glandular structures are formed in the hyperplastic epithelium. Note transitional zone to normal ductal epithelium.

Early/Active Inflammatory Phase

In these patients, dense lymphoplasmacytic infiltration of the periductal connective tissue extending into the region of the venous plexus is associated with edema and resultant narrowing of the ductal lumen. In these patients with the most severe inflammatory process, the duct remains patent but is severely narrowed by soft tissue compression (Fig. 10-17). In many of these ducts, foci of erosion with varying degrees of infiltration by polymorphonuclear leukocytes were encountered (Fig. 10-12). Granulation tissue with a mixed inflammatory infiltrate is sometimes seen. We rarely see extensive areas of acute inflammation in any patient with PANDO, but very early biopsies have not been available for examination.

The histologic findings in early PANDO suggest that the obstruction may be a reversible process. In most patients in this group, typically biopsied less than 1 year after the onset of epiphora, the ductal lumen remains functionally patent. Because edema and inflammatory cellular infiltration are a factor in luminal narrowing, it is conceivable that obstruction might be reversed with antiinflammatory agents, although we have not yet proven this hypothesis.

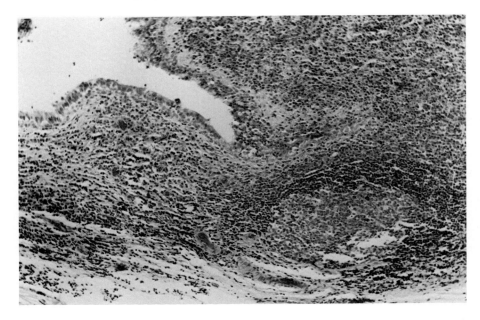

Fig. 10-15 Lymphoid follicles, (lower right) are encountered infrequently even in cases of severe and long-standing ductal inflammation.

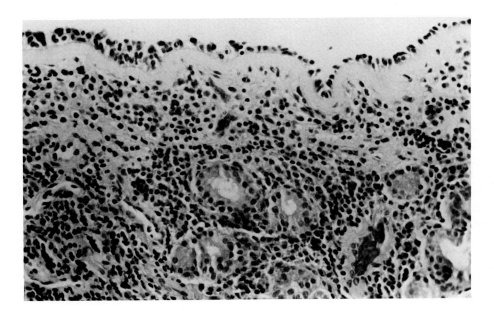

Fig. 10-16 A dense lymphoplasmacytic inflammatory infiltrate is seen beneath a markedly thickened basement membrane (hyalinized zone immediately subjacent to epithelium).

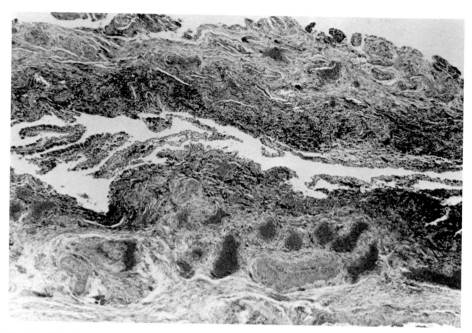

Fig. 10-17 Dense, chronic inflammatory infiltrates, periductal edema and fibrosis, and venous congestion are typical of the early/active inflammatory phase of PANDO. The lumen (longitudinal section) is markedly narrowed, and the mucosa is ragged in many areas.

Intermediate Phase

We have defined a category of patients in whom focal fibrous obliteration of the duct is seen. Clinically, the duration of symptoms prior to biopsy overlaps that of the early and late phases. Histopathologically, chronic and sometimes focal acute inflammation persists in some regions in the periductal tissue, but less intensely than in the early phase (Fig. 10-18). In the intermediate phase, the inflammatory process appears to be gradually resolving, and in scarred areas very few inflammatory cells are present. Typically, the mid-portion of the ductal lumen is replaced by dense, collagenized scar tissue. In a few cases we observed tiny islands of trapped epithelial cells within this tissue (Fig. 10-19), suggesting that synechiae had formed between apposed, eroded luminal walls, leading to the obstructing scar (Fig. 10-20).

The periductal connective tissue in these cases also usually shows increased collagenization in regions without luminal obliteration, probably resulting from the chronic edema and low-grade chronic inflammatory infiltration around the venous plexus.

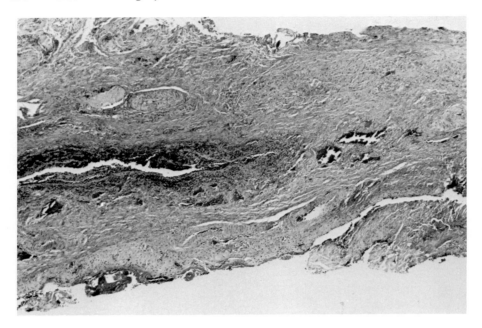

Fig. 10-18   In the intermediate phase of PANDO, chronic inflammation begins to subside. There is focal obstruction of the duct by dense fibrosis (right).

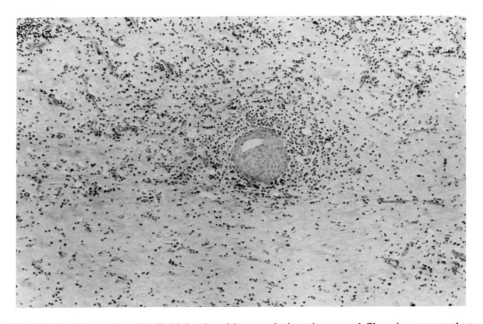

Fig. 10-19   Trapped epithelial islands with granulation tissue and fibrosis suggest that synechia formation may be important in the pathogenesis of fibrous ductal obstruction.

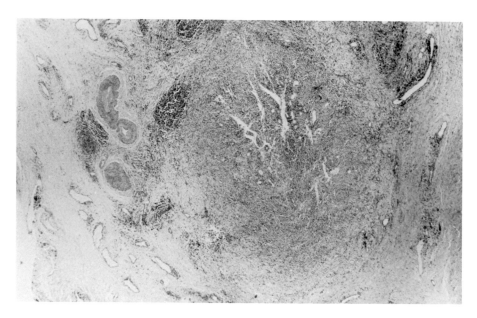

Fig. 10-20 Cross section of duct focally obliterated by granulation tissue and fibrosis. Other parts of the duct were patent.

Late/Fibrotic Phase

Generally by 2 to 3 years after the onset of symptoms, but in some cases earlier, the chronic inflammatory process has progressed so that nearly the entire ductal lumen is replaced by fibrous scar tissue (Figs. 10-21 and 10-22). No ductal epithelium or periductal epithelial structures remain, and only scattered inflammatory cells are seen. Capillary proliferation is occasionally present in the central portion of the scar tissue in the region of the obliterated duct, further suggesting that granulation tissue formation and synechial formation underlie the pathogenesis of the obstruction (Fig. 10-22). Hemosiderin-laden macrophages are encountered in some specimens, suggesting that hemorrhage may also play a role in the formation and progression of the scar tissue.

As stated above, focal obstruction in the intermediate phase typically involves the mid-portion of the duct. By the fibrotic phase, the cicatrizing process has progressed proximally to the junction of the sac and duct. Distal progression is less consistent. The membranous portion of the duct typically remains patent. These observations further support the contention that soft-tissue compression of the ductal lumen underlies the pathogenesis of nasolacrimal duct obstruction, because the membranous portion of the duct does not lie within the confines of the osseous canal. Although the same inflammatory changes affect this portion of the duct, soft-tissue compression of the duct and fibrous obliteration

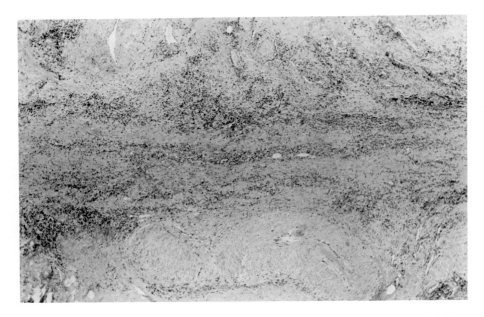

Fig. 10-21   In the late phase of PANDO, luminal obliteration is complete, and inflammation has largely subsided, with maturation of the scar tissue. Fibrous tissue replaces the duct (center), shown here in longitudinal section.

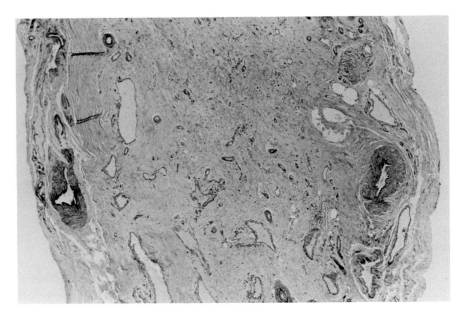

Fig. 10-22   In this specimen, capillary proliferation is prominent in the region of ductal obliteration.

are not usually seen, presumably because the periductal tissues can "swell" into the nasal cavity.

Secondary Acquired Nasolacrimal Duct Obstruction

By performing routine excisional biopsy of the nasolacrimal duct during DCR, we have had the opportunity to study the ductal tissues from patients with a variety of known causes of nasolacrimal duct obstruction. The basic histopathologic changes observed are usually as we have described. Generally, only the initial etiology or inciting cause differs. We present here our recent experience with cases of secondary nasolacrimal duct obstruction, although our findings obviously do not represent all possible causes.

Radiation

We studied the ductal tissues of a 23-year-old woman who had mid-facial radiation therapy for nasopharyngeal carcinoma. Although the carcinoma was successfully treated, the patient developed epiphora secondary to common canalicular obstruction. DCR and canalicular repair were performed 4 years after radiation.

The excisional biopsy specimen showed a markedly stenotic but patent ductal lumen. A moderate, primarily plasmacellular infiltrate was present in the subepithelial stroma. Increased numbers of mast cells were present, a finding we have not otherwise seen. The epithelium was disorganized and varied in thickness, although maturation was intact in most areas. The connective tissue stroma was hyalinized, but the fibrocytes were prominent and irregular, as is usually seen in radiation fibrosis. Further, many of the vessels of the congested vascular plexus had thickened intima and media with vacuolar change (Fig. 10-23), a finding typically seen in radiation damage.[33]

Functional obstruction of the duct and canaliculus from the hyalinizing fibrosis induced by radiation was the probable pathogenetic mechanism in this patient. We have not otherwise seen this degree of periductal fibrosis and luminal stensosis without fibrous ductal obliteration.

Trauma

In fractures of the nasolacrimal canal, mechanical obstruction of the duct frequently occurs. Because of the osseous abnormality, the biopsy is difficult if not impossible to perform. Therefore, we have not had the opportunity to study complete specimens from patients with trauma.

However, we have seen duct obstruction following surgical trauma in a 63-year-old man who developed functional nasolacrimal duct obstruction immediately following nasal polypectomy. During DCR surgery 7 months later,

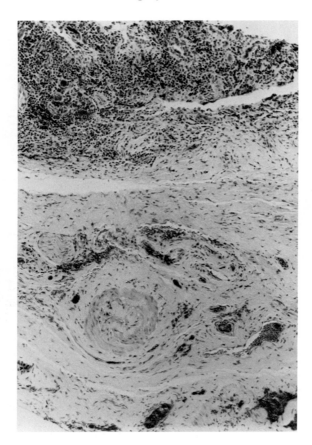

Fig. 10-23 Radiation-damaged ducts showing dense fibrosis with reactive fibroblasts, vacuolar degeneration within vessel walls, and chronic inflammation.

the duct was excised. Patency of the duct was demonstrated by inserting a probe through the entire length of the specimen. There was moderately severe periductal chronic inflammation in the distal segment, and reactive changes and epithelial proliferation were noted in the membranous portion of the duct (Fig. 10-24). Although the epithelium was largely denuded artefactually by the probing, intact areas were normal. In this case, the surgical trauma appears to have incited an inflammatory reaction heaviest in the membranous (nasal) portion of the duct, which resulted in soft-tissue compression and functional obstruction of the duct.

Leukemia

A 72-year-old man with a 2-year history of chronic lymphocytic leukemia presented clinically with acute left dacryocystitis and nasolacrimal duct obstruction. Tissue examination revealed a dense atypical lymphocytic infiltrate along nearly the entire length of the specimen (Fig. 10-25). This infiltrate caused

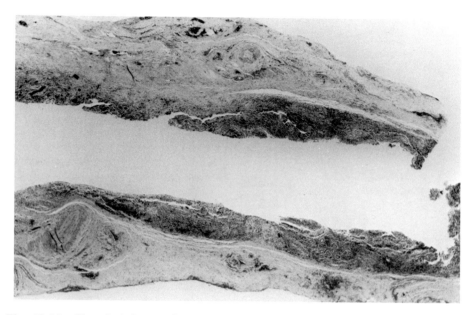

Fig. 10-24   Chronic inflammation is most severe in the distal segment (right) of this longitudinally sectioned specimen. The specimen was fixed after a probe was inserted in the freshly excised specimen, thereby artificially enlarging the lumen.

severe stenosis of the ductal lumen by soft tissue compression. However, the lumen of the specimen was probe patent.

   Nasolacrimal duct obstruction in leukemia has been previously reported,[34] but documentation of ductal involvement and soft tissue compression of the duct by the atypical infiltrate has not been published previously. Our patient's disease was stable on medical therapy, but nasolacrimal duct obstruction developed nevertheless. It is well recognized that the neoplastic infiltrates of hematologic malignancies can appear in mucosal tissues with an "adenoid" layer (mucosal-associated lymphoid tissue). We believe that the mucosa of the nasolacrimal duct serves a similar function. Diagnostic biopsy of the duct should be performed in any patient with hematologic malignancy who presents with dacryocystitis and/or nasolacrimal duct obstruction to determine whether there is neoplastic involvement at this site.

Noncaseating Granulomatosis (Presumed Sarcoidosis)

   We unexpectedly encountered diffuse noncaseating granulomatous inflammation (Fig. 10-26) involving the nasolacrimal duct of a 52-year-old white woman who presented with PANDO. Numerous sarcoidal granulomas with many Langhans-type multinucleated giant cells and several typical asteroid

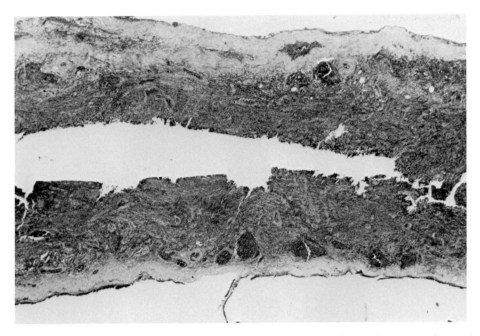

Fig. 10-25   Duct with a diffuse leukemic infiltrate that caused ductal compression and obstruction. The lumen was artificially enlarged with a probe after excision.

bodies filled the periductal tissues and compressed the ductal lumen. Subsequent laboratory evaluation revealed elevated serum levels of angiotensin converting enzyme and lysozyme. Complete physical examination including chest roentgenograms revealed no evidence of systemic sarcoidosis. No causative agents (organisms, organic material, etc.) were identified in special histologic studies. We have reported this case as an example of presumed localized sarcoidosis limited to the lacrimal duct.[35] The patient has shown no evidence of systemic disease after 2 years of follow-up.

Atypical Lymphoid Infiltrates

One 78-year-old woman, in whom excisional biopsy could not be completed during DCR because of intraoperative medical complications, showed a thickened, gray lacrimal sac mucosa. The sac and the tissue from the upper canal were biopsied. These showed an atypical, monotonous lymphoid infiltrate throughout the stromal tissues (Fig. 10-27). Immunohistologic studies revealed a monotypic (λ light chains) population of B lymphocytes. Systemic evaluation revealed no evidence of leukemia or lymphoma, and neither obstruction nor a mass lesion has recurred after 1 year of follow-up. We believe this lesion

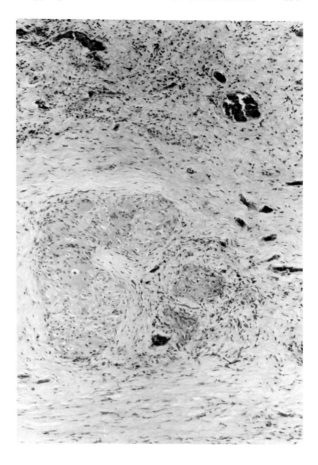

Fig. 10-26 Numerous periductal sarcoidal granulomas caused ductal obstruction in this case. Langhans giant cells, some of which contain asteroid bodies, are prominent in these granulomas.

represents an atypical lymphoid infiltrate of the ocular adnexa, akin to similar orbital lesions, limited to involvement of the lacrimal excretory system. No orbital lesions have developed in this patient.

Congenital Nasolacrimal Duct Obstruction

Congenital atresia of the nasolacrimal duct is relatively common compared to atresia of other segments of the excretory system. It was present in 73 percent of stillborn, full-term fetuses in one study.[36] Canalization of the canal is normally complete by the end of gestation, but a distal impatency may persist into infancy. This thin membrane often consists only of basally apposed nasolacrimal and nasal epithelia with minimal intervening stroma. This explains why probing with or without the placement of stents has such a high success rate.[37–39]

Attempts to use similar techniques in adult patients with PANDO have

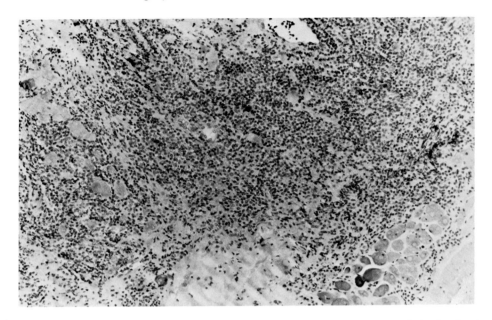

Fig. 10-27 An atypical, monoclonal lymphoid infiltrate in the region of the lacrimal sac led to ductal obstruction in this patient. The infiltrate has aggressive features, including destruction of adjacent musculature (left).

had variable results.[40] The pathologic alterations described above readily explain why this is so. Probing a completely fibrosed nasolacrimal canal in the late phase of PANDO should be difficult and cannot be expected to result in a permanent lumen. Likewise, if congenital obstruction is not treated and/or does not resolve spontaneously (usually in the first year of life), probing and similar therapies are much less successful. We believe that the pathogenesis of chronic congenital obstruction may be similar to PANDO. This may explain why probing is less successful in congenital cases of long duration.

We examined the canal contents from a 4-year-old boy who had had obstruction since birth. The lumen was patent but markedly narrowed on pathologic examination. In some areas there was intense periductal chronic inflammation, multiple foci of erosion, and granulation tissue. Intact epithelium showed striking squamous metaplasia. Generally, these findings were identical to the early phase of PANDO. However, this patient showed multiple blind-ended branches from the main ductal lumen that were lined largely by squamous epithelium. Some arborizations extended through the venous plexus almost to the periosteal surface (Fig. 10-28). We have not encountered these in any other patient, and are unsure of their prevalence or significance in the pathogenesis of congenital obstruction. However, these branches might result from aberrant canalization, which may be associated with the underlying defect.

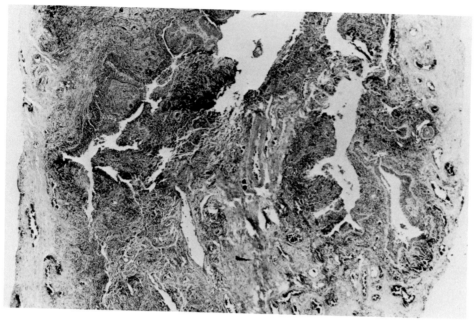

Fig. 10-28 The duct branches abnormally in this patient with congenital obstruction. Tortuous luminal arborizations extend into the periductal vascular plexus in several areas. Left and right edges of the specimen represent periosteal margins.

SUMMARY

From our pathologic studies of nasolacrimal canal tissues from a wide variety of patients with nasolacrimal duct obstruction, a clinically relevant classification scheme based on pathogenesis is immediately suggested (see Table 10-2).

To our knowledge, routine biopsy of nasolacrimal tissues during DCR has not previously been employed. In only a few years, with a relatively modest number of patients, we have learned a great deal about the pathology of this region by utilizing the excisional biopsy technique presented here. This technique, which adds less than 10 minutes to the routine surgical procedure, is safe and simple. We have encountered no postoperative complications.

We urge other lacrimal surgeons to consider using this biopsy technique routinely and to submit tissues for pathologic examination. Only with such study will understanding of the pathogenesis of primary acquired nasolacrimal duct obstruction be advanced. Further, such study is likely to reveal a variety of clinically unsuspected, specific underlying pathologies, such as we have encountered in 3 of 40 patients with the clinical syndrome of PANDO.

Table 10-2. Clinicopathologic Classification of Nasolacrimal Duct Obstruction

I. **Congenital nasolacrimal duct obstruction**
   A. Early—amenable to probing
   B. Late/complicated—obstruction progresses to fibrosis

II. **Primary acquired nasolacrimal duct obstruction**
   A. Early—may be amenable to anti-inflammatory agents
   B. Intermediate—focal fibrous obstruction
   C. Late—complete fibrosis of nasolacrimal canal

III. **Secondary acquired nasolacrimal duct obstruction**
   A. Primary neoplasms
   B. Secondary involvement of canal by extrinsic neoplasms
   C. Specific infectious etiologies
   D. Specific inflammatory etiologies (e.g. sarcoidosis, pseudotumor)
   E. Trauma
   F. Radiation
   G. Others

REFERENCES

1. Traquair HM: Chronic dacryocystitis: Its causation and treatment. Arch Ophthalmol 26:165, 1941
2. Scott GI, Summerskill WH: Discussion on treatment of chronic dacryocystitis. Trans Ophthalmol Soc UK 69:477, 1949
3. McLachlan DL, Shannon GM, Flanagan JC: Results of dacryocystorhinostomy: Analysis of reoperations. Ophthalmic Surg 11:427, 1980
4. Welham RAN, Henderson PH: Results of dacryocystorhinostomy: Analysis of cases of failure. Trans Ophthalmol Soc UK 93:601, 1973
5. Linberg JV, McCormick SA: Primary acquired nasolacrimal duct obstruction: A clinicopathologic report and biopsy technique. Ophthalmology 93:1055, 1986
6. Font RL: Eyelids and lacrimal drainage system. p. 2314. In Spencer WH (ed): Ophthalmic Pathology: An Atlas and Textbook. WB Saunders, Philadelphia, 1986
7. Demant E, Hurwitz JJ: Canaliculitis: Review of 12 cases. Can J Ophthalmol 15:73, 1980
8. Sacks E, Jakobiec FA, Dodick J: Canaliculops. Ophthalmology 94:78, 1987
9. Hornblass A, Jakobiec FA, Bosniak S, Flanagan J: The diagnosis and management of epithelial tumors of the lacrimal sac. Ophthalmology 87:476, 1980
10. Ryan SJ, Font RL: Primary epithelial neoplasms of the lacrimal sac. Am J Ophthalmol 76:73, 1973
11. Peretz WL, Ettinghausen SE, Gray GF: Oncocytic adenocarcinoma of the lacrimal sac. Arch Ophthalmol 96:303, 1978
12. Biggs SL, Font RL: Oncocytic lesions of the caruncle and other ocular adnexa. Arch Ophthalmol 95:474, 1977
13. McKee SH: The pathologic histology of the lacrimal sac in chronic purulent dacryocystitis. Int Clin 3:64, 1925; also Trans Am Ophthalmol Soc 23:54, 1925
14. Rollet, Bussy: Recherches anatomo-pathologiques sur cent cas de dacryocystites avec extraction du sac et du canal. Arch Ophthalmol (Paris) 40:321, 1923
15. Seidenari R: Ricerche sul dotto osseo naso-lacrimale e sulla mucosa nasale circostante alla papilla lacrimale. Minerva Med 38:176, 1947

16. Jones DB, Robinson NM: Anaerobic ocular infections. Trans Am Acad Ophthalmol Otolaryngol 83:309, 1977
17. Ghose S, Mahajan VM: Microbiology of congenital dacryocystitis—its clinical significance. J Ocul Ther Surg 4:54, 1985
18. Weinstein GS, Biglan AW, Patterson JH: Congenital lacrimal sac mucoceles. Am J Ophthalmol 94:106, 1982
19. Sasaki T, Tanaka N, Odagiri Y, et al.: Microbial flora in dacryocystitis. Acta Soc Ophthalmol Jap 77:644, 1973
20. Sood NN, Ratnaraj A, Balaraman G, Madhavan, HN: Chronic dacryocystitis—a clinico-bacteriological study. All-India Ophthalmol Soc 15:107, 1967
21. Hornblass A, Gabry M: Diagnosis and treatment of lacrimal sac cysts. Ophthalmology 86:1655, 1979
22. Meller J: Diseases of the lacrymal apparatus. Trans Ophthalmol Soc UK 49:233, 1929
23. Jones LT, Boyden GL: The lacrimal apparatus, In Coates GM, Schenck HP (eds): Otolaryngology. Vol 3. WF Prior, Hagerstown, PA, 1962
24. Santos-Fernandez J: The measurements of the nasal canal according to the race. Am J Ophthalmol 4:32, 1921
25. Heinonen O: Klinische Untersuchungen uber die Bedeutungg der Nasenkrankheiten und einigen disponierenden Momenten in der Aetiologie der Dakrystenose (schwedisch). Klin Monatsbl Augenheilkd 65:601, 1920
26. Avasthi P, Misra RN, Sood AK: Clinical and anatomical considerations of dacryocystitis. Int Surg 55:200, 1971
27. Whitnall SE: The nasolacrimal canal: The extent to which it is formed by the maxilla, and the influence of this upon its caliber. Ophthalmoscope 10:557, 1912
28. Phillips CI, George M: Epiphora and the bony naso-lacrimal canal. Br J Ophthalmol 40:673, 1956
29. Hurwitz JJ: Failed dacryocystorhinostomy in Paget's disease. Can J Ophthalmol 14:291, 1979
30. Stranc MF: The pattern of lacrimal injuries in naso-ethmoid injuries. Br J Plastic Surg 23:339, 1970
31. Duke-Elder S: The ocular adnexa. p. 5302. In Textbook of Ophthalmology. Vol. 5. Kimpton, London, 1952
32. Pine L, Shearin WA, Gonzales CA: Mycotic flora of the lacrimal duct. Am J Ophthalmol 52:619, 1961
33. Fechner, RE: The surgical pathology of iatrogenic lesions. p. 87. In Silverberg SG (ed): Principles and Practice of Surgical Pathology. John Wiley & Sons, New York, 1983
34. Kincaid MC, Green WR: Ocular and orbital involvement in leukemia. Surv Ophthalmol 27:211, 1983
35. Vasquez R, Linberg JV, McCormick SA: Nasolacrimal duct obstruction secondary to presumed localized sarcoidosis. Ophthalmic Plast Reconstr Surg (submitted for publication)
36. Cassady JV: Developmental anatomy of nasolacrimal duct. Arch Ophthalmol 47:141, 1952
37. Petersen RA, Robb RM: The natural course of congenital obstruction of the nasolacrimal duct. J Pediatr Ophthalmol Strabismus 15:246, 1978
38. Dortzbach RK, France TD, Kushner BJ, Gonnering RS: Silicone intubation for obstruction of the nasolacrimal duct in children. Am J Ophthalmol 94:585, 1982

39. Durso F, Hand SI Jr, Ellis FD, Helveston EM: Silicone intubation in children with nasolacrimal obstruction. J Pediatr Ophthalmol Strabismus 17:389, 1980
40. Angrist RC, Dortzbach PK: Silicone intubation for partial and total nasolacrimal duct obstruction in adults. Ophthalmic Plast Reconstr Surg 1:51, 1985
41. Khalil MK, Lorenzetti DWC: Epidermoid carcinoma of the lacrimal sac: a clinicopathologic case report. Can J Ophthalmol 15:40, 1980
42. Gurney N, Chalkey T, O'Grady R: Lacrimal sac hemangiopericytoma. Am J Ophthalmol 71:757, 1971
43. Cole SH, Ferry AP: Fibrous histiocytoma (fibrous xanthoma) of the lacrimal sac. Arch Ophthalmol 96:1647, 1978
44. Farkas TG, Lamberson RE: Malignant melanoma of the lacrimal sac. Am J Ophthalmol 66:45, 1968
45. Yamade S, Kitagawa A: Malignant melanoma of the lacrimal sac. Ophthalmologica 177:30, 1978
46. Howcroft MJ, Hurwitz JJ: Lacrimal sac fibroma. Can J Ophthalmol 15:196, 1980
47. Carlin R, Henderson JW: Malignant lymphoma of the nasolacrimal sac. Am J Ophthalmol 78:511, 1974
48. Stokes WH: Dacryocystitis in lymphatic leukemia. Arch Ophthalmol 20:85, 1938
49. Spalton DJ, O'Donnell PJ, Graham EM: Lethal midline lymphoma causing acute dacryocystitis. Br J Ophthalmol 65:503, 1981
50. Barton D: A case of basal-cell carcinoma of the lacrimal sac presenting as chronic dacryocystitis. Trans Ophthalmol Soc UK 69:523, 1949
51. Milder B: Neurofibroma of the lacrimal sac. Am J Ophthalmol 53:1016, 1962
52. Campbell CH, Apt RK, Schimek RA. Compression of lacrimal sac by inverted papilloma arising in the maxillary sinus. South Med J 67:773, 1974
53. Cole JG, Brackup A, Hanley JS, Higgins GK: Pseudotumor of the lacrimal sac. Am J Ophthalmol 55:136, 1963
54. Radnot M, Gall J: Tumoren des Tranensackes. Ophthalmologica 151:1, 166
55. Harris GJ, Williams GA, Clarke GP: Sarcoidosis of the lacrimal sac. Arch Ophthalmol 99:1198, 1981
56. Haynes BF, Fishman ML, Fauci AS, Wolff SM: The ocular manifestations of Wegener's granulomatosis: Fifteen years' experience and review of the literature. Am J Med 63:131, 1977
57. Tabbara KF, Bobb AA: Lacrimal system complications in trachoma. Ophthalmology 87:298, 1980
58. Postic S: Remarques sur le trachome lacrymal: etude comparative. Arch Ophthalmol (Paris) 17:749, 1957
59. Weerekoon L: Ocular leprosy in Ceylon. Br J Ophthalmol 53:457, 1969
60. Andersen SR: Tuberculous dacryocystitis and lupus of the nose diagnosed as Boeck's disease. Acta Ophthalmol 25:455, 1947
61. Jain SC, Darban BS, Bhatnagar BS. Ocular rhinosporidiosis. Eye Ear Nose Throat Month 47:380, 1968

11 | Lacrimal Sac Tumors: Surgical Management

Joseph C. Flanagan
Christine L. Zolli

The most common causes of a medial canthal mass are inflammation or mucocele that cause lacrimal obstruction and resulting distention of the lacrimal sac. Lacrimal sac neoplasms are extremely rare, yet they must be considered when evaluating a medial canthal mass. A malignancy in this area, whether epithelial or mesenchymal, has an unfavorable prognosis; it is apt to recur, and after recurrence has less than a 50 percent 5-year survival rate.[1-3] The fact that 60 percent of noninflammatory lacrimal sac neoplasms are malignant[3-6] makes prompt diagnosis and timely treatment very important.

On a less somber note, it is our impression from the Wills Eye Hospital experience and reports during the last 20 years[6-9] that the survival rate for the epidermoid malignant tumors of the lacrimal sac is improving. In our estimate, the survival rate for squamous cell carcinoma of the sac is approximately 85 to 90 percent. Better diagnostic modalities, including dacryocystogram and CT scan, have resulted in earlier diagnosis and more accurate tumor staging. Radical surgery, radiation therapy, and now chemotherapy employed in a combined modality approach have also helped improve the survival rate.

After histology, early diagnosis is the second most important factor in the prognosis for lacrimal sac malignancies. Patients whose tumors have spread to the orbit or sinuses, or patients who initially refuse treatment, are more likely to have recurrences and metastases even when the neoplasms appear to be completely excised.

Three characteristics of lacrimal sac tumors are documented in the literature: (1) rarity, (2) a disproportionately high prevalence of malignancies, and (3) a high prevalence of epithelial carcinomas.[1,4–6]

In 1951 Ashton and Choyce[10] reviewed nine cases of lacrimal sac carcinoma and reported two of their own, emphasizing the similarities between carcinomas found in the lacrimal sac and corresponding tumors in the nasal and paranasal cavities. They suggested that papillomas, epitheliomas, and carcinomas represent a spectrum of histologic change in the lacrimal epithelium; once an epithelial tumor has arisen, it may progress through a series of stages to become malignant.

In a review of 117 cases of lacrimal sac tumor, Duke Elder[1] found that 26 (22 percent) were pseudotumors and 91 were neoplasms, of which 73 (80 percent) were malignant. The total percentage of neoplasms in the series was 60 percent. Carcinomas were the most common, comprising 33 percent of the entire series.

In a review of 189 cases, Radnot and Gall[4] found 46 (25 percent) pseudotumors. Epithelial carcinomas comprised 69 cases (34 percent) and were three times as frequent as benign epithelial lesions. There were 26 mesenchymal malignancies; these tumors were five times more common than benign mesenchymal tumors. Schenck et al.[6] presented their analysis of 205 lacrimal sac tumors and also found a high prevalence of malignant lesions.

It is possible that benign tumors of the lacrimal sac are not being reported as consistently as malignancies. Benign lesions become more prevalent if granulomas, pseudotumors, and cysts are included in a series. An informal survey of the Wills Eye Hospital oculoplastic staff concerning the lacrimal sac masses treated from 1982 to 1986 showed that granuloma was a common diagnosis (Table 11-1).

Histologically, the lacrimal drainage apparatus is lined with mucosa of various types in different areas of its pathway[11–13] (see Chs. 1 and 10). Tumors that arise in the lacrimal sac or adjacent tissues present a gamut of histopathologic types (Table 11-2). The confined position of the sac behind the anterior lacrimal crest and under several soft-tissue layers makes the clinical diagnosis difficult; diagnosis must be established with biopsy.

Table 11-1. Lacrimal Sac Masses Treated by Wills Eye Hospital Oculoplastic Staff between 1982 and 1986

Diagnosis	No. of Patients
Granuloma	5
Sarcoid	2
Dacryoliths	2
Actinomyces infection	1
Inverted papilloma	1
Squamous cell carcinoma	1
Transitional cell carcinoma	0
Lymphoma	2
Melanoma of the canaliculus	1
Metastatic carcinoma	1

Table 11-2. Primary Lacrimal Sac Tumors
Benign
Mucocele of the sac
Granuloma and pseudotumor
Dacryoliths
Squamous papilloma
Cysts
Diverticula
Polyps
Nevi
Potentially malignant
Transitional cell (inverted) papilloma
Fibrous histiocytoma
Reactive lymphoid hyperplasia
Hemangiopericytoma
Malignant
Epithelial carcinoma
Squamous cell carcinoma
Transitional cell carcinoma
Anaplastic carcinoma
Adenocarcinoma
Malignant melanoma
Mesenchymal tumors
Malignant lymphomas
Undifferentiated sarcoma
Malignant histocytic
Reticulous fibrosarcoma
Metatastic carcinoma

COMMON LACRIMAL SAC TUMORS

Benign Lacrimal Sac Masses

Lacrimal sac granulomas, sarcoid, actinomyces infection, squamous papillomas, polyps, cysts, dacryolyths, neurilemmomas, fibroids, and nevi have been described.[14–18]

Granulomas

Sarcoid and other granulomas occasionally occur in the lacrimal sac area, either involving the sac wall or overlying the sac as an infiltrate. In an informal survey, the Wills Eye Hospital oculoplastic staff ranked granuloma the most common lacrimal sac mass treated during the past 5 years (Fig. 11-1).

Squamous Papillomas

Squamous papillomas appear as cauliflower-like growths with a central fibrovascular stroma. The stratified squamous epithelium is hypertrophic. The epithelium rests on an intact basement membrane; few, if any, mitoses are seen in these cells.

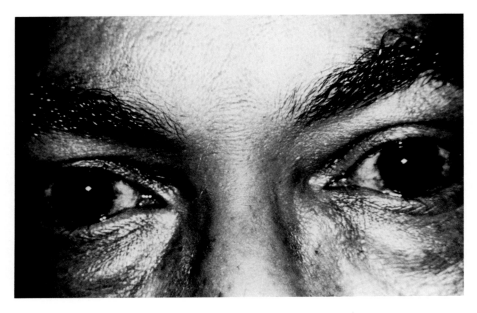

Fig. 11-1   Lacrimal sac granuloma. A painless, firm medial canthal mass of 5 months duration in a 37-year-old man. Biopsy under local anesthesia disclosed a sarcoid granuloma.

Lacrimal Sac Polyps

Lacrimal sac polyps usually arise in chronically inflamed sacs. They are typically small and are often discovered during a routine dacryocystorhinostomy (DCR). These round, smooth masses are attached by a pedicle to the lacrimal sac wall.

The stroma of the polyp is immature fibrovascular tissue, and the epithelium is similar to the sac mucosa. Irritation often results in pseudopolyps—immature connective tissue-like polyps without an epithelium covering.

Actinomyces Infection

Actinomyces, once considered a fungus, is now placed systematically between the bacteria and the fungi. It is a weakly acid-fast staining, quasianaerobic microorganism with a thin, filamentous structure. It produces sulfur granules. It is often part of the normal flora of the tonsils (personal communication, N. Muriani, United Hospitals Medical Center, Newark, NJ).

In the eye, *Actinomyces* may cause a chronic canaliculitis. Clinically this condition may present as a thickening of the canalicular wall or as a chalazion-like swelling adjacent to the canaliculus. These lesions have a soft center of

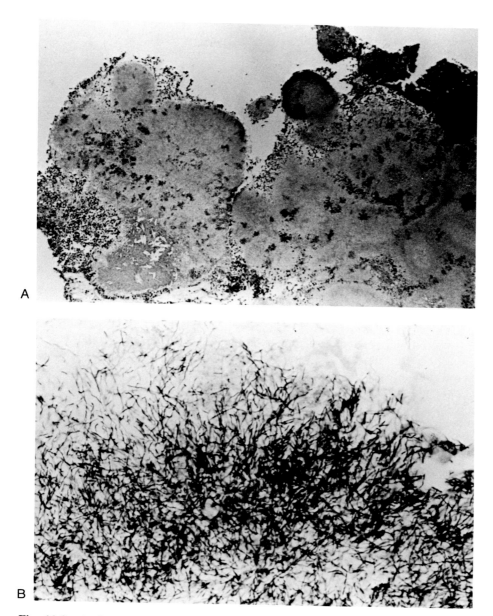

Fig. 11-2 *Actinomyces* infection. Histology of a biopsy specimen from a 73-year-old woman who presented with an indolent swelling of both canaliculi and a pea-sized mass under the medial canthal tendon of the right eye.

green, cheesy material. An *Actinomyces* infection responds slowly to standard antimicrobial therapy, but clears promptly when the concretions are removed surgically. This lesion is included in the discussion of lacrimal sac tumors because it sometimes presents as a firm mass under the medial canthal tendon (Fig. 11-2).

MALIGNANCIES

Transitional Cell (Inverted) Papillomas and Carcinomas

Fibroepithelioma, epithelial papilloma, inverted papilloma, Schneiderian papilloma, and malignant papilloma are synonyms for a group of nasal cavity neoplasms.[19] These papillomas and carcinomas can arise from the lacrimal epithelium. In these tumors the cells lose their pseudostratified cylindrical or cuboidal shape and become fusiform and stratified. Interspersed between this "transitional epithelium" are many large goblet cells, an identifying feature of these tumors. Grossly the tumors appear cauliflower-shaped and have a densely corrugated surface. The thick, multilayered epithelium is thrown into tight folds over a soft, spongy fibrovascular tissue core. These tumors are called *inverted* because the epithelium infolds into the stroma instead of growing exophytically.

Areas of altered and mixed cytology are characteristic of these tumors. Areas of squamous or adenoid metaplasia may lie next to benign-appearing transitional cell segments. Three pathologic types have been recognized by Harry and Ashton:[5] (1) transitional cell papilloma (inverted benign papilloma), (2) intermediate precancerous transitional cell tumor, in which an active cellular pleomorphism and frequent mitotic figures are seen but the basement membrane is intact, and (3) transitional cell carcinoma. In this last type, all features of the tumor are exaggerated. There is more anaplasia and actual tumor invasion through the basement membrane.

Ryan and Font[20] combine the transitional cell epithelioma with squamous cell epithelioma as one type of epithelial neoplasm, seeing little difference in their behavior. Both transitional papillomas and carcinomas behave aggressively, are prone to recurrence after apparently complete excision, and can invade contiguous structures. The literature suggests that they may have a better prognosis in the lacrimal sac and nasal cavity than in the paranasal sinuses.

Epidermoid Squamous Cell Papilloma and Carcinoma

Epidermoid squamous cell papillomas and carcinomas are characteristic primary tumors of the lacrimal sac. The growth of squamous cells is exophytic, into the lumen of the sac. Tumor invades the stroma of the sac and can cause ulceration of the overlying tissue (Figs. 11-3A and 11-4).

These tumors are composed of nonkeratinizing squamous epithelium over-

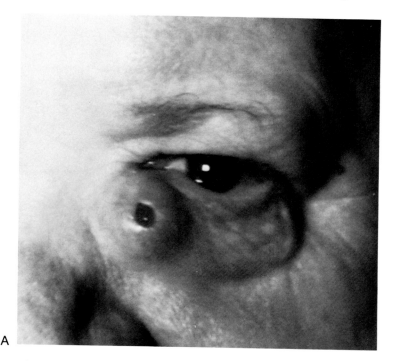

A

Fig. 11-3 Squamous cell carcinoma of the lacrimal sac in a 63-year-old man. **(A)** Clinical presentation of the tumor mass. (*Figure continues*).

lying papillomatous connective tissue. The epithelial cells are large and pale and have a central nucleus and eosinophylic cytoplasm.

Pathologists often diagnose squamous cell epitheliomas and transitional cell (Schneiderian) papillomas and carcinomas as the same entity. Radical surgery with radiation therapy offers the best prognosis.

Hemangiopericytoma

Hemangiopericytoma is a mesenchymal tumor thought to arise from pericytes. It grows slowly within the lacrimal sac stroma and is usually well circumscribed. Most hemangiopericytomas have a low malignancy potential.[21] Although rare, this tumor has been reported as a primary neoplasm of the lacrimal drainage system.

Malignant Melanoma of the Lacrimal Sac

Malignant melanoma is extremely rare in the lacrimal system; only 12 cases have been reported in the world literature.[22] Melanomas may arise primarily in the canaliculi or in the lacrimal sac mucosa. A benign nevus[23] and a metastatic melanoma[18] have also been reported.

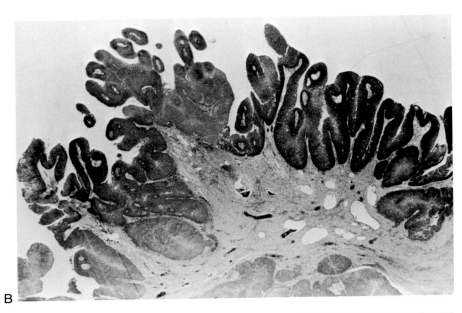

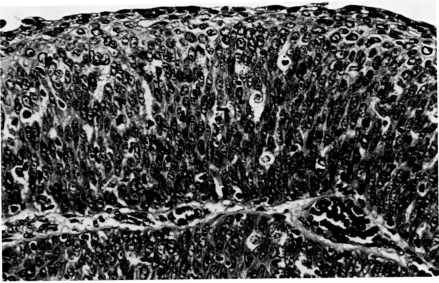

Fig. 11-3 (*Continued*).   (**B, C**) Histology of the tumor shows areas of exophytic and inverted growth patterns. Anaplasia and frequent mitoses are present. (H & E; B × 50, C × 400.)

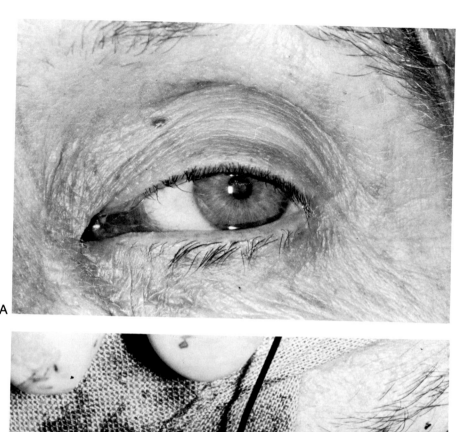

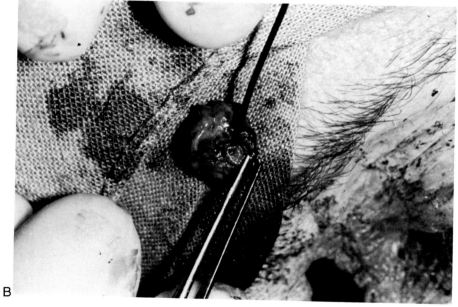

Fig. 11-4 Squamous cell carcinoma of the lacrimal sac. **(A)** Cylindrical mass in left medial canthus; caruncle is erythematous. Bleeding from the puncta has occurred on three occasions. **(B)** Specimen obtained by dacryocystectomy shows the tumor involving the wall of the sac. (*Figure continues.*)

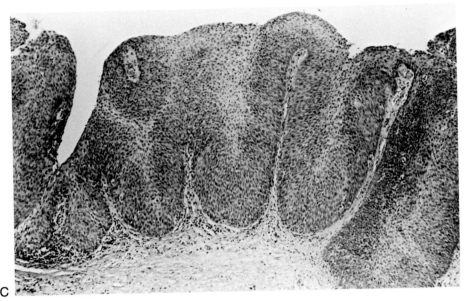

C

Fig. 11-4 (*Continued*). (**C**) Histology shows parakeratosis, acanthosis, and an enormous increase in the numbers of cell layers (H & E; ×200). Patient subsequently had ethmoidectomy, lacrimal bone removal, and medial canthal maxillectomy, and is now tumor free.

How a melanoma arises in the lacrimal sac is unclear. The lacrimal drainage system is derived from downgrowth of embryonic ectoderm, and one author[24] postulates that this tissue harbors melanocyte-like cells that can give rise to a malignant melanoma.

The tumor usually presents as a soft, dark, globular mass protruding into the sac lumen. By the time of diagnosis it has usually invaded the stroma of the lacrimal sac as well. Malignant melanoma is composed of large pleomorphic cells with vesicular nuclei and melanin granules. The symptoms are similar to those of other lacrimal sac tumors. Bleeding from either the puncta or nose is frequent. An important but rare diagnostic sign is a dark discharge from the puncta. The patient may also occasionally report black sputum.[22]

Treatment is wide resection of the tumor and radiation therapy. Wide resection means the removal of the sac, nasolacrimal duct, adjoining bones, nasal mucosa, the portion of the eyelids containing the canaliculi, and the soft tissues of the anteriomedial orbit. If incompletely excised, the tumor tends to recur rapidly.[25]

Lymphoproliferative Disorders and Lymphomas

Lymphomas in the lacrimal sac may cause symptoms of lacrimal obstruction and dacryocystitis,[26] but these lymphoid tumors more commonly present in the medial canthal area, external to the sac (Fig. 11-5A, B). Sometimes they

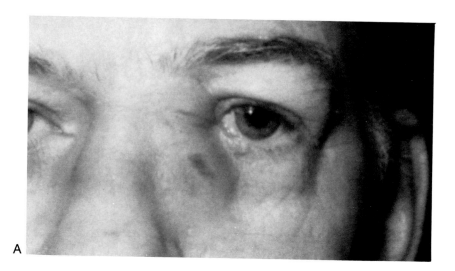

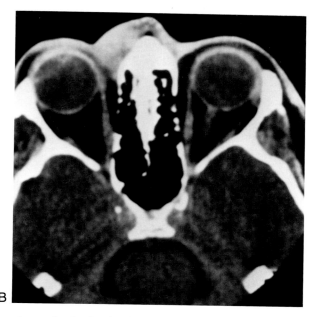

Fig. 11-5 Lymphoma in the lacrimal sac of a 56-year-old man. **(A)** Rapidly growing mass in the left medial canthus, 8 months after DCR for nasolacrimal duct obstruction. **(B)** CT scan shows a lesion in the medial canthus, external to the orbit.

will occur in the medial aspect of the anterior orbit. On CT scan these tumors demonstrate typical "contouring" of the neoplasm around adjacent structures. Lymphomas are friable, have no fibrous stroma, and do not bleed.

Lymphoid tumors are composed of proliferative, immunologically active lymphocytes or their precursors. The pathology can range from a benign lymphoid hyperplasia to frank lymphoblastic sarcoma. Knowles and Jakobiec[27,28] proposed a classification for orbital lymphoid neoplasms based on histopathology and clinical correlation.

Histopathologic and immunocytochemical diagnosis of lymphatic infiltrates is necessary for tumor staging (Ann Arbor Staging System) and for planning therapy.[29–33]

In addition to histocytologic classification, the clinical staging of lymphoma is an important factor in planning treatment. An oncologist should coordinate the patient's tumor workup and therapy, even if the lymphoma appears to originate primarily in the lacrimal sac. Surgery is performed to obtain a tissue diagnosis and debulk the tumor, but is not definitive therapy. Radiation is employed for small conjunctival and anterior orbital lesions.[34] A combination of local radiotherapy and chemotherapy has been recommended as definitive treatment. Lymphomas involving the paranasal sinuses are treated with immunological drugs for CNS prophylaxis, because spread of the tumor to the central nervous system is common. Many protocols exist for combination chemotherapy. One of the most recently developed protocols, MACOP-B, comes from Canada and is becoming very popular in the U.S.[35]

Metastatic Malignancies of the Lacrimal Sac

Metastatic malignancies involving the medial canthus and the anterior medial orbit are relatively common, although they seldom involve the lacrimal sac. (Fig. 11-6). The tumor cells do not respect fascia planes and are not circumscribed.

SIGNS AND SYMPTOMS OF LACRIMAL SAC TUMORS AND THE DIAGNOSTIC WORKUP

Epiphora, a firm mass in the lacrimal sac area, and bleeding from the puncta are characteristic signs of lacrimal sac tumors.

Initially, a lacrimal sac neoplasm may mimic an indolent dacryocystitis, with epiphora being the earliest and most constant symptom. However, irrigation will often demonstrate a patent lacrimal pathway. A painless, hard mass (sometimes feeling as hard as bone to palpation) is a cardinal sign, especially if it extends above the medial canthal tendon.[7] Most patients complain of tearing long before a mass appears in the medial canthal region.

Other signs of lacrimal sac tumor are bleeding from the lacrimal puncta, hemoptysis, increased vascularity of the skin overlying the mass, and injection

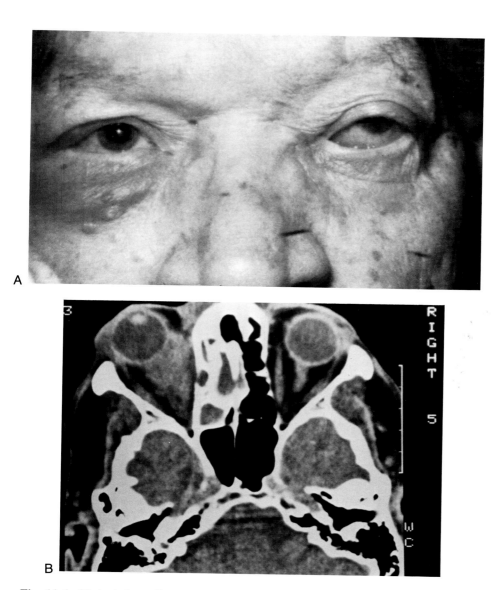

Fig. 11-6 Metastatic malignancy. **(A)** Medial canthal mass of 6 months' duration in a 69-year-old man, associated with upward and lateral displacement of the globe and restriction of motility. **(B)** CT scan shows large infiltrative lesion in the inferomedial orbit.

Table 11-3. Signs and Symptoms of Lacrimal Sac Tumors

Epiphora (especially when the lacrimal passages are patent to irrigation)
Bleeding from the puncta, purulent or black discharge (malignant melanoma)
Epistaxis
Hard mass in the lacrimal sac area
Vascularity of skin and caruncle
Lower eyelid swelling
Displacement of globe
Diplopia and extraocular muscle disturbances (late sign)
Pain (late symptom)

of the tissues in the medial canthus. The globe and ocular motility are usually unaffected. If the tumor has invaded the orbit the globe will be upward and laterally displaced as a result of restriction of motility (Table 11-3).

Tumor Workup

The workup for a suspected lacrimal sac tumor should begin with a thorough medical history of sinus disease, systemic disorders, and malignancy. History of tearing, bleeding from the puncta, nasal obstruction, or epistaxis should be sought. Palpation of the mass should provide information on tumor size and firmness, and on whether it is adhering to the periosteum. Any discharge produced by compressing the sac should be cultured. Pap smears may be prepared and sent for cytology.

Important tests in the tumor workup are the dacryocystogram and the CT scan.[11,12] A normal dacryocystogram will show a wide vertical line of dye, descending in a continuous stream from the medial canthal area to the floor of the nose (see Ch. 2, Fig. 2-7). With a lacrimal sac tumor, the dacryocystogram often reveals a dilated lacrimal sac containing dye in a mottled (honeycombed) pattern (Fig. 11-7). It is helpful to obtain films 15 to 30 minutes later, checking for retention of dye in the sac, and to use a dense formula of water-soluble contrast material, such as Hypaque 76 percent solution. A supine Waters' view is taken. The radiographic image can be magnified ($\times 1.5$) by positioning the head on a 3-inch block of sponge.

Axial and coronal CT scans will delineate the size of the tumor and show bony erosion, nasolacrimal duct enlargement, and extension of the tumor into the surrounding tissues. These scans provide fundamental data for tumor staging and planning of therapy.

If the medial canthal mass is large, readily palpable, and elevates the skin, an incisional biopsy of the sac wall may be performed under local infiltration anesthesia.

TREATMENT

If the tumor is confined within the lacrimal fascia, an "in fascia" dacryocystectomy with frozen section control is performed. The lacrimal sac is removed with the surrounding periorbita. During surgery the sac is opened and

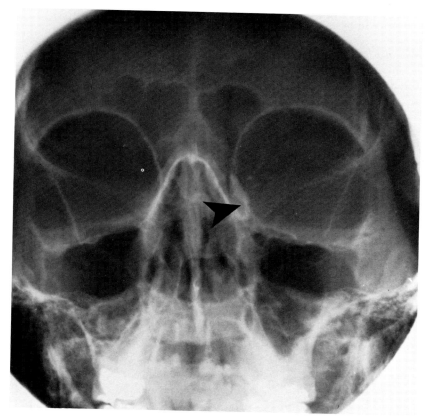

Fig. 11-7 Dacryocystogram with a lacrimal sac mass. The column of dye is curved, with a filling defect in the concavity (arrow).

tumor specimens are taken for frozen section analysis. After dacryocystec-tomy, the margins of the surrounding tissues are also sent for frozen sectioning. If the canaliculi show tumor cells in the plane of transection, the medial one third of each lid is resected. The caruncle and the medial conjunctiva are also removed. The resulting defect is closed by suturing each lid to the stump of the medial canthal tendon. Horizontal tension is relieved by canthotomy and cantholysis.

If the tumor extends into the nasolacrimal duct or is invading the bone of the lacrimal fossa, then the lateral wall of the nose, the anterior ethmoids, the maxillae containing the nasolacrimal duct, and the corresponding nasal mucosa must be widely excised. The tip of the middle turbinate is removed as well. Such extensive surgery usually requires the combined efforts of an ophthal-mologist and otorhinolaryngologist. The Webber-Ferguson incision provides excellent exposure of this entire area and gives an excellent cosmetic result (personal communication, M. T. Brennan, Mercy Catholic Medical Center, Philadelphia, PA).

When a malignant tumor is diagnosed, the patient should be referred to an oncologist for metastatic workup and tumor staging. A radiologist may be consulted for postoperative radiation therapy. In our therapeutic protocol, all malignant lacrimal sac tumors receive postoperative radiation therapy. We also believe that the combination of chemotherapy and radiation improves the survival rate for some tumors, especially the lymphomas. The amount of radiation is determined by the radiologist, in a range of 2,500 to 6,000 rads. Complications of radiation therapy include radiation dermatitis, loss of lashes, atrophy of orbital fat, and cataract.

A combination therapy—surgery/radiation or surgery/radiation/chemotherapy—is employed for many tumors. Cis-platinum, which is used in the treatment of squamous and transitional cell tumors of the paranasal sinuses, may also be used for transitional epidermoid lacrimal sac carcinomas. (personal communication, J. Orsini, University of Medicine and Dentistry of New Jersey, Newark, NJ). Cis-platinum, an alkylating agent, is a chelated complex of platinum.

Dacryocystectomy Technique

An "in fascia" extirpation of the lacrimal sac may be used for tumors limited to the sac.

Anesthesia

Local or general anesthesia may be employed. Adequate local anesthesia can be achieved with regional nerve blocks and subcutaneous infiltration. The infratrochlear nerves are blocked 8 mm above the medial canthal tendon at the superomedial angle of the orbit. The trochlea of the superior oblique muscle is palpated, a blunt, long, 25-gauge needle is then introduced 1.5 cm into the orbit just below the trochlea, and 1 ml of anesthetic solution is injected. The terminal branches of the nasociliary nerve are blocked by injecting another 1 ml of solution 1 cm deep to the upper edge of the medial canthal tendon. The infraorbital nerve is blocked 6 to 8 mm inside the infraorbital foramen. The infraorbital block may also be accomplished by injecting over the infraorbital foramen, followed by massage. Adding Wydase to the anesthetic solution will enhance the effect of local massage. The soft tissues over the incision site are also injected. A one-to-one mixture of bupivacaine 0.5 percent and lidocaine 2 percent containing epinephrine 1:100,000 is a good mixture for anesthesia. The addition of Wydase to these anesthetic agents is helpful.

Nasal Packing

For vasoconstriction and additional anesthesia, the nasal cavity is packed with cottonoid strips moistened in 4 percent cocaine solution. When the patient's health precludes the use of cocaine, oxymetazoline 1 percent nasal solution is used instead. With a bayonet forceps and nasal speculum, three half-inch neurosurgical cottonoid strips are moistened with cocaine and guided up into the middle meatus. One strip is placed along the nasal septum, one against the lateral wall of the nose, and one along the floor, with the lower portion of each strip extending from the nares. A quarter-inch ribbon gauze, also moistened with cocaine or oxymetazoline, is packed tightly into the central space between the cottonoids. The ribbon gauze packing presses the cottonoids against the contours of the nasal passages, improving hemostasis.

Incision

If the angular vein is visible, a marking pen is used to outline it on the skin surface before local anesthetic is injected. The bulge of the tumor mass is also marked on the skin surface. A vertical skin incision is made with a #15 Bard Parker blade, medial to the angular vessels and parallel to the base of the nose (Fig. 11-8). The incision begins 5 mm above the medial canthal tendon

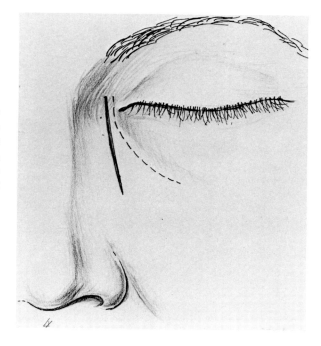

Fig. 11-8 Two commonly employed skin incisions: incision vertical and medial to the angular vessels (solid line), and incision lateral to the vessels and curved along the orbital rim, 3 mm external to the anterior lacrimal crest ridge (dashed line).

and descends for about 25 to 30 mm. The scalpel incises all the tissues down to bone with one controlled cut. Alternatively, a curved incision may be positioned 3 mm outside the orbital rim (Fig. 11-8).

Mobilization of the Lacrimal Sac

Using a Freer elevator, the periosteum is elevated toward the anterior lacrimal crest. The superficial head of the medial canthal tendon is elevated. At the anterior lacrimal crest the periosteum adheres firmly to the ridge and may tear if care is not taken. It may be helpful to elevate the periosteum on the frontal process of the maxillae, below the lacrimal crest, where the orbital rim is rounded. The orbit may be entered easily in this area. Then, with the elevator already inside the orbit, the periosteum is lifted off the lacrimal crest in a retrograde fashion. The lacrimal fossa is exposed back to the posterior lacrimal crest (Fig. 11-9). Dissection beyond the posterior lacrimal crest is not advised because significant bleeding may result, occasionally causing a retro-

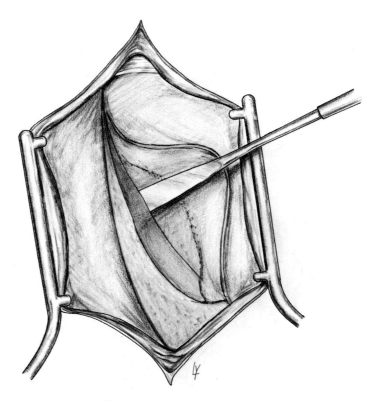

Fig. 11-9 Elevating the periosteum from the anterior lateral crest and lacrimal sac fossa.

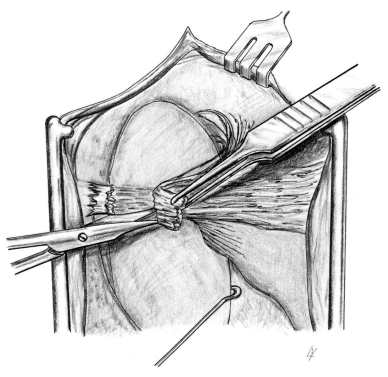

Fig. 11-10 Incising partially the medial canthal tendon (2/3 thickness) to begin a plane of dissection around the lateral sac wall.

bulbar hemorrhage. The medial sac wall is incised, creating an anterior flap. A segment of the tumor including the wall of the sac is excised and sent for frozen section diagnosis. One 4-0 silk mattress suture is used to close the sac. With the medial wall separated from the lacrimal fossa, dissection around the lateral wall of the sac is initiated (Figs. 11-10 and 11-11). In dacryocystectomy for malignancies, a wide resection is required. To expose the lateral wall of the sac, the plane of dissection is carried external to the lacrimal fascia. If the tumor mass distends the sac, then the dissection may be external to the plane of the orbicularis muscle. Under the medial canthal tendon, sharp and blunt dissection are used to develop an artificial plane slightly external to the lacrimal fascia (Fig. 11-10). A Bowman probe is placed in each canaliculus until it is identified in the dissection. It may be helpful to place the tip of a blunt Stevens tenotomy hook along the posterior lacrimal crest, and then twist the hook laterally. This maneuver will delineate the posterior limits of the lacrimal sac. The lacrimal canaliculi are transected midway between the puncta and the sac. An additional 1 to 2 mm of each canaliculus is removed and sent for frozen section analysis to determine if the plane of resection is tumor free. The fundus

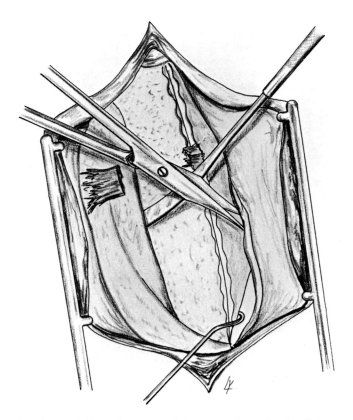

Fig. 11-11 The plane of dissection around the anterolateral wall of the sac is located external to the lacrimal fascia, following the contours of the tumor.

of the sac is dissected free and pulled forward. The plane of dissection is extended inferior to the resected canaliculi, as far as the entrance to the nasolacrimal canal. When the entire lacrimal sac is isolated, it is transected close to the opening of the nasolacrimal duct (Fig. 11-12). Tissue from the nasolacrimal duct mucosa is sent for frozen section analysis, and biopsies of surrounding tissues are similarly submitted. The nasolacrimal duct is curetted thoroughly (Fig. 11-13) and the contents sent for pathologic examination. Hemostasis is achieved with cautery and strips of Gelfoam dipped in thrombin. After the entire tumor has been resected and clean margins have been verified by analysis of frozen sections, the wound is closed. The lateral deep tissues are sutured to the periosteum at the medial edge of the incision with 5-0 Vicryl. The skin and orbicularis muscle are closed with 5-0 or 6-0 nylon interrupted vertical mattress sutures.

If the tumor is not confined to the lacrimal sac, then the help of an otorhinolaryngologist will be needed in order to accomplish a wider resection.

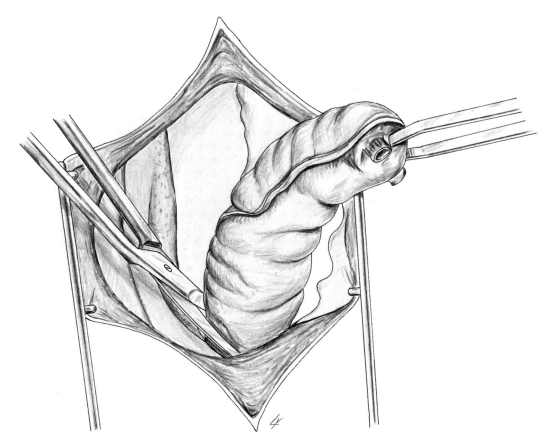

Fig. 11-12   The freed lacrimal sac is transected at the entrance of the bony nasolacrimal canal.

SUMMARY

Malignant lacrimal sac tumors can extend into the maxillary, lacrimal, and ethmoidal bones, involve the orbit, and penetrate the cranium. They also spread through the lymphatic and blood vessels to produce regional and distal metastases; lung metastases are especially common.

Radical surgery combined with other cancer treatment modalities can effect a cure in a good majority of cases of primary malignancy of the lacrimal sac. The prognosis for metastatic tumors is less favorable.

ACKNOWLEDGMENTS

We wish to thank Dr. Ralph C. Eagle, Director of Pathology, Wills Eye Hospital, Philadelphia, PA; Dr. Neena Muriani, Director of Laboratories,

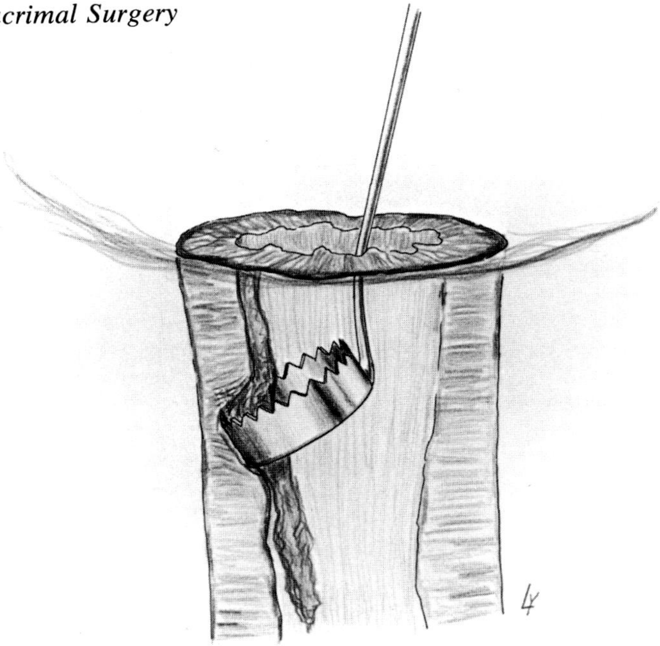

Fig. 11-13 The nasolacrimal duct is curetted thoroughly and the specimen is sent as another frozen section specimen in order to determine if the tumor has extended into the nasolacrimal duct.

United Hospitals Medical Center, Newark, NJ: Dr. Martin T. Brennan, otolaryngologist, Mercy Catholic Medical Center, Philadelphia, PA; Dr. James Orsini, M.D., oncologist, University of Medicine and Dentistry of New Jersey, Newark, NJ: and Dr. Merrill J. Solan, radiation therapist, Lankenau Hospital, Philadelphia, PA for reading and preparing the slides and sharing their knowledge and techniques with us.

Special thanks go to Marie Moore, executive coordinator of our oculoplastic service, Patricia Moore, and Laura Webb for their help in the preparation of the manuscript.

REFERENCES

1. Duke-Elder S: Tumors of the lacrimal passages. pp. 5345–5358. In Duke-Elder S (ed): System of Ophthalmology. Vol. 5. CV Mosby, St. Louis, 1952

2. Milder B, Weil BA: Tumors of the lacrimal excretory system. In Milder B: The Lacrimal System. Appleton-Century-Crofts, Norwalk, CT, 1983

3. Spaeth EB: Carcinomas and tumors of the lacrimal sac. Arch Ophthalmol 57:689, 1952

4. Radnot M, Gall J: Tumoren des traensackes. Ophthalmologica 151:1, 1966. Cited in Schenck NJ, Ogura JH, Pratt LL: Cancer of the lacrimal sac. Presentation of five cases and review of the literature. Ann Otol Rhinol Laryngol 82:153, 1973

5. Harry J, Ashton N: The pathology of tumors of the lacrimal sac. Trans Ophthalmol Soc UK 88:19, 1969

6. Schenck L, Ogura JH, Pratt LL: Cancer of the lacrimal sac. Presentation of five cases and review of the literature. Ann Otol Rhinol Laryngol 82:153, 1973

7. Hornblass A, Jakobiec FA, Bosniak S, et al: The diagnosis and management of epithelial tumors of the lacrimal sac. Ophthalmology 87:476, 1980

8. Milder B, Smith ME: Notes, cases, instruments. Carcinoma of lacrimal sac. Am J Ophthalmol 65:782, 1968

9. Stokes DP, Flanagan JC: Dacryocystectomy for tumors of the lacrimal sac. Ophthalmic Surg 8:85, 1977

10. Ashton N, Choyce DP, Fison LG: Carcinoma of the lacrimal sac. Br J Ophthalmol 35:366, 1951

11. Russell EJ, Czervionke L, Huckman M, et al: CT of the inferomedial orbit and the lacrimal drainage apparatus. Normal and pathologic anatomy. Am J Radiol 145:1147, 1985

12. Spira R, Mondshine R: Demonstration of nasolacrimal duct carcinoma by computed tomography. Ophthalmic Plast Reconstr Surg 2:159, 1986

13. Whitnall ES: The Anatomy of the Human Orbit. Oxford University Press, London, 1932

14. Nolan J: Granuloma of lacrimal sac: Simulating a neoplasm. Am J Ophthalmol 62:756, 1966

15. Bouzas A: Polyps of the lacrymal sac. Arch Ophthalmol 66:236, 1961

16. Karcioglu ZA, Caldwell DR, Reed HT: Papillomas of lacrimal drainage system: A clinicopathologic study. Ophthalmic Surg 15:670, 1984

17. Hornblass A, Gabry JB: Diagnosis and treatment of lacrimal sac cysts. Ophthalmology 86:1655, 1980

18. Eitrem E: Innocent, pigmented nevus-cell tumor (melanoma) of the lacrimal sac. Acta Ophthalmologica 31:283, 1953

19. Verner FL, et al: Epithelial papillomas of the nasal cavities and sinuses. Ann Otolaryngol 70:574, 1959

20. Ryan SJ, Font RL: Primary epithelial neoplasms of the lacrimal sac. Am J Ophthalmol 76:73, 1973

21. Gurney N, Chalkley T, O'Grady R: Lacrimal sac hemangiopericytoma. Am J Ophthalmol 71:757, 1971

22. Yamade S, Kitagawa A: Malignant melanoma of the lacrimal sac. Ophthalmologia (Basel) 177:30, 1978

23. Economides NG, Page RC: Metastatic melanoma of the lacrimal sac. Ann Plast Surg 15:244, 1985

24. Duguid IM: Malignant melanoma of the lacrimal sac. Br J Ophthalmol 48:394, 1964

25. Farkas TG, Lamberson RE: Malignant melanoma of the lacrimal sac. Am J Ophthalmol 66:45, 1968

26. Benger RS, Frue BR: Lacrimal drainage obstruction from lacrimal sac infiltration by lymphocytic neoplasia. Am J Ophthalmol 101:242, 1986

27. Knowles DM, Jakobiec FA: Orbital lymphoid neoplasms: A clinicopathologic study of 60 patients. Cancer 46:576, 1980

28. Knowles II DM, Jakobiec FA, Halper JP: Immunologic characterization of ocular adnexal lymphoid neoplasms. Am J Ophthalmol 87:603, 1979

29. Bennett CL, Putterman A, Bitran JD, Recant W: Staging and therapy of orbital lymphomas. Cancer 57:1204, 1986

30. Rappaport H: Tumors of the hematopoietic system. In: Atlas of Tumor Pathology, Washington DC, Armed Forces Institute of Pathology, 1966
31. Lukes RJ, Taylor CR, Chir B et al: A morphologic and immunologic surface marker study of 299 cases of non-Hodgkin lymphomas and related leukemias. Am J Pathol 90:461, 1978
32. Rosenberg SA et al: National Cancer Institute sponsored study of classification of non-Hodgkin's lymphomas. Summary and description of a working formulation for clinical usage. Cancer 49:2112, 1982
33. Ellis JH, Banks PM, Campbell RJ, et al: Lymphoid tumors of the ocular adnexa: Clinical correlation with the working formulation classification and immunoperoxidase staining of paraffin sections. Ophthalmology 92:1311, 1985
34. Jereb B, et al: Radiation therapy of conjunctival and orbital lymphoid tumors. J Radiat Oncol Biol Phys 10:1013, 1984
35. Klimo P, Connors JM: MACOP-B chemotherapy for the treatment of diffuse large-cell lymphoma. Ann Intern Med 102:596, 1985

12 | Lacrimal Gland Fossa Masses

Don S. Ellis
Peter S. Levin
William B. Stewart

The spectrum of inflammatory and neoplastic lesions involving the lacrimal gland is broad and includes malignant neoplasms of epithelial origin. The significant incidence of these malignant tumors, combined with their very aggressive nature and dismal prognosis, mandate that all masses in the region of the lacrimal gland be considered potentially malignant until proven otherwise. If the devastating course of these tumors is to be altered, early diagnosis and prompt treatment is essential. It is also important to diagnose benign mixed tumors since if managed appropriately, patients with this condition can usually be cured of their disease.

The need for early incisional biopsy in the diagnosis of malignant neoplasms must be tempered by the potential complications that may follow inappropriate incisional biopsy of a benign mixed tumor. This dilemma highlights the need for prompt and accurate clinical diagnosis of lacrimal gland lesions to determine optimal management.

The management of lacrimal gland masses is further complicated by the complex regional anatomy. The gland is intimately associated with the conjunctival cul-de-sac, levator aponeurosis, lateral rectus muscle, lateral and superior orbital bones, and the globe. Neoplastic extension can involve these structures as well as contiguous periorbital tissues.

The lacrimal gland is considered a minor salivary gland. The understanding and classification of benign and malignant epithelial tumors of the lacrimal gland has been greatly aided by the analogy that has been drawn with the histologic classification of major salivary gland lesions.[1] However, the incidence, aggressiveness, and management of tumors of the lacrimal gland can differ from those of salivary gland tumors.

CLINICAL PRESENTATION

Many lesions of the lacrimal gland fossa have a classical clinical presentation;[2] however, it must be remembered that there are exceptions to the rules and characteristic findings. The duration of symptoms, the presence or absence of pain, and the findings on orbital imaging studies, such as computer tomography (CT), are probably the most important features for distinguishing inflammatory from neoplastic processes and benign from malignant tumors (Table 12-1).

Clinical signs of a lacrimal gland fossa mass include upper lid lateral fullness, ptosis, and an S-shaped contour of the upper lid. Globe displacement or motility disturbance may be present. The presence of inflammatory signs such as swelling, erythema, and discharge must also be considered (Fig. 12-1). Systemic findings may also contribute to the clinical diagnosis.

The differential diagnosis of lacrimal gland fossa lesions is varied. Acute dacryoadenitis sets in rapidly, over days to a few weeks, and is often painful,

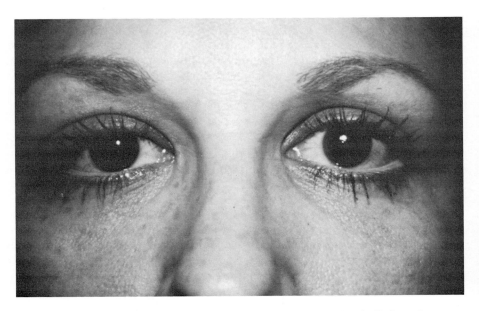

Fig. 12-1 Patient with superotemporal fullness, ptosis, and classic S-shaped curve to right upper eyelid characteristic of a lacrimal gland fossa mass.

Table 12-1. Guidelines To Management of Lacrimal Gland Fossa Masses

Etiology	Symptoms	Duration	CT Findings	Treatment
Inflammatory/infectious	Pain, swelling, erythema, discharge	Usually acute, but several conditions are chronic	Diffuse gland involvement, conforming to bone without lytic or pressure changes	Medical treatment; incisional biopsy[a] if diagnosis not secure or signs not regressing
Lymphomatous (ranging from idiopathic pseudotumor to malignant lymphoma)	Variable	Variable	Diffuse gland involvement, conforming to soft tissue and usually without bony changes	Medical treatment may include x-ray therapy or chemotherapy. Incisional biopsy[b] to confirm diagnosis
Benign mixed tumor	Lid fullness or droop, globe displacement; pain usually absent	Usually >12 months	Rounded globular mass with sharp borders. May cause bony pressure changes and displacement of orbital structures	En bloc excision[c] of entire lacrimal gland without preliminary incisional biopsy
Malignant epithelial tumors	Usually painful	Usually <12 months	Rounded globular mass with indistinct borders. Usually causes bony destructive changes and displacement of orbital structures	Incisional biopsy[a] followed by radical excision, including biopsy tract, involved bone and orbital soft tissues

[a] Incisional biopsy done via transcutaneous transseptal approach.
[b] Incisional biopsy done via transcutaneous transseptal approach or transconjunctival route.
[c] En bloc excisional biopsy done via lateral orbitotomy.

with periorbital swelling and erythema. It tends to be unilateral and to occur in younger patients, but may occur at any age. Proptosis, inferior displacement of the globe, and motility disturbances may be seen. There may be associated conjunctival chemosis and discharge. Preauricular adenopathy may be present. Systemic findings such as pyrexia, malaise, and abnormal blood studies may be present.[2] Ocular inflammation, localized lid infections, and preseptal and orbital cellulitis must be considered in the differential diagnosis. Computed tomography (CT) will show diffuse lacrimal gland enlargement with contouring to orbital structures without bony changes. A well-defined mass in the gland is usually absent. Chronic dacryoadenitis may follow acute dacryoadenitis and will show similar findings.

Many infectious and noninfectious inflammatory processes can affect the lacrimal gland; it has been said that inflammatory lesions are at least five times as common as epithelial tumors.[3] These processes include viral, bacterial, and fungal infections; Sjögren's syndrome; lymphomatous lesions; and granulomatous inflammation such as sarcoidosis. The histologic spectrum of lymphomatous lesions ranges from idiopathic inflammatory pseudotumor to malignant lymphoma.

Lacrimal gland inflammation may also be secondary to systemic diseases such as infectious mononucleosis, mumps, or herpes zoster. These forms of infection should be readily recognizable by the associated systemic abnormalities. Infection, sarcoidosis, or Graves' disease may result in chronic lacrimal gland inflammation.[4]

Patients with Sjögren's syndrome may demonstrate lacrimal gland enlargement. Systemic findings of connective tissue disease may be present, or the abnormality may be limited to the exocrine glands with resultant dry eye and dry mouth. Sjögren's syndrome tends to be bilateral in middle-aged women. Acute inflammatory signs are absent, although symptoms of ocular irritation from dry eye are common. Orbital imaging may show diffuse lacrimal gland enlargement without bony changes. Benign lymphoepithelial lesion, a distinct entity, is characterized by diffuse infiltration of the lacrimal and salivary glands by lymphocytes, with some reactive and proliferative changes. It is not associated with dry eye or systemic disease.

Sarcoidosis may cause painless subacute, or chronic lacrimal gland enlargement. These lesions are extremely firm on palpation and may be quite bulky. Sarcoidosis may involve the lacrimal gland bilaterally, but it is often asymmetric. Sarcoid granulomas tend to localize within the lacrimal gland rather than in other orbital soft tissues, although other signs of orbital, ocular, or systemic disease may be present. "Sarcoid-like" lesions can occur in leprosy, syphilis, lymphogranuloma venereum, other infectious conditions without evidence of systemic involvement, and in idiopathic orbital pseudotumor.[5]

Lymphomatous lesions of the lacrimal gland range from idiopathic inflammatory pseudotumor to malignant lymphoma, and vary widely in clinical presentation. Acquired immunodeficiency syndrome-related lymphomatous lesions may also present as a lacrimal gland fossa mass. Inflammatory pseudotumor often presents with findings of acute dacryoadenitis, whereas true lym-

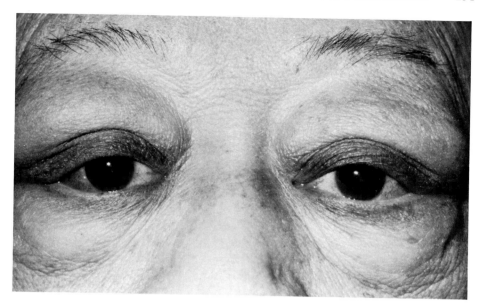

Fig. 12-2 Patient with bilateral lymphomatous lesions of the lacrimal gland. Note the marked upper eyelid fullness and proptosis.

phomas appear as a progressively enlarging orbital mass without associated pain or inflammatory signs (Fig. 12-2). The spectrum of lymphomatous lesions typically shows a diffuse enlargement of the lacrimal gland with contouring to adjacent tissue planes and without bony change (Fig. 12-3),[6] although bony disruption has been reported.[7] Systemic abnormalities may be present initially or may develop subsequently.

The vast majority of neoplasms of the lacrimal gland are of epithelial origin. The benign mixed tumor represents approximately one half of these epithelial neoplasms. Patients with this tumor generally give a history of lacrimal gland enlargement lasting more than 12 months; pain is unusual.[2] Fullness, droop, or deformity of the lid may be the presenting complaint. The mean age on presentation is 39 years with a range of 7 to 77 years.[3] Orbital imaging techniques typically show a rounded or globular soft tissue mass (Fig. 12-4).[6] Enlargement of the osseous lacrimal gland fossa may result from the pressure of slow tumor growth.

It is widely accepted that the benign mixed tumor has the potential for malignant change and that this degeneration may take place over a 20- or 30-year period.[3] Thus, a patient with a long-standing mass (over 12 months) that suddenly alters, for example by an increase in size or the onset of pain, should be suspected of harboring a malignancy in a benign mixed tumor. Seeding of an incision after biopsy or incomplete excision may lead to recurrence of a benign mixed tumor. These recurrences may be associated with subsequent

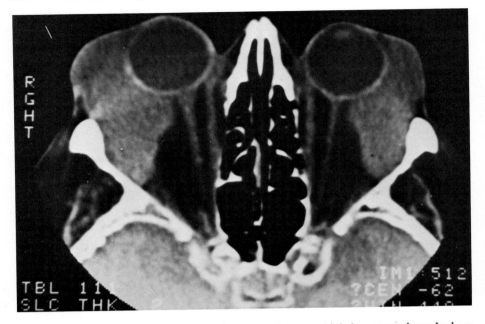

Fig. 12-3 CT scan of extensive lymphomatous lesion which has caused marked exophthalmos without bony changes or deformation of the globe.

malignant transformation and display aggressive behavior with infiltration of adjacent soft tissues and bone.[3]

Patients with malignant epithelial tumors of the lacrimal gland classically present with symptoms of short duration—usually less than 12 months.[2,8] Pain is present in most patients and is thought to be caused by perineural, periosteal, or bony invasion. The age of patients with epithelial malignancies has a wide range but the incidence tends to be higher in children, adolescents, and the elderly. Benign mixed tumors tend to be seen more commonly in "middle age." CT of benign mixed tumors shows a globular mass that may displace orbital structures and indent the sclera (Fig. 12-5). Radiologic evidence of bony pressure erosion or destructive change is seen in the majority of tumors; however, the bone may be normal, particularly in lesions of short duration. Clinical evaluation may reveal signs of cavernous sinus involvement and/or perineural extension beyond the apparent radiologic extent of the tumor.[8,9] Calcium may be present within the malignant tumor, although this can also be seen in benign lesions.[10] Statistically, adenoid cystic carcinoma is the most common lacrimal gland malignancy, followed by malignant mixed tumor and then adenocarcinoma. These tumors can be further classified by histologic subtype.[3] In the series reported by Wright,[8] 7 of 24 patients who underwent excision of a localized malignancy of the lacrimal gland have survived free of tumor for 5 years or more; these results are encouraging, although longer follow-up is needed. It has been suggested that 15 years must elapse before the final outcome can

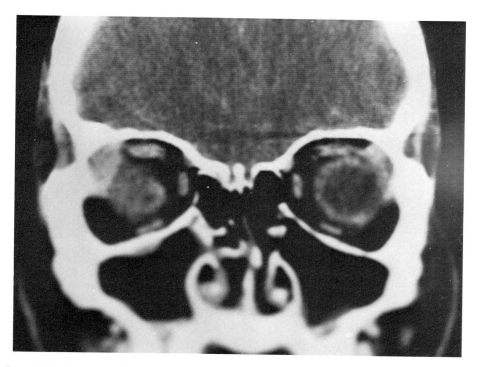

Fig. 12-4 Coronal reformatted CT image of a lacrimal gland epithelial neoplasm shows a globular mass with bony pressure erosion.

be determined in patients with lacrimal gland malignancies.[11] It is generally agreed that despite aggressive treatment, the prognosis is dismal for all epithelial malignancies.[2,8,12,13] Rare lesions of the lacrimal gland fossa include cavernous hemangioma,[14] eosinophilic granuloma, cholesterol granuloma, oncocytoma, monomorphic adenoma, schwannoma, neurofibroma, mucoepidermoid carcinoma, squamous cell carcinoma, and metastatic carcinoma.[3]

Dermoid cysts (ectodermal inclusion cysts) usually present in childhood as a smooth, nontender palpable mass at the superolateral orbital rim. Usually, these lesions are easily distinguished from lesions of the lacrimal gland. Radiologic evaluation may reveal a localized indentation of the bony orbital rim or a deeper orbital involvement.

Childhood malignancy may present as an orbital mass, often in association with local inflammatory signs. Granulocytic sarcoma, a tumor which is often misdiagnosed on initial histopathologic evaluation, may arise during an acute leukemic process or precede the development of leukemia.[15] Orbital metastases of neuroblastoma have a propensity for the zygomatic bone and are bilateral in 50 percent of patients; most of whom have advanced systemic disease or a palpable abdominal mass. The most common childhood orbital malignancy is

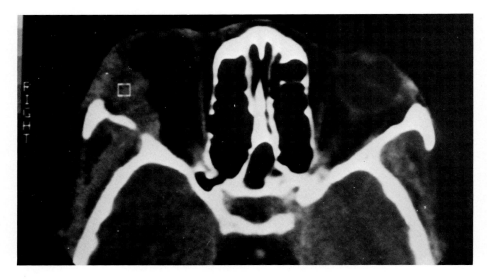

Fig. 12-5 CT image of a patient with a lacrimal gland epithelial neoplasm demonstrates a globular mass which deforms the globe and has caused proptosis. There is adjacent bony destruction.

rhabdomyosarcoma. It may appear as a drooping of the upper lid or an upper lid mass, although involvement of the superotemporal orbit is rare.

MANAGEMENT

The key to management of lacrimal gland lesions is a prompt clinical diagnosis based on all the available information. The clinical diagnosis guides decisions on whether and how to biopsy or resect lacrimal gland fossa masses (Table 12-1). A management protocol based on duration of symptoms and radiographic findings was proposed by Wright, Stewart, and Krohel in 1979[2] and has subsequently been augmented by others.[4,6,16] The goal is to make a prompt histopathologic diagnosis of malignant lesions for early treatment, while avoiding the inappropriate incisional biopsy of benign mixed tumors.

It is important to recognize the clinical picture of benign mixed tumor. Incisional biopsy of a benign mixed tumor is contraindicated because it increases the potential for orbital seeding, recurrence, and subsequent malignant transformation. The treatment of choice for a benign mixed lacrimal gland tumor is complete excision of the tumor en bloc with the entire lacrimal gland through a lateral orbitotomy. Excision will be incomplete if tumor extending beyond the pseudocapsule is not excised or if the disease is multifocal and the entire lacrimal gland is not excised.

Lateral orbitotomy may be accomplished in standard fashion (Fig. 12-6).[16,17] The superior bone cut on the orbital rim is made as high as possible in

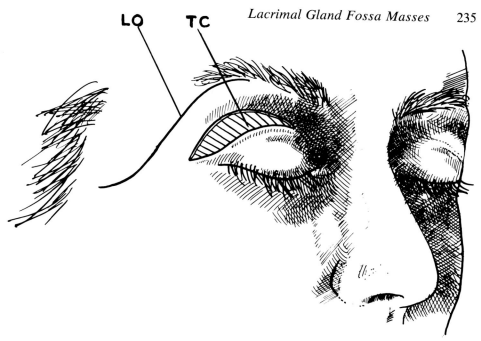

Fig. 12-6 Incision sites for standard lateral orbitotomy (LO) and transcutaneous transseptal biopsy (TC). The lateral orbitotomy incision is placed along the illustrated line. Its length may vary depending on the situation. The zone for transcutaneous, transseptal biopsy is depicted. The incision may be placed in the upper eyelid skin crease or directly overlying the mass.

order to maximize the superior aspect of the osteotomy and enhance exposure of the lacrimal gland and tumor mass. In selected patients, improved cosmesis may be obtained by using a bicoronal scalp flap to gain access to the lateral orbit and then proceeding in standard fashion[18] (Fig. 12-7). This approach allows greater superior and posterior exposure, which may be helpful. When diagnosis is uncertain and malignant lesions are strongly suspected, this approach should be avoided since seeding of the incisions may be anticipated.

Lesions suspected of malignancy should undergo prompt transcutaneous, transseptal incisional biopsy to obtain early histologic diagnosis (Fig. 12-6). This route is selected in order to preserve intact the periorbita and its theoretical barrier to disease spread.

The role of needle biopsy in the management of lacrimal gland fossa masses is still unclear,[19] although it has been useful in the management of salivery gland tumors. In cases likely to be benign mixed tumors, the procedure is contraindicated. Needle biopsy may allow the physician to distinguish lymphomatous from epithelial lesions, but may not accurately place a lesion in the lymphomatous spectrum. Because of the possibility of coexisting benign and malignant epithelial lacrimal gland tumors, a needle biopsy may not be as definitive as a large incisional or excisional biopsy.

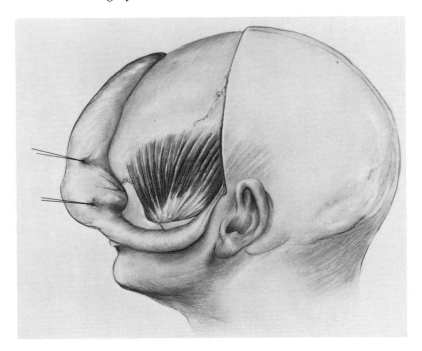

Fig. 12-7   Coronal scalp flap for approach to lateral orbitotomy.

Histologically confirmed malignant lesions that are confined to the orbit should undergo complete en bloc excision, including involved contiguous soft tissue and bone. There is controversy over the optimal surgical approach and extent of excision. Henderson has suggested that the optimal treatment for malignant lesions is en bloc excision of the lesion and surrounding bone through an anterolateral orbitotomy without preliminary biopsy.[11] Although the prognosis is generally poor despite extensive surgical resection, Wright has reported seven patients in whom excision of malignant tumors confined to the orbit has resulted in survival without tumor recurrence after 5 years (two patients received postoperative radiotherapy).[8] The extent of surgery for lacrimal gland malignancies in Wright's series ranged from total excision of the lacrimal gland with tumor capsule intact, in a patient clinically suspected of benign mixed cell tumor, to orbital exenteration with excision of the orbital roof and lateral wall. Others have recommended a radical resection involving the multidisciplinary team of ophthalmic surgeon, neurosurgeon, and plastic surgeon.[9,12,20,21] Marsh suggests an initial craniotomy to explore the anterior and middle cranial fossa in order to confirm resectability (with frozen section evaluation of orbital cranial nerves), followed by en bloc resection including the superolateral bony orbit, entire orbital contents, and eyelids. The surgical resection is followed by postoperative radiotherapy.[21] Currently there is no large series available with adequate data defining preoperative extent of lesions and including sufficient follow-up to provide guidelines on the proper surgical management of malignant lacrimal gland tumors. Long-term survival, however, is clearly the exception in patients with malignant epithelial lacrimal gland neoplasms.

The value of postoperative radiation is under debate. It has been advocated as adjunctive therapy in the immediate postoperative period[8,21] but has also been implicated as a cause of tumor recurrence.[13] Radiation therapy may be used as palliative treatment in certain patients with metastatic disease, patients with extension outside the orbit, or those who are unwilling to undergo extensive disfiguring surgery. The prognosis for these patients is very poor. Radiation therapy may also be useful in the treatment of local recurrences. There is general consensus that chemotherapy is of little benefit in the management of these lesions, although it has been used as an adjunct to surgery and radiation therapy.

Lesions suspected of being inflammatory or lymphomatous should also undergo transcutaneous transseptal incisional biopsy (Fig. 12-6) if they do not respond rapidly to medical management with a decrease in inflammatory signs and mass size. Occasionally, a lacrimal gland mass will appear in the superior cul-de-sac, allowing a transconjunctival approach to biopsy. Incisional biopsy will usually secure an accurate histologic diagnosis and allow the initiation of appropriate local therapy, or guide further evaluation and management. Many patients with lymphomatous lesions will respond, often dramatically, to radiation therapy (Fig. 12-8). Patients with lymphomatous lesions of the lacrimal gland must be both evaluated for the presence of lymphoma or other systemic disease and followed for the subsequent development of systemic disease.

Only patients with a short history (3 weeks or less), associated inflammatory signs, and benign findings on imaging studies may safely be observed for a short period with medical treatment. Patients with infectious signs should receive a course of oral antibiotics, and those who have findings consistent with inflammatory pseudotumor and develop visual loss, intractable pain, or diplopia should receive a short course of oral corticosteroids. Corticosteroids should be used only when the diagnosis is secure without biopsy and not as a diagnostic clinical trial, since the results may be misleading in certain malignant lesions. Incisional biopsy should be performed on presumed inflammatory lesions that do not show progress toward resolution.

These guidelines provide an approach to lacrimal gland fossa masses, based initially on clinical history, examination, and radiologic findings. A prompt, accurate clinical diagnosis will guide the physician toward proper initial medical or surgical management for most patients, although some will be atypical. Management is then determined by a histologic diagnosis.

ACKNOWLEDGMENT

Supported in part by a grant from the Pacific Vision Foundation, San Francisco.

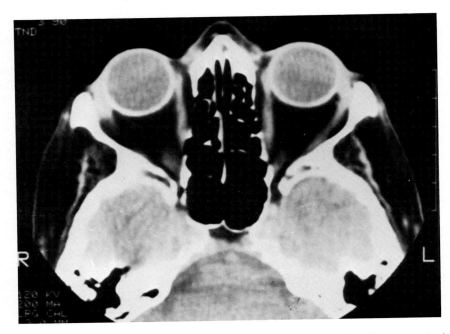

Fig. 12-8 CT scan of the patient in Fig. 12-3, with bilateral lymphomatous lesion, demonstrates marked response to radiotherapy to the orbit.

REFERENCES

1. Forrest AW: Epithelial lacrimal gland tumors: Pathology as a guide to prognosis. Trans Am Acad Ophthalmol Otolaryngol 58:848, 1954
2. Stewart WB, Krohel GB, Wright JE: Lacrimal gland and fossa lesions: An approach to diagnosis and management. Ophthalmology 86:886, 1979
3. Jakobiec FA, Font RL: Lacrimal gland tumors. p. 2496. In Spencer WG (ed): Ophthalmic Pathology. An Atlas and Textbook. Vol 3. WB Saunders, Philadelphia, 1986
4. Hurwitz JJ: A practical approach to the management of lacrimal gland lesions. Ophthalmic Surg 13:829, 1982
5. Jones IS, Jakobiec FA: Diseases of the Orbit. Harper & Row, Hagerstown, MD, 1979, p. 227
6. Jakobiec FA, Yeo JH, Trokel SL, et al. Combined clinical and computed tomographic diagnosis of primary lacrimal fossa lesions. Am J Ophthalmol 94:785, 1982
7. Harris GJ, Dixon TA, Haughton VM: Expansion of the lacrimal gland fossa by a lymphoid tumor. Am J Ophthalmol 96:546, 1983
8. Wright JE: Factors affecting the survival of patients with lacrimal gland tumors. Can J Ophthalmol 17:3, 1982
9. Janecka I, Housepian E, Trokel S, et al. Surgical management of malignant tumors of the lacrimal gland. Am J Surg 148:539, 1984
10. Portis JM, Krohel GB, Stewart WB: Calcifications in lesions of the fossa of the lacrimal gland. Ophthalmic Plast Reconstr Surg 1:137, 1985

11. Henderson JW, Farrow GM: Primary malignant mixed tumors of the lacrimal gland. Report of 10 cases. Ophthalmology 87:466, 1980
12. Jakobiec FA, Henderson JW, Farrow GM: Discussion of primary malignant mixed tumors of the lacrimal gland. Ophthalmology 87:473, 1980
13. Perzin KH, Jakobiec FA, Livolsi VA, Desjardins L: Lacrimal gland malignant mixed tumors (carcinomas arising in benign mixed tumors). Cancer 45:2593, 1980
14. Seiff SR, McFarland JE, Shorr N, Simons KB: Cavernous hemangioma of the lacrimal fossa. Ophthalmic Plast Reconstr Surg 2:21, 1986
15. Davis JL, Parke DW, Font RL: Granulocytic sarcoma of the orbit. Ophthalmology 92:1758, 1985
16. Krohel GB, Stewart WB, Chavis RM: Orbital Disease: A Practical Approach. Grune & Stratton, New York, 1981, p. 129
17. Wright JE: Surgical exploration of the orbit. p. 312. In Stewart WB (ed): Ophthalmic Plastic and Reconstructive Surgery. American Academy of Ophthalmology, San Francisco, 1984
18. Stewart WB, Levin PS, Toth BA: Orbital surgery: the coronal scalp flap approach to the lateral orbitotomy. Arch Ophthalmol. In press
19. Alper MG: Fine needle aspiration biopsy of the lacrimal gland. In Bosniak SL (ed): Advances in Ophthalmic Plastic and Reconstructive Surgery. Vol. 3. Pergamon Press, Elmsford, New York, 1984
20. Jones IS: Surgical considerations in the management of lacrimal gland tumors. Clin Plast Surg 5:561, 1978
21. Marsh JL, Wise DM, Smith M, Schwartz H: Lacrimal gland adenoid cystic carcinoma: intracranial and extracranial en bloc resection. Plast Reconstr Surg 68:577, 1981

13 | Trauma of the Lacrimal Drainage System

Michael J. Hawes
Richard K. Dortzbach

CANALICULAR LACERATIONS

Diagnosis

Suspicion is a key element in diagnosis of canalicular injury. Until proven otherwise, all lacerations in the medial eyelid and medial canthal area should be presumed to involve the lacrimal drainage system. The distal canaliculus is located very superficially along the lid margin; even trivial injuries within 6 mm medial of the punctum can lacerate the canaliculus. The severity of the injury can vary greatly (Figs. 13-1 to 13-5). Passage of a lacrimal probe through the punctum will confirm canalicular involvement when the probe emerges from the lacerated end of the canaliculus (Fig. 13-6).

Dog bites, fist fights, fingernail scratches, and falls are among the more common causes of injury to the canaliculi,[1] and children and young adults are the most common victims.

Necessity of Repair

There is controversy over the need to repair isolated upper (especially) or lower canalicular lacerations. A single patent canaliculus is said to be adequate to drain tears in most patients.[2] Iatrogenic injury to the uninjured canaliculus,

241

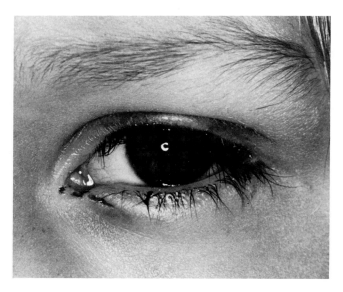

Fig. 13-1 Four-year-old boy who sustained a dog bite injury to the left lower lid with an apparently minor laceration that did involve the inferior canaliculus.

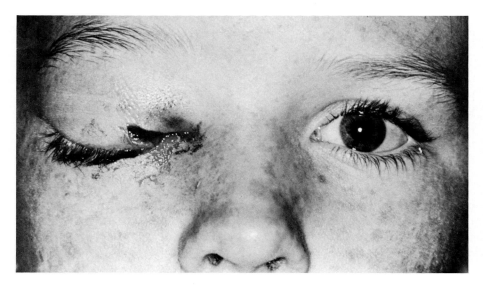

Fig. 13-2 Thirteen-year-old boy who ran into a tree while jogging and lacerated the right superior canaliculus.

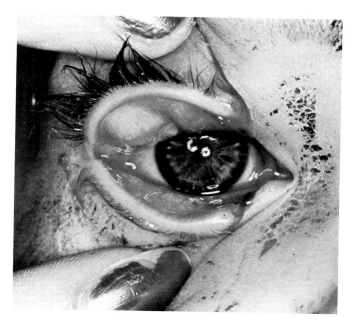

Fig. 13-3 Five-year-old boy with a dog bite injury to the right upper and lower lids involving both canaliculi.

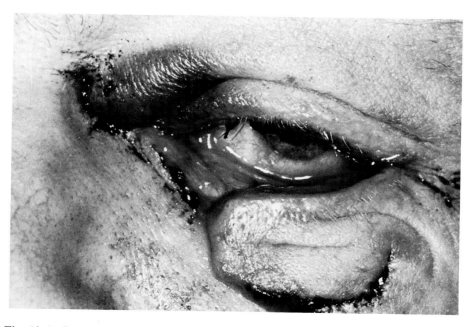

Fig. 13-4 Forty-nine-year-old man who sustained left lower lid and inferior canalicular injury from a skiing accident where ski tip lacerated eyelid.

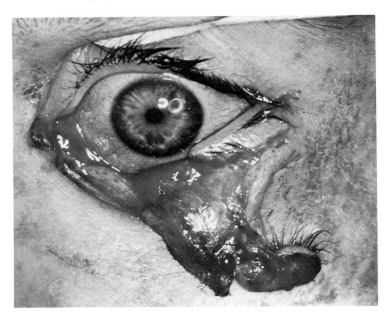

Fig. 13-5   Eight-year-old girl who sustained dog bite injury with inferior canalicular laceration and eyelid avulsion.

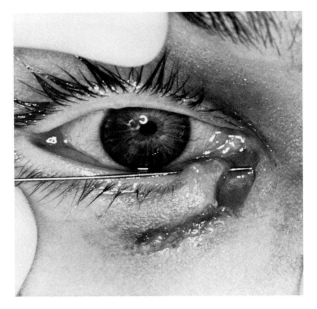

Fig. 13-6   Probe passed through inferior canaliculus emerges from distal end of severed canaliculus. (Hawes MJ, Segrest DR: Effectiveness of bicanalicular silicone intubation in the repair of canalicular lacerations. Ophthalmic Plast Reconstr Surg 1:185, 1985. Raven Press, NY.)

the common internal punctum, or both, is a potential complication of repair. Such injuries are most common when the pigtail probe is used.[3]

In a study of student nurses,[2] Jones showed that transit time of tears through the superior and inferior canaliculi is nearly equal. This study casts some doubt on the commonly held notion that the superior canaliculus is of little consequence in tear drainage.

Most patients sustaining these injuries are young (average age 18 years[1]), and the possibility exists for future injury or disease affecting the uninjured canaliculus. Furthermore, surgeons using proper instrumentation and techniques in repairing lacerated canaliculi have reported a high success rate.[1,4] It is therefore our opinion that repair of recent canalicular lacerations should be attempted by experienced surgeons using appropriate technique. If the surgeon is not familiar with repair of this type of injury, it may be best to avoid manipulation of the lacrimal drainage system, particularly when one canaliculus is intact, and only repair the lid laceration.

Timing of Repair

Trauma often occurs at night or on weekends. Canalicular lacerations need not be repaired immediately. Delay of repair may allow time to obtain an operating team familiar with surgery of this nature. Repair within 24 to 48 hours of injury is preferable; however, surgical correction usually is successful if performed within 5 days of injury.[1,2]

Late repair (weeks to months) is far less likely to be successful because of scarring and consequent difficulty in locating the canaliculus.

Location of Repair

The magnification provided by an operating microscope is very helpful in locating the canaliculus and providing better visualization for suturing it. Sedation, anesthesia, suitable stents, fine sutures, suction, and operating microscopes are most readily available in a hospital or ambulatory surgery facility. Off-hours repair in a minor surgery room, without assistance, is often frustrating and unsuccessful.

Anesthesia

The choice of general or local anesthesia will depend on the age of the patient, the location and extent of injury, the type of stent, and the surgeon's experience. For placement of a bicanalicular stent, general anesthesia is customary in children and anxious adults.

For some patients, a local anesthesia is suitable. A regional nerve block may be obtained by injecting the anesthetic (equal portions of lidocaine 2 per-

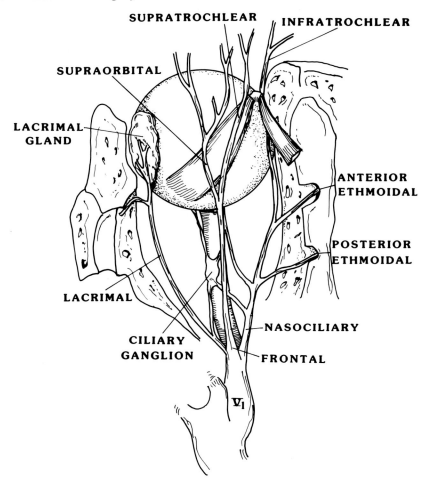

SUPRATROCHLEAR

INFRATROCHLEAR

SUPRAORBITAL

LACRIMAL GLAND

ANTERIOR ETHMOIDAL

POSTERIOR ETHMOIDAL

LACRIMAL

NASOCILIARY

CILIARY GANGLION

FRONTAL

V_1

Fig. 13-7 Branches of nasociliary nerve that supply sensory innervation to medial eyelids, canaliculi, and lacrimal sac.

cent with epinephrine 1:100,000 and bupivicaine 0.75 percent with 150 units added hyaluronidase) above the medial canthal tendon and then passing the needle along the medial wall of the orbit to a point about 20 mm posterior to the tendon. Two to three ml injected in this area will block the anterior ethmoidal and infratrochlear branches of the nasociliary nerve (Figs. 13-7 and 13-8). Excellent anesthesia of the medial canthus is obtained with this injection. A cotton ball containing cocaine 4 percent solution is placed inferiorly in the nasal passage, especially around the inferior turbinate. This provides nasal hemostasis and anesthesia, but some discomfort can still be expected during efforts to retrieve the stent from the nose. Direct injection of the local anesthetic mixture around the inferior turbinate gives more profound anesthesia.

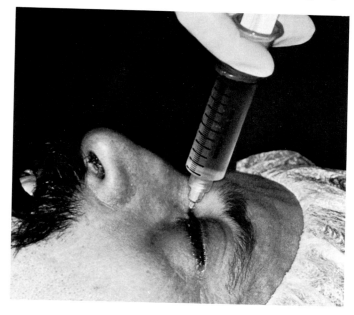

Fig. 13-8   Regional nerve block for repair of medial canthal injuries.

Technique

Finding the Canaliculus

The distal end of the lacerated canaliculus is usually identified by passing a probe through the punctum and noting where the probe emerges from the laceration. Locating the proximal end of the canaliculus is more difficult. Magnification and illumination from an operating microscope are excellent aids; retraction by a skilled assistant is particularly helpful. Cotton applicators, forceps, and gentle suction should be used to explore the area. Probes tend to create false passages that complicate localization of the canaliculus. The cut end of the canaliculus has rolled white edges and a shiny epithelial lining (Fig. 13-9). If the laceration is close to the punctum, the proximal canaliculus will be easier to locate; it will be found near the lid margin. For lacerations close to the lacrimal sac, the surgeon must look deeper for the proximal canaliculus, keeping in mind that the common canaliculus is deep to the medial canthal tendon. A lacrimal probe placed in the intact canaliculus can help the surgeon judge where to seek the common canaliculus. Irrigation of fluorescein, air, sterile milk, or a steroid through the intact canaliculus has been suggested, but we have found this technique neither necessary nor useful. Irrigation with methylene blue is not recommended; it will stain the entire operative field. Use of a pigtail probe is not advised, because of the risk of iatrogenic damage to the intact canaliculus, the common canaliculus, or both.[3] In situations where the

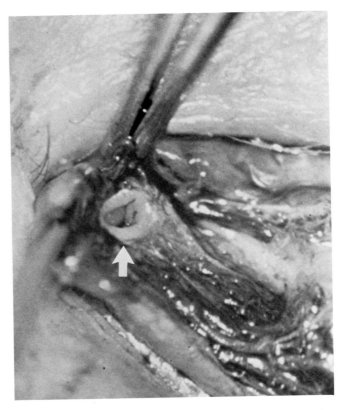

Fig. 13-9   Arrow indicates view of proximal canaliculus through operating microscope. (Hawes MJ, Segrest DR: Effectiveness of bicanalicular silicone intubation in the repair of canalicular lacerations. Ophthalmic Plast Reconstr Surg 1:185, 1985. Raven Press, NY.)

proximal canaliculus is not identifiable, it is wisest to cease the attempt at canalicular repair and try to achieve good closure and alignment of the lid margin.

Stents

Monocanalicular stents minimize the risk of injury to the intact canaliculus, but retention can be a problem.[5] Veirs rods can rust, are subject to loss from suture breakage or erosion through the lid tissues, and are easily displaced. Johnson rods and Beyer rods avoid the breakage problem, but still have bulky ends that can be caught on a finger or garment. A suture (i.e., 0 chromic) or piece of silicone tubing can be used to stent the canaliculus when no more suitable device is available. Monocanalicular silicone stents can be obtained

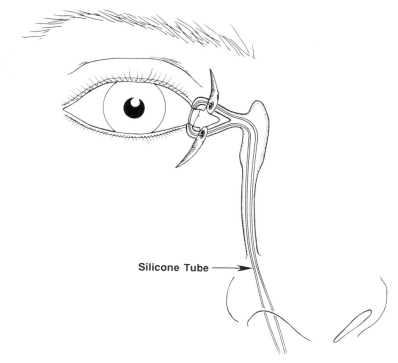

Silicone Tube ⟶

Fig. 13-10 Schematic view of silicone tubing in proper position for repair of canalicular laceration.

(Storz Instrument Company, St. Louis, MO, designed by Dr. Brad Lemke, #SP7 24359), but cause moderate irritation where they rest against the bulbar conjunctiva.

Our preferred stent is silicone tubing passed through both the canaliculi and down the nasolacrimal duct (Fig. 13-10). This type of stent is well tolerated and effective.[1,4,6,7] Silicone is softer than polyethylene tubing;[8] the smooth surface of the silicone tube allows epithelialization of the injured canaliculus.[9] Punctal erosion, slitting of the canaliculus, corneal irritation, granuloma formation, and tube displacement can occur with silicone tubing.[10,11] Punctal erosion and a slit canaliculus may force early removal of the tubing but usually do not result in epiphora[12] (Fig. 13-11). A corneal abrasion usually resolves promptly after tube removal. Granulomata can be excised with the tube in place, or will resolve with tube removal (Fig. 13-12). Displaced tubing can generally be repositioned[13,14] (Fig. 13-13).

Intubation with silicone tubing can be technically difficult.[15] The injured canaliculus should be intubated prior to intubation of the intact canaliculus. Probes should never be forced through resistant areas. Surgeons should abandon bicanalicular intubation if they experience unusual difficulty with intu-

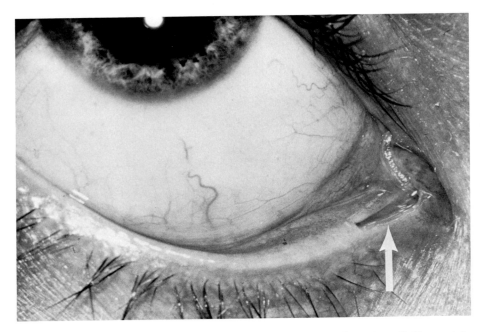

Fig. 13-11   Arrow indicates inferior canaliculus slit because of erosion of silicone tube through tissue.

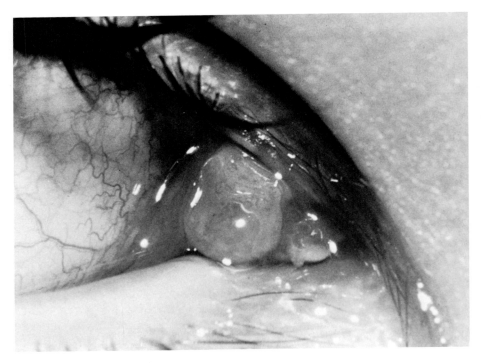

Fig. 13-12   Granuloma around silicone tubing.

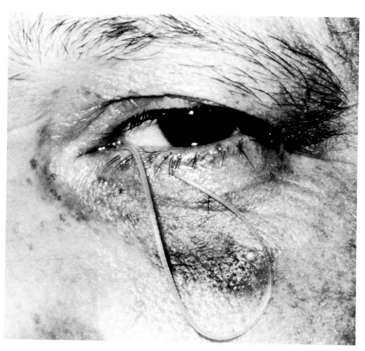

Fig. 13-13 Displaced silicone tubing after patient had caught tubing with finger and pulled loop of tubing onto his cheek.

bation of the injured canaliculus. By following these guidelines, iatrogenic injury to the intact portions of the system can be avoided.

Locating the probe in the nose and retrieving it are usually the most difficult aspects of intubation. The nasolacrimal duct opening is located anteriorly beneath the inferior turbinate in the vault of the inferior meatus (Fig. 13-14). Ophthalmologists unfamiliar with nasal anatomy may require assistance in locating the probe. A key point is to look along the extreme lateral wall of the nose beneath the inferior turbinate. We prefer the probes originally described by Quickert and Dryden[16] because they come in a variety of sizes and are both reusable and inexpensive. The cost of the intubation sets varies considerably (Table 13-1).

Once the tubing is placed, it should be adjusted for proper tension, and the ends of the tube joined in the nose. Our preferred technique is to tie six single knots with the tubing and pass a 4-0 nylon suture into the loop of tubing. The nylon suture is then secured with a deep bite inside the ala of the nose, and the suture is tied with a loose loop to avoid undue traction on the silicone tubing (Fig. 13-15). The nylon suture is used to prevent superior displacement of the tube and to keep the silicone tubing in an anterior position in the nose to facilitate later removal. Alternative techniques include use of a retinal sponge as a bolster[17] and gluing a suture into the lumen of the tubing.[18]

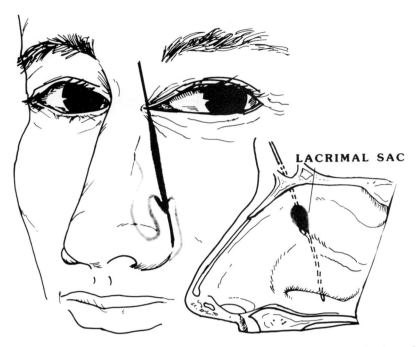

Fig. 13-14 Nasolacrimal duct opening beneath inferior turbinate on the lateral wall of the nose.

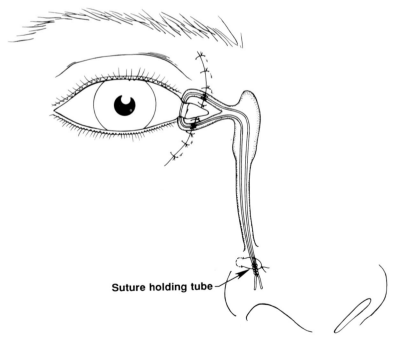

Fig. 13-15 Detail of suture securing silicone tubing to nasal mucosa.

Tabe 13-1. Bicanalicular Silicone Intubation Sets

Type of Set	Source	Catalog No.	Cost per 10 Intubations
Quickert	Storz[a,b]	E-4220-00 N-5941-1 E-4220-15 N-5890	$60.00
Crawford	Jedmed[c]	28-0185 28-0186	$406.00
Jackson	Storz	E-5651	$420.00
Pilling	Pilling[d]	42-6010 42-6020	$450.00
Visitec	Visitec[e]	5013	$455.00
Catalano	Storz	E-5654	$585.00
Guibor	Concept[f]	9035	$628.00
Concept	Concept	9045	$833.00
Concept Fiberoptic	Concept	9055	$955.00

[a] Storz Instrument Company, 3365 Tree Court Industrial Blvd., St. Louis, Missouri 63112.
[b] Reusable.
[c] Jedmed Instrument Company, 1430 Hanley Industrial Court, St. Louis, Missouri 63144.
[d] Narco Scientific, Pilling Division, 420 Delaware Drive, Fort Washington, PA 19034.
[e] Visitec, 2043 Whitfield Park Drive, Sarasota, FL 33580.
[f] Concept, 12707 U.S. 19 South, Clearwater, FL 33516.

Closure

We prefer to anastomose the canalicular ends directly with two or three sutures of 8-0 polyglycolic acid on a half-circle spatula needle under visualization with the operating microscope (Fig. 13-16). These small sutures may not be able to withstand the tension if a large gap exists between the lacerated ends of the canaliculus; it is helpful to tighten the silicone tube temporarily to relieve the tension. Some surgeons believe that direct suturing of the canaliculus is unnecessary, provided a stent is in place and the surrounding tissues are brought together.[19]

In canalicular lacerations, the attachment of the tarsus to the medial canthal tendon is often disrupted. McCord has emphasized the importance and difficulty of restoring the posterior crus of the medial canthal tendon attachment[20] (Fig. 13-17). The medial lid should be attached to the posterior lacrimal crest to allow proper apposition of the lid to the probe. Inadequate canthal tendon repair can result in a medial ectropion and epiphora, despite successful canalicular repair (Fig. 13-18). A polyglycolic acid suture (4-0 or 5-0) is used to join the medial lid or tarsus to the posterior medial canthal tendon stump at the posterior lacrimal crest. The anterior crus of the tendon is found just anterior to the common canaliculus, and the posterior crus is posterior to the common canaliculus.

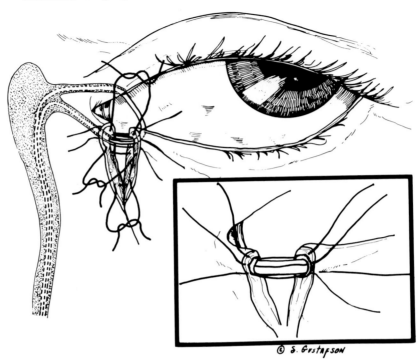

© S. Gustafson

Fig. 13-16 Detail of direct anastomosis of proximal and distal canalicular ends. (Hawes MJ, Segrest DR: Effectiveness of bicanalicular silicone intubation in the repair of canalicular lacerations. Ophthalmic Plast Reconstr Surg 1:185, 1985. Raven Press, NY.)

Tubing Removal

The silicone stent is left in place for 6 to 12 months. It is usually well tolerated during this time, and epiphora resolves within a few weeks after the initial repair. Extubation is performed by cutting the tube between the eyelids, cutting the suture in the nose, and removing the tubing and suture from the nose.

Evaluation of Repair

Probing or irrigation of the repaired canaliculus to confirm anatomic patency is the best technique for evaluating the surgical result in each canaliculus. Saunders et al. reported a series of 51 canalicular lacerations repaired by the pigtail probe method.[3] Although only 36 percent of the repaired canaliculi were patent to probing or irrigation, 80 percent of the patients were asymptomatic. Inquiry as to the presence of tearing is thus not an adequate test for success

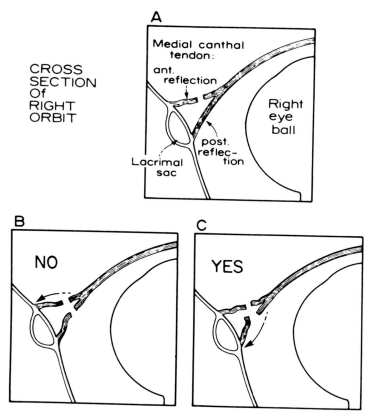

Fig. 13-17 Correct placement of medial canthal fixation suture. **(A)** Location of posterior reflection of the medial canthal tendon behind the lacrimal sac. **(B,C)** Posterior direction of the correct fixation point. (McCord, CD Jr. (ed): Oculoplastic Surgery. Raven Press, New York, 1981.)

of repair. Two published studies report 94 to 95 percent success in early repair of canalicular lacerations with bicanalicular silicone intubation.[1,4]

LACRIMAL SAC INJURIES

Diagnosis

The lacrimal sac is sheltered from minor trauma by its location in the bony lacrimal fossa posterior to the anterior lacrimal crest and the anterior crus of the medial canthal tendon. Lacrimal sac injuries should be suspected in the setting of nasoethmoidal fractures, deep medial canthal soft tissue trauma, or both (Fig. 13-19). Motor vehicle accidents and chain saw, corn picker, hatchet,

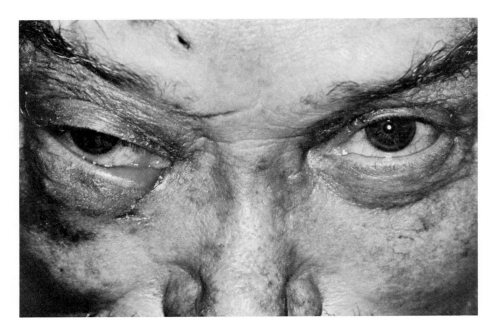

Fig. 13-18 Cicatricial ectropion of right lower lid following canalicular laceration repair with inadequate reattachment of tarsus to medial canthal tendon.

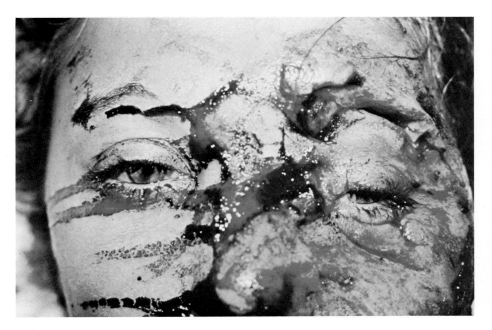

Fig. 13-19 Female victim of motorcycle accident who had craniofacial dysjunction (Le Fort III), left orbital blowout fracture, left tripod fracture, avulsion of medial canthal tendon, and nasoethmoidal fractures.

or dogbite injuries are examples of trauma that may cause disruption of the lacrimal sac. Most often the diagnosis is confirmed by exploration of the canthus after the patient is anesthetized for repair of associated injuries.

Associated Injuries

Neurologic

Neurologic evaluation overrides other concerns in the acutely injured patient. Penetrating bone fragments and other brain injuries are treated by a neurosurgeon. About 20 percent of patients with naso-orbital fractures will have a cerebrospinal fluid leak.[21] Chemical analysis of a clear fluid leaking from the nose or into the posterior pharynx will confirm its nature. The leak usually stops spontaneously within 7 to 10 days, and does not necessarily contraindicate early fracture repair, provided the patient is neurologically stable.[22]

Ocular

Injuries of the globe are frequently associated with major medial canthal trauma.[23] Scleral lacerations, hyphema, uveitis, corneal lacerations, retinal edema, and detachment may be seen.

Midface Fractures

Disruption of the nasal, lacrimal, and maxillary bones may result in traumatic telecanthus, or abnormally increased distance between the medial canthi (Figs. 13-20 and 13-21). Medial orbital wall, orbital floor blowout, and Le Fort fractures may be seen. An acutely injured patient with telecanthus and a foreshortened, depressed nose should prompt radiologic studies, followed by appropriate neurosurgical, otorhinolaryngological, and plastic surgical consultations.

Early Repair of Lacrimal Sac Injuries

Early repair requires a team approach, with neurologic and ocular repair taking precedence over facial fracture and lacrimal repair. Ideally, a disrupted lacrimal sac may be operated on at the time of fracture reduction and tendon restoration.[22] Silicone intubation, with or without suture closure of the sac, may suffice for lesser injuries. A dacryocystorhinostomy (DCR) is indicated when the sac is grossly disrupted. Scar formation may impair the usually satisfactory result.[24]

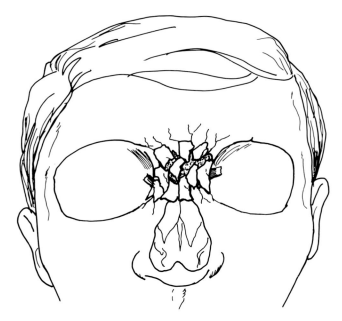

Fig. 13-20 Interorbital comminuted fractures with disruption of medial canthal tendons and their bony attachments, causing traumatic telecanthus.

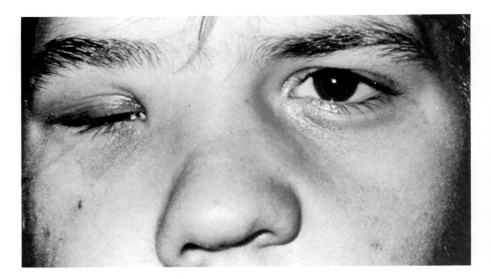

Fig. 13-21   Traumatic telecanthus following naso-orbital fracture.

Late Repair of Lacrimal Sac Injury and Telecanthus

Dacryocystography may be helpful in planning the repair of complicated cases involving the sac, the nasolacrimal duct, or both.[25] If one or both canaliculi are patent, a DCR is the operation of choice.[26] Acute infections of the sac should be treated with systemic antibiotics prior to DCR. Often the nasal mucosa is scarred to the adjacent bone and flaps are difficult to fashion. Lacrimal sac flaps may be sewn to periosteum if nasal mucosal flaps are inadequate. The use of a silicone stent will improve the success rate in difficult cases.[27]

If the canaliculi are destroyed, a conjunctivodacryocystorhinostomy with placement of a Pyrex tube is necessary.[2] For proper tube function, intranasal space is mandatory.

Late repair of traumatic telecanthus is difficult. Transnasal wiring and osteotomies may be done at the time of DCR.[28]

NASOLACRIMAL DUCT TRAUMA

Diagnosis

Like the lacrimal sac, the nasolacrimal duct is protected from injury by its bony surroundings. However, when the medial maxilla is fractured, the membranous nasolacrimal duct may be disrupted. Motor vehicle accidents are the leading cause of such injuries. Iatrogenic trauma to the duct may also occur with poor and/or repeated probings, antrostomy, or intranasal or maxillary sinus surgery.

Early diagnosis is made on the basis of clinical and x-ray evidence of midfacial fractures involving the medial maxilla. At this point the patient may not have epiphora, or associated injuries may demand priority care.

Late diagnosis is made when epiphora and/or dacryocystitis develop. Attempted irrigation of the lacrimal drainage system reveals fluid reflux from the canaliculus opposite the irrigated one.

Early Repair of Nasolacrimal Duct Injury

Multiple specialites may be involved in the acute care of the patient with midfacial fractures. Airway and neurologic problems receive highest priority. Silicone intubation of the lacrimal system may be performed at the time of fracture repair (Fig. 13-22). A successful early intubation will prevent the need for later, more extensive surgery.[29]

Late Repair of Nasolacrimal Duct Injury

Epiphora and dacryocystitis may appear within weeks to months after trauma. Infection is best treated with systemic antibiotics; DCR is then performed to bypass the nasolacrimal duct obstruction.

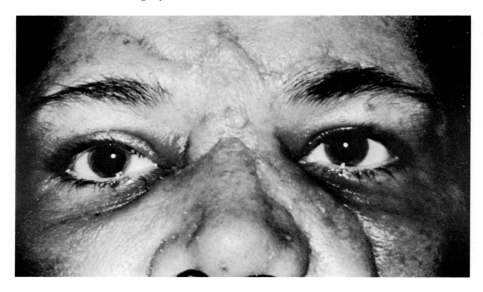

Fig. 13-22 Victim of Moped accident who sustained midfacial fractures involving the medial wall of the maxilla on both sides. Early silicone intubation of the lacrimal drainage system was performed.

EDITOR'S COMMENTS

The need for the repair of single canalicular lacerations is controversial. The older ophthalmic literature suggests that canalicular repair often fails and that a single canaliculus is adequate for tear drainage. Both of these facts have been challenged in the recent literature.

The editor has recently completed a study of the symptoms associated with experimental canalicular obstruction.[30] Hydroxypropyl cellulose plugs were used to temporarily occlude a single canaliculus in 20 normal adults. These volunteers then reported symptoms of epiphora, watery eye, blurred vision, or mattering of the eyelashes. The upper and lower canaliculus of each eye were experimentally occluded on separate days, so that symptoms could be compared.

More than 60 percent of all monocanalicular obstructions resulted in subjective symptoms. There was no significant difference in the rate of symptoms associated with upper versus lower canalicular obstruction. Thus, a majority of normal volunteers did report symptoms with monocanalicular obstruction. The upper and lower canaliculus seem to have an equal role. Symptoms were often intermittent, and varied with environmental conditions.

Unfortunately we do not have any test that allows us to predict which patient with a canalicular laceration will subsequently be symptomatic. The only way to avoid symptomatic patients is to repair all canalicular lacerations. With modern microsurgical techniques, as described by Drs. Hawes and Dortzbach, a very high success rate has been documented. Since late repair of canalicular obstruction has a lower success rate, primary repair of single canalicular lacerations seems appropriate.

If the ophthalmic surgeon is not comfortable with modern techniques of canalicular repair, then referral to an oculoplastics specialist will improve the prognosis. Even if this referral delays treatment for several days, the prognosis for a successful surgical result is excellent.

REFERENCES

1. Hawes MJ, Segrest DR: Effectiveness of bicanalicular silicone intubation in the repair of canalicular lacerations. Ophthalmic Plast Reconstr Surg 1:185, 1985
2. Jones LT, Wobig JL: Surgery of the Eyelids and Lacrimal Adnexa. Aesculapius Publishing Co, Birmingham, AL, 1976
3. Saunders DH, Shannon GM, Flanagan JC: The effectiveness of the pigtail probe method of repairing canalicular lacerations. Ophthalmic Surg 9:33, 1978
4. Dortzbach RK, Angrist RA: Silicone intubation for lacerated lacrimal canaliculi. Ophthalmic Surg 16:639, 1985
5. Beyer-Machule CK: Lacrimal stents. p. 171. In Bosniak SL (ed): Advances in Ophthalmic Plastic and Reconstructive Surgery. Vol 3. Pergamon Press, Elmsford, NY, 1984
6. Pashby RC, Rathbun JE: Silicone intubation of the lacrimal drainage system. Arch Ophthalmol 97:1318, 1979
7. Keith CG: Intubation of the lacrimal passages. Am J Ophthalmol 65:70, 1968
8. Crawford JS: Intubation of obstructions in the lacrimal system. Can J Ophthalmol 12:289, 1977
9. Snead JW, Rathbun JE, Crawford JB: Effects of the silicone tube on the canaliculus: An animal experiment. Ophthalmology 87:1031, 1980
10. Dortzbach RK, France TD, Kushner BJ, et al.: Silicone intubation for obstruction of the nasolacrimal duct in children. Am J Ophthalmol 94:585, 1982
11. Anderson RL, Edwards JJ: Indications, complications, and results with silicone stents. Ophthalmology 86:1474, 1979
12. Hurwitz J: The slit canaliculus. Ophthalmic Surg 13:572, 1982
13. Gonnering RS: Gentle, technically simple repositioning of displaced lacrimal tubing. Ophthalmic Surg 16:307, 1985
14. Beyer RW, Levine M: A method for repositioning or extraction of lacrimal system tubes. Ophthalmic Surg 17:496, 1986
15. Lauring L: Silicone intubation of the lacrimal system: Pitfalls, problems, and complications. Ann Ophthalmol 8:489, 1976
16. Quickert MH, Dryden R: Probes for intubation in lacrimal drainage. Trans Am Acad Ophthalmol Otolaryngol 74:431, 1970
17. Neuhaus R, Shorr N: Modified lacrimal system intubation. Ophthalmic Surg 14:1026, 1983
18. Rutherford S, Crawford J, Hurwitz J: Silicone tubing used in intubating the lacrimal system. Ophthalmology 91:963, 1984
19. Zolli CI: Microsurgical technique of lacrimal canalicular repair in the management of traumatic medial canthal eyelid avulsions. p. 197. In Bosniak SL (ed): Advances in Ophthalmic Plastic and Reconstructive Surgery. Vol 3. Pergamon Press, Elmsford, NY, 1984

20. McCord CD, Nunery WR: Reconstructive procedures of the lower eyelid and outer canthus. p. 201. In McCord CD (ed): Oculoplastic Surgery. Raven Press, New York, 1981
21. Lewin W: Cerebrospinal fluid rhinorrhea in closed head injuries. Br J Surg 42:1, 1954
22. Beyer CK, Fabian R, Smith B: Naso-orbital fractures, complications, and treatment. Ophthalmology 89:456, 1982
23. Beyer CK, Smith B: Naso-orbital fractures: Their complications and treatment. p. 107. In Tessier P, Callahan A, Mustardé JC, Salyer KE (eds): Symposium on Plastic Surgery in the Orbital Region. CV Mosby, St. Louis, 1976
24. McLachlan DC, Shannon GM, Flanagan JC: Results of dacryocystorhinostomy: Analysis of the reoperations. Ophthalmic Surg 11:427, 1980
25. Hawes MJ: Dacryocystography. p. 191. In Wesley RE (ed): Techniques in Ophthalmic Plastic Surgery. John Wiley & Sons, New York, 1986
26. Dortzbach RK: Dacryocystorhinostomy. Ophthalmology 85:1267, 1978
27. Older JJ: Routine use of a silicone stent in dacryocystorhinostomy. Ophthalmic Surg 13:911, 1982
28. Converse JM, Smith B: Naso-orbital fractures and traumatic deformities of the medial canthus. Plast Reconstr Surg 38:147, 1966
29. Harris GJ, Fuerste FH: Lacrimal intubation in the primary repair of midfacial fractures. Ophthalmology 94:242, 1987
30. Moore CA, Linberg JV: A evaluation of upper and lower lacrimal canalicular obstruction. Invest Ophthalmol Vis Sci, 28 (ARVO Suppl):308, 1987

14 | Canaliculodacryo-cystorhinostomy

Jeffrey J. Hurwitz
Kathleen F. Archer

The terms regarding operations involving the canaliculus vary and are sometimes confusing. We will begin by defining a useful terminology, which will be used throughout this chapter. The term *canaliculodacryocystorhinostomy* covers two separate operations: first, anastomosis of the common canaliculus to the tear sac followed by dacryocystorhinostomy (DCR), and second, anastomosis of either the lower or upper canaliculus to the tear sac followed by dacryocystorhinostomy. *Canaliculodacryocystorhinostomy* should not refer to the removal of a membrane covering the common internal punctum in conjunction with a DCR; this should be called a dacryocystorhinostomy with a common internal punctoplasty.

The anastomosis between the common canaliculus and the nasal mucosa, bypassing the tear sac, should be called a *common canalicular rhinostomy*. The anastomosis of a canaliculus directly to the nasal mucosa bypassing the lacrimal sac should be called a *canaliculorhinostomy*. The term *conjunctivo-dacryocystorhinostomy* is used only when the whole lacrimal system is bypassed either with an artificial tube or with a mucosal graft.

PERTINENT ANATOMY

Several anatomic characteristics are important in discussing the canaliculodacryocystorhinostomy operation. First, the lower canaliculus is more important in tear drainage than the upper canaliculus; 65 percent of tears are believed to go through the lower canaliculus and 35 percent through the upper canaliculus.[1] However, in some patients the upper canaliculus may drain more tears than the lower canaliculus, so individual variation must be considered. The canaliculi drain into the common canaliculus, which is 2 to 5 mm long. The common canaliculus empties into the tear sac through the common internal punctum, which sits on the inner wall of the tear sac. The distance from the punctum to the beginning of the common canaliculus is about 8 to 12 mm, but also varies from patient to patient. If an obstruction is located less than 8 mm from the punctum it is usually situated within the lid, whereas if the obstruction is more than 8 mm from the punctum it is usually within the medial canthus.

PATTERNS OF CANALICULAR DISEASE

Common Canaliculus

Obstruction in the common canaliculus may occur at its medial end (at the common internal punctum), where the common canaliculus drains into the tear sac. A common internal punctum obstruction is usually secondary to a primary obstruction at the lower end of the sac and is caused by a membrane obstructing the opening of the common canaliculus into the tear sac. This can be approached from within the sac as the dacryocystorhinostomy is performed. Common canalicular obstruction may also occur within the common canaliculus or at its lateral end, where the upper and lower canaliculus join the common canaliculus. It is in this latter situation that the canaliculodacryocystorhinostomy operation becomes important because it is extremely difficult to dissect out these more lateral membranes in the common canaliculus from within the sac.

Individual Canalicular Obstructions

Individual canalicular obstructions may occur in the proximal or distal ends of the canaliculi. If an obstruction occurs in the proximal part of the canaliculus (less than 8 mm in from the punctum), it is difficult to dissect out the canaliculus and attach it to the tear sac. Therefore, in these situations a bypass procedure with an artificial tear duct tube is the operation of choice. In distal obstructions located more than 8 mm from the punctum, the surgeon can dissect the individual canaliculus or both canaliculi and anastomose these to the tear sac with a canaliculodacryocystorhinostomy operation. Complete canalicular obstruction may occur in the upper canaliculus, the lower canaliculus, or both. When an obstruction occurs in the upper canaliculus with a normal lower canaliculus, common canaliculus, sac, and duct, the patient usually does not experience tearing, and no treatment is usually necessary. However, if the obstruction is in the lower canaliculus with a normal upper canaliculus, common canaliculus, sac, and duct, the patient usually has tearing. Many of these patients may be cured merely by a dacryocystorhinostomy,

Table 14-1. Canalicular Obstruction

Site of Obstruction	Other Factors	Recommended Surgery
Medial common canaliculus only		DCR with common internal punctoplasty
Lateral common canaliculus only		Canaliculodacryocystorhinostomy
Lower canaliculus only, more than 8 mm from punctum	Upper canaliculus patent Upper canaliculus obstructed	DCR Canaliculodacryocystorhinostomy
Lower canaliculus only, less than 8 mm from punctum	Upper canaliculus patent Upper canaliculus obstructed	DCR Conjunctivodacryocystorhinostomy
Upper canaliculus only, more than 8 mm from punctum	Lower canaliculus patent Lower canaliculus obstructed	Surgery usually not needed Canaliculodacryocystorhinostomy
Upper canaliculus only, less than 8 mm from punctum	Lower canaliculus patent Lower canaliculus obstructed	Surgery usually not needed Conjunctivodacryocystorhinostomy
Combined upper/lower canalicular obstruction	Either canaliculus patent for more than 8 mm from punctum	Canaliculodacryocystorhinostomy
	Neither canaliculus patent for more than 8 mm from punctum	Conjunctivodacryocystorhinostomy

which increases tear drainage through the upper canaliculus by eliminating the resistance of the nasolacrimal duct.[2] The canalicular obstructions may be complete or incomplete. Because repeated dilation of an incomplete obstruction may produce a complete obstruction, it should not be done. Treatment of an incomplete obstruction should follow the same principles as treatment of a complete obstruction (Table 14-1).

INDICATIONS FOR CANALICULODACRYOCYSTORHINOSTOMY

Indications for canaliculodacryocystorhinostomy are as follows:

Canalicular obstruction involving both the upper and lower canaliculus with at least 8 mm of patent canaliculus, measured from the punctum.
Lateral common canalicular obstruction.
Failed DCR surgery with a small residual sac or no residual sac.
Following dacryocystectomy or trauma with a scarred sac. (This is really a common canaliculorhinostomy.)
Obstruction following removal of a tumor or a dermoid at the inner canthus.
Following extrusion of a Jones tube if sufficient patent canaliculi remain for re-anastomosis.

HISTORY OF CANALICULODACRYOCYSTORHINOSTOMY

Jones and Corrigan first described canaliculodacryocystorhinostomy in the British literature in 1959.[3] At that time, the operation was popular in Britain and to a lesser extent in Europe. In 1970, Tenzel published an article in the *Archives of Ophthalmology* entitled "Canaliculodacryocystorhinostomy."[4] What he described is really a dacryocystorhinostomy with common internal punctoplasty for a membrane occurring at the junction of a common canaliculus and the tear sac. The operation was described in the Canadian literature in 1975,[5] but was not mentioned in the American literature until 1982, when Doucet and Hurwitz published two articles describing the procedure for canalicular obstructions and failed lacrimal surgery.[6,7] A modification of the procedure was described by Rodgers and Hurwitz in the European literature in 1983.[8]

SELECTION OF PATIENTS FOR CANALICULODACRYOCYSTORHINOSTOMY

Candidates for canaliculodacryocystorhinostomy are patients with canalicular obstruction at least 8 mm in from the punctum. A patient's history might include the use of miotics, antiviral agents, or antimetabolites, and possibly a history of viral infections such as herpes simplex, herpes zoster, vaccinia, or varicella. Evidence of trichoma or any injury, either traumatic or iatrogenic, is important. The ophthalmologist also should try to ascertain whether the obstruction is intracanalicular or extracanalicular because this distinction may have some therapeutic significance.

Syringing of the lacrimal system is important. If there is no reflux through the upper canaliculus when the lower canaliculus is syringed, the surgeon can assume that there is an obstruction in the lower canaliculus. The next step is to slide a probe through the punctum until the obstructing membrane is reached, thus ascertaining the exact location of the obstruction. The upper canaliculus must then be syringed to determine whether it is indeed blocked or whether one can syringe into the common canaliculus, sac, or nose. If the upper canaliculus is blocked, the distance of the obstruction from the punctum should be measured as well. With a blocked lower canaliculus and a patent upper canaliculus, a dacryocystogram[9] is useful to determine exactly where the obstruction lies in the system. If syringing the lower canaliculus produces reflux through the upper canaliculus, a dacryocystogram is useful to determine whether the obstruction lies within the sac-duct, or whether the obstruction is more proximal, e.g., in the common canaliculus. An obstruction within the common canaliculus where it joins the tear sac, (Fig. 14-1) is best treated by a DCR plus common internal punctoplasty and not by a canaliculodacryocystorhinostomy. An obstruction within the common canaliculus or on its lateral aspect where the upper and lower canaliculi join it is best treated by a canaliculodacryocystorhinostomy (Fig. 14-2). A nuclear lacrimal scan[10] is only

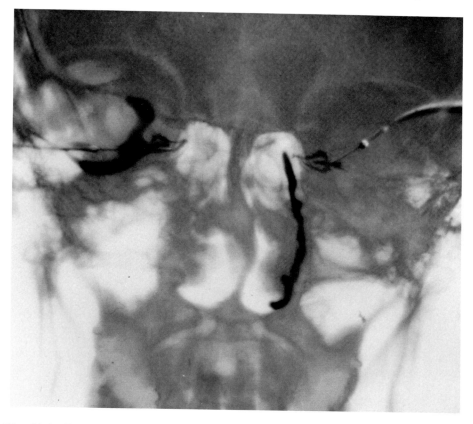

Fig. 14-1 Dacryocystogram showing right-sided medial end of common canaliculus obstruction necessitating dacryocystorhinostomy plus common internal punctoplasty.

useful where there is a stenosis of the system with patency to syringing; in these situations the scan may reveal the significance of the stenosis. The scan cannot localize the point of obstruction nor is it of any value when the system is completely obstructed to syringing.

TECHNIQUE OF DCR PLUS COMMON INTERNAL PUNCTOPLASTY

DCR plus common internal punctoplasty is performed for obstructions within the sac at the internal ostium where the common canaliculus drains into the sac. A standard DCR is performed. The sac is opened, and when a probe is placed within the common canaliculus the obstructing membrane may be tented over the probe. This membrane may be excised. The dacryocystorhinostomy is completed by placing indwelling Silastic stent tubes for approxi-

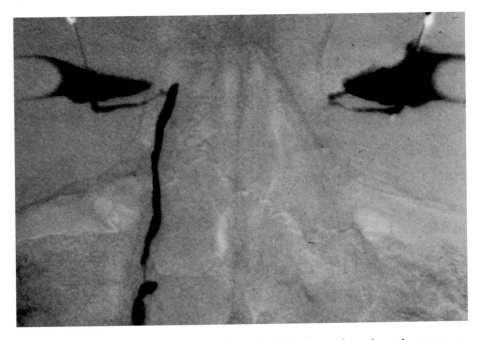

Fig. 14-2 Dacryocystogram demonstrating left-sided obstruction where the upper canaliculus and lower canaliculus join the common canaliculus necessitating canaliculodacryocystorhinostomy.

mately 6 weeks. The operation has a success rate for long-term patency of 85 to 90 percent.[11]

TECHNIQUE OF CANALICULODACRYOCYSTORHINOSTOMY[3,6,7]

Standard Canaliculodacryocystorhinostomy

Using the standard DCR incision, the orbicularis muscle and subcutaneous tissues are dissected and retracted. Then the medial canthal tendon is identified, incised at its periosteal attachment, and retracted laterally. The common canaliculus lies immediately posterior. Probes are then passed into each canaliculus for identification. With microscopic visualization, the common canaliculus is separated from the posterior limb of the medial canthal tendon with a sharpened periosteal elevator. The canaliculus is then opened over the medial aspect of the probes. Scar tissue (obstructed common canaliculus) between this area and the lacrimal sac is excised. A silicone or polyethylene tube is passed through each punctum and out the newly formed, but shortened, common canaliculus. The freely mobilized common canaliculus is retracted laterally, away from the

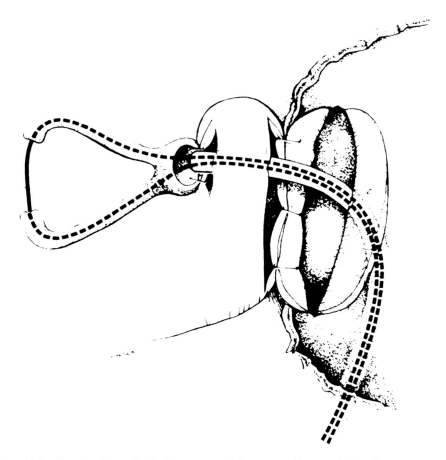

Fig. 14-3 Standard canaliculodacryocystorhinostomy diagram indicating anastomosis of anterior and posterior flaps of common canaliculus to lateral wall of tear sac and anterior and posterior lacrimal nasal mucosa flaps anastomosed to medial, anterior, and posterior lacrimal sac flaps.

field. A rhinostomy is then created larger than in the standard DCR procedure to ensure large, mobile nasal flaps. Posterior nasal mucosal-lacrimal sac flaps are fashioned and anastomosed (Fig. 14-3). A small, vertical incision is created on the lateral aspect of the lacrimal sac at the original cite of the common canaliculus, creating small anterior and posterior flaps. The intubation tubes are carried through this incision, as well as through the rhinostomy and out the nares. The anterior and posterior flaps of the common canalicular mucosa are then anastomosed to the lateral flaps of the lacrimal sac with 5-0 polyglycolic acid suture (Dexon), and the anterior nasal mucosal-lacrimal sac flaps are sutured. The subcutaneous tissue and skin are closed in layers. The intubation tubes are removed in 3 to 4 months.

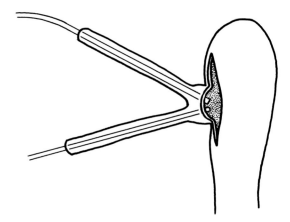

Fig. 14-4 Modified canaliculo-dacryocystorhinostomy. A vertical incision made as lateral as possible within the tear sac where the probes enter the common canaliculus.

Modified Canaliculodacryocystorhinostomy[8]

A standard DCR incision is made on the side of the nose. The subcutaneous tissues and the anterior crux of the medial canthal tendon are retracted. Probes are placed in the upper and lower canaliculi until the obstruction is encountered (Fig. 14-4) Using the operating microscope, all scar tissue medial to the probes is excised and the opened lateral common canaliculus is dissected free anteriorly, superiorly, and inferiorly. A vertical incision is then made in the anterior part of the tear sac, as lateral as possible, immediately adjacent to the freed lateral end of common canaliculus. (Fig. 14-5) The anterior part of the sac,

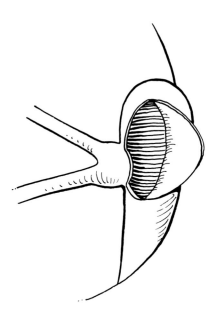

Fig. 14-5 Anterior tear sac is reflected as far medially as possible to become part of the new posterior lacrimal sac flap.

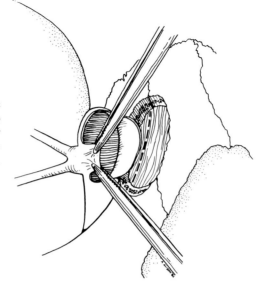

Fig. 14-6 The posterior lacrimal sac flap is anastomosed to the posterior flap of nasal mucosa, and a large anterior common canalicular flap will be sutured to the anterior flap of nasal mucosa.

medial to the incision, is then reflected medially so that the whole of the tear sac becomes the new posterior flap. (Fig. 14-6)

Attention is then directed to the rhinostomy. The canalicular system is retracted laterally, and a large bony rhinostomy requiring removal of bone around the nasolacrimal duct as well as around the fundus of the nasolacrimal sac is made. The nasal mucosa is then incised in such a way as to form a large anterior mucosal flap and a small posterior flap. The posterior flaps of nasal mucosa and lacrimal sac are then anastomosed, i.e., the posterior flap of sac mucosa is sutured to the small posterior flap from nasal mucosa using three interrupted 5-0 absorbable sutures. The upper and lower canaliculi are intubated with Silastic tubes that are passed through the rhinostomy and into the nose. The anterior canalicular flap is then anastomosed to the anterior nasal mucosa (Fig. 14-7). It is useful to place the anterior flap sutures before tying them in order to facilitate precise anastomosis of the large anterior nasal mucosal flap to the small anterior common canalicular flap. The Silastic tubes are left in place for 3 to 4 months.

The standard procedure necessitates double anterior and posterior anastomoses. Obtaining enough mucosa to bridge the gap between canaliculi and lacrimal sac is often a problem, as is the suturing of the lateral flaps (canaliculi to sac), especially those that are posterior. With the modified technique, the difficulty of insufficient posterior flap tissue is circumvented by making the incision of the sac wall laterally and reflecting the anterior flap medially so that the whole of the sac becomes a posterior flap that can be anastomosed to the posterior nasal flap. When the whole lacrimal sac is used to form most of the posterior wall of the epithelial-lined channel, only a small posterior nasal flap

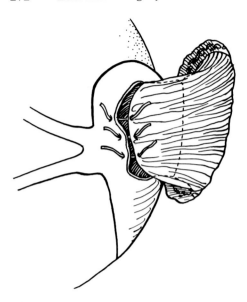

Fig. 14-7 Anterior flap of common canaliculus sutured to anterior flap of nasal mucosa.

is necessary, making a correspondingly larger anterior nasal flap available to form the major part of the anterior wall of the epithelial-lined channel. Mobilization of the nasal mucosal flap tissue is facilitated by making a large rhinostomy. In some cases, infracturing of the nasal turbinate may be necessary if the nasal mucosal incision is made too far posterior, but this does not usually present a problem.

The difficult posterior canalicular anastomosis of the standard canaliculodacryocystorhinostomy is thus avoided because during dissection of the common canaliculus, the posterior attachment of the common canaliculus to the nasolacrimal sac is not disturbed. An anterior flap can then be fashioned from the anterior part of the common canaliculus and anastomosed to the large anterior flap of nasal mucosa. The operation thereby necessitates single rather than the double anterior and posterior anastomoses necessary in the standard canaliculodacryocystorhinostomy.

Lower and Upper Canaliculodacryocystorhinostomy

In this situation, each canaliculus is obstructed lateral to the junction at the common canaliculus. Probes are placed in each canaliculus to identify the obstruction. Scar tissue (obstructed lower, upper, and common canalicular system) between the obstructions and the lacrimal sac is excised. The tissue between the inferior wall of the upper canaliculus and the superior wall of the lower canaliculus is excised for 2 to 3 mm. Incisions oriented in the long axis of the two walls create anterior and posterior flaps (at the medial end of this "new common canalicular channel") that are now available for anastomosis with either the lacrimal sac or nasal mucosa, as in the previous description. This same procedure may be performed if a scarred sac is to be removed or following a dacryocystectomy where the individual canaliculi or common canaliculus may be anastomosed directly to the nasal mucosa.

Following Unsuccessful DCR

When a small sac or no sac is identified, the patient may be cured with a canaliculodacryocystorhinostomy rather than the classical approach of inserting Jones bypass tubes.[7] A canaliculodacryocystorhinostomy is more advisable in this situation than the direct approach to the obstructed anastomosis. The dissection begins in fresh, undisturbed tissue and progresses toward the scarred, often unidentifiable, sac, thus facilitating flap formation that otherwise would be extremely difficult.

A standard DCR incision is made along the side of the nose. The subcutaneous tissue and anterior crus of the medial canthal tendon are retracted, and probes are placed into each canalicular system until the obstruction is encountered. With microscopic visualization, the common canaliculus is dissected from the posterior limb of the medial canthal tendon. Its most medial patent aspect can be identified by visualizing the probe tips and then opened. The patent canaliculus is dissected circumferentially, intubated with silicone tubes, and retracted laterally away from the surgical field. The scar remaining medial to this, which includes the scarred lacrimal system, is excised. The existing rhinostomy is always enlarged to enable the creation of larger, mobile nasal mucosal flaps. The canalicular system is then anastomosed to whatever patent lacrimal sac remains, and the medial sac flaps are sutured. If no sac remains, the residual patent common canaliculus is anastomosed directly to nasal mucosal flaps. This procedure is facilitated by making small longitudinal incisions in the long axis of the common canalicular remnant, creating anterior and posterior canalicular flaps. These flaps are then anastomosed to the corresponding nasal mucosal flaps with 5-0 absorbable sutures. Silicone tubes are passed through the rhinostomy and out the nares before the anterior flaps are completed. The tubes are left in place for 3 to 4 months. If the obstruction lies lateral to the common canaliculus, then the canaliculi may be sutured individually to the residual sac or nasal mucosa in a similar manner.

INTUBATION TECHNIQUE

Silastic Intubation

For intubation, two tubes are utilized: the stent and the sleeve. The preferred materials are Silastic medical grade tubing sizes 0.51 mm inner diameter and 0.94 mm outer diameter for the canalicular tubing, and for the sleeve, 1.57 mm inner diameter and 2.41 mm outer diameter.

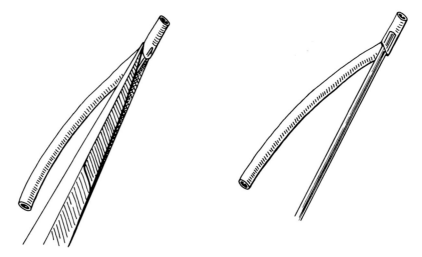

Fig. 14-8   Silastic intubation with insertion of probe along the tube wall.

The Silastic is cut to a length of approximately 20 cm and gas autoclaved. A 3-cm piece of the Silastic sleeve is included in the package.

Technique of Insertion

About 3 mm from each end of the smaller Silastic tubing, an oblique cut is made halfway through the tube's diameter. A small lacrimal probe is snugly fit into this cut and inserted 2 mm into the tube's lumen toward the end of the

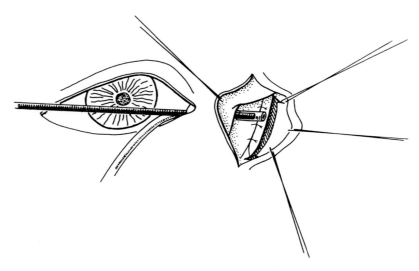

Fig. 14-9   Passage of tube along lower canaliculus into sac.

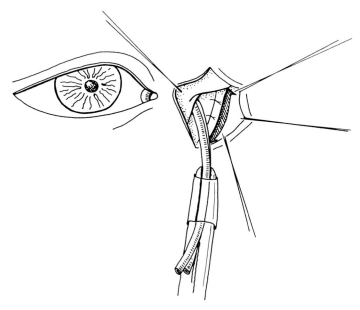

Fig. 14-10 Tubes passed into sac. Silastic sleeve placed around the tubes.

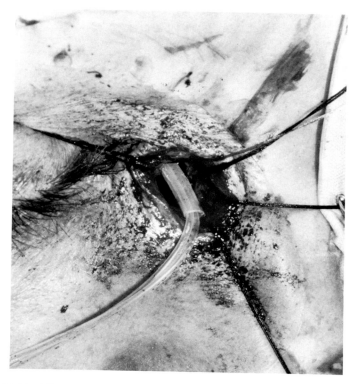

Fig. 14-11 Silastic sleeve passed up snug against the common canaliculus.

tube. (Fig. 14-8) After the posterior flaps of sac and nasal mucosa are sutured, the inferior punctum is dilated, and the tubing, with the probe positioned inside the lumen, is carefully passed into the punctum through the canaliculus until visualized as it passes through the common internal punctum (Fig. 14-9). The tubing is held with a hemostat, the probe pulled back through the punctum, and the end tag easily pulled off. The other end is similarly passed through the superior punctum and canaliculus.

A 1- to 1.5-cm length of the larger Silastic tubing is cut as the sleeve and stretched over the jaws of a hemostat. The two ends of the smaller tubing are passed through the sleeve simultaneously (Fig. 14-10). Under direct visualization, the sleeve position is adjusted around the smaller tubing up to the common internal punctum. (Figs. 14-11 and 14-12) Since the sleeve fits snugly around the free ends of the canalicular tubes, they need not be sutured. A hemostat is passed through the external nares into the rhinostomy; the two free ends of the canalicular tubing are grasped and pulled out of the nose. (Fig. 14-13)

The anterior flaps are then anastomosed over the tubing without including the tubing in the flap sutures. A black silk suture is tied snugly around the ends of the tube just inside the external nares, and the two ends of the tube are cut, allowing no protrusion from the nose.

The tube is left in place for the desired time. The patient is informed that tearing may be experienced while the tube is in place. When removing the tubes, the Silastic tubing visible at the medial canthus is cut. The patient is asked to blow his nose several times, and the free ends are grasped in the nares and gently removed.

Polypropylene Intubation

When the upper canaliculus is totally obliterated and it is impossible to pass bicanalicular Silastic tubes, intubation of the lower canaliculus may be beneficial in order to place a stent between the flaps of the canalicular anastomosis.[12] A small polypropylene tube has been designed with an inner diameter of 1.25 mm and an outer diameter of 2 mm, which may be inserted in the lower canaliculus. The ocular flanged end is sutured to the punctum after a one-snip procedure is performed on the punctum. This tube will not only act as a stent, but will also allow tear drainage while it is in place. To remove the tube, the surgeon merely snips the stitch at the punctum and withdraws the tube from the punctum. (Fig. 14-14)

RESULTS OF SURGERY

In most cases of canalicular or common canalicular obstruction, the previous treatment of choice has been the insertion of a permanent tear duct bypass tube. Anyone performing lacrimal surgery on a regular basis is familiar with

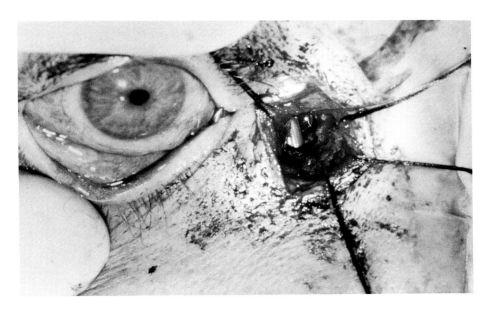

Fig. 14-12 Tubes passed into nose. Silastic tube within sac.

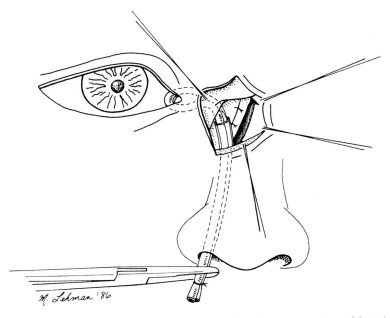

Fig. 14-13 Tubes passed down into nose and sutured to each other with a 4-0 black silk suture.

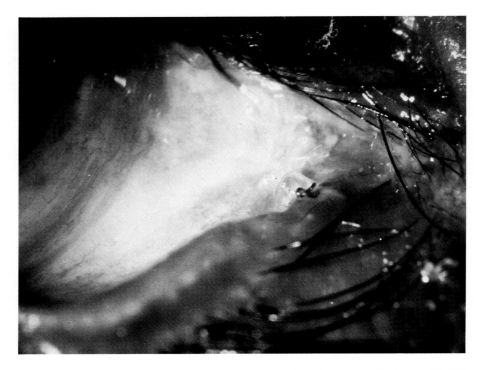

Fig. 14-14 Small polypropylene stent tube placed along lower canaliculus and held in place with a 6-0 nylon suture.

the potential complications of a bypass tube. It is greatly to the patient's advantage if epiphora can be relieved without the need for these tubes. In all situations where a canaliculodacryocystorhinostomy is possible, we believe it should be attempted. A large rhinostomy provides adequate room in the nose for the possibility of a secondary Jones tube or bypass tube insertion, should the canaliculodacryocystorhinostomy fail. The success rate for canaliculodacryocystorhinostomy is 75 to 80 percent when performed for common canalicular obstruction and 50 to 60 percent when performed for more proximal obstructions.[11] With less than 8 mm of patent canaliculus, the success rate for canaliculodacryocystorhinostomy is below 50 percent, and therefore a bypass tube is the preferred procedure.

We believe that when one performs anastomosis between the common canaliculus and the sac or between the individual canaliculi and the sac, one achieves better drainage of the sac by also performing a DCR. Even with intubation, we believe there is a tendency for the sac to close if a DCR is not performed in conjunction with the canalicular operation. Performing a DCR makes it simple to insert a bypass tube secondarily, should the canalicular operation fail.

INTUBATION WITHOUT OPEN SURGERY

Some controversy exists as to whether canalicular obstruction should be treated primarily with probing and intubation or whether primary canaliculo-dacryocystorhinostomy should be performed. Certainly if the surgeon cannot probe a canalicular obstruction, it will be impossible to insert tubes without performing open surgery. If an attempt is made to insert tubes without performing open surgery, the surgeon must be able to perform open surgery should it be impossible to probe the system and pass tubes.

CONCLUSION

The canaliculodacryocystorhinostomy is an effective way of treating patients with epiphora due to canalicular obstructions, without the inherent problems of a permanent prosthetic bypass tube. The procedure has a very acceptable success rate considering both the difficult nature of the problem and the fact that this procedure allows patients to be cured without a prosthetic device. Therefore, we suggest that the armamentarium of the lacrimal surgeon include the canaliculodacryocystorhinostomy operation.

REFERENCES

1. Rabinovitch J, Hurwitz JJ, Chin-Sang H: Quantitative evaluation of canalicular flow using lacrimal scintillography. ORBIT 1985
2. Jones BR: The surgical cure of obstruction in the lacrimal canaliculus. Trans Ophthalmol Soc UK 80:343, 1960
3. Jones BR, Corrigan MJ: Obstruction of the Lacrimal Canaliculi in Proceedings of the Second International Corneo-Plastic Conference, London, 1967. Pergamon Press, Oxford, 1969, p. 101
4. Tenzel RR: Canaliculodacryocystorhinostomy. Arch Ophthalmol 84:765, 1970
5. Hurwitz JJ, Welham RAN, Lloyd GAS: The role of intubation macrodacryocystography in management of problems of the lacrimal system. Can J Ophthalmol 10:361, 1975
6. Doucet TW, Hurwitz JJ: Canaliculodacryocystorhinostomy in the treatment of canalicular obstruction. Arch Ophthalmol 100:306, 1982
7. Doucet TW, Hurwitz JJ: Canaliculodacryocystorhinostomy in the management of unsuccessful lacrimal surgery. Arch Ophthalmol 100:619, 1982
8. Rodgers KJA, Hurwitz JJ: A simplified canaliculodacryocystorhinostomy. ORBIT 2:231, 1983
9. Hurwitz JJ, Victor WH: The role of sophisticated radiological testing in the assessment and management of epiphora. Ophthalmology 92:407, 1985
10. Hurwitz JJ, Welham RAN, Maisey MN: Intubation macrodacryocystography and quantitative scintillography—the complete lacrimal assessment. Trans Am Acad Ophthalmol Otolaryngol 81:575, 1976

11. Hurwitz JJ, Rutherford S: Computerized survey of lacrimal surgery patients. Ophthalmology 93:14, 1986
12. Hurwitz JJ: New polypropylene tube to stent or bypass the lacrimal system. Can J Ophthalmol 19:261, 1984
13. Hurwitz JJ, Rodgers J, Doucet TW: Dermoid tumor involving the lacrimal drainage pathway: A case report. Ophthalmic Surg 100:377, 1982

15 Conjunctivodacryo-cystorhinostomy

Allen M. Putterman

A conjunctivodacryocystorhinostomy (CDCR) is performed if the upper and lower ipsilateral canaliculi are completely obstructed. One of the most common causes of canalicular obstruction is the unsuccesssful repair of traumatic eyelid lacerations. Chronic infections of the conjunctiva and lacrimal excretory system are another cause of canalicular obstruction. Viral infections are included in this etiology, and I have had several patients with conjunctival herpetic infections that have resulted in canalicular obstruction. Inflammatory disease such as sarcoidosis is another cause. The use of miotics in the treatment of glaucoma is a well-known cause of canalicular obstruction. Finally, many of these obstructions occur without an obvious cause.

STANDARD CDCR TECHNIQUE

A DCR is performed according to the standard techniques through the step of suturing the posterior nasal mucosal and lacrimal sac flaps to each other (Fig. 15-1A).[1,2] Then, the anterior tip of the middle turbinate is resected with a rongeur if it rises above the closed posterior flaps. (This must be done almost routinely.) The anterior aspect of the caruncle is excised with Westcott scissors (Fig. 15-1B).

A 19-gauge needle is bent slightly and inserted 2 mm posterior to the medial canthal skin-mucosal junction and is passed in a 30- to 40-degree inferior direction over the sutured posterior nasal mucosal-lacrimal sac flaps (Fig. 15-1C). A Von Graefe knife is passed along and adjacent to the needle, and the needle is withdrawn (Fig. 15-1D). The knife end is pushed and pulled with short movements in a superior and inferior direction to enlarge the track. A No. 1

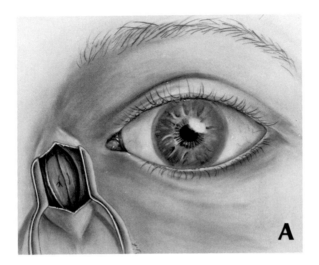

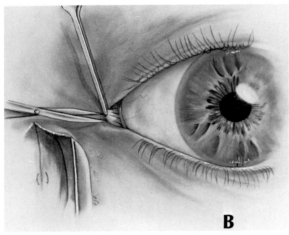

Fig. 15-1 Standard technique for CDCR. **(A)** Posterior flaps of the nasal mucosal and lacrimal sac have been connected with 5-0 Dexon suture. **(B)** The anterior aspect of the caruncle is excised. **(C)** A 19-gauge needle is passed 2 mm posterior to the medial canthal skin-mucosal junction. (*Figure continues.*)

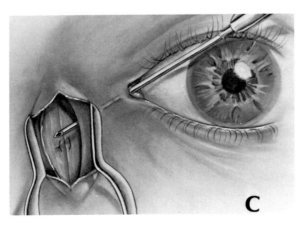

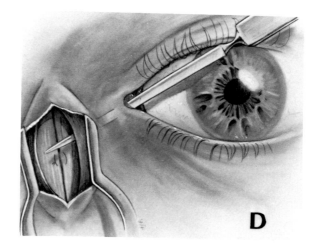

Fig. 15-1 (*Continued*). (D) A Von Graefe knife is passed through the previous tunnel and is moved upward and downward. (E) A Bowman probe is passed through the ostium until it meets the nasal septum. A hemostat grasps the probe at the medial canthus. (F) The distance from hemostat to the Bowman probe end is measured. (*Figure continues.*)

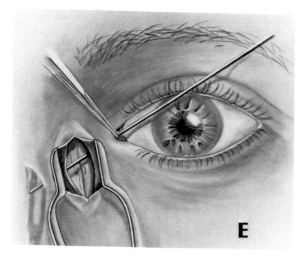

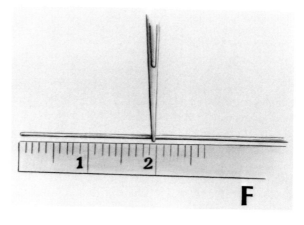

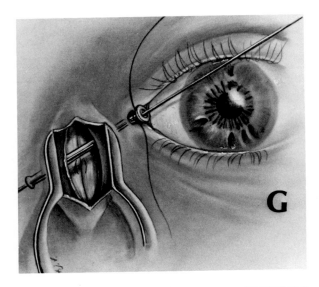

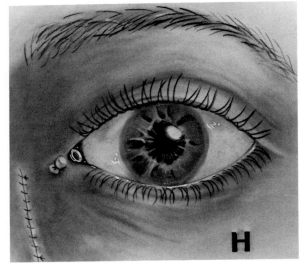

Fig. 15-1 (*Continued*). (**G**) A Jones tube with a 3- to 4-mm collar and a length 3 mm less than the measurement determined in **F** is placed over a Bowman probe and slid into the ostium. A 6-0 black silk double-armed suture is wrapped around the Jones tube several times. (**H**) The 6-0 black silk suture is brought out through the medial canthus, where it is tied over a cotton pledget. Jones tube remains in place after closure of the anterior lacrimal sac and nasal mucosal flaps, periosteum, orbicularis, and skin.

or 2 Bowman probe is passed along the shaft of the knife until it meets the nasal septum (Fig. 15-1E). The Von Graefe knife is then carefully withdrawn. The Bowman probe is grasped with a hemostat where it enters the caruncle and is then withdrawn. The distance from the probe end to the hemostat is measured, and a Jones Pyrex tube 3 to 4 mm shorter than this length is chosen from the various tubes available from Gunther Weiss, Inc. (available through Weiss Scientific Glass Blowing Co., Portland, OR) (Fig. 15-1F). In most of my cases, I prefer to use a tube that has a 4-mm collar. At times, however, if the collar is obviously too large, I will use a 3.5- or 3-mm collar.

The selected Jones tube is slid onto the Bowman probe, and the probe is passed through the CDCR ostium. The Jones tube is next slid through the ostium with pressure on its collar by the surgeon's thumbnail until the collar rests at the medial canthus; the distal end of the tube should be within the nasal cavity but at least 3 mm from the nasal septum (Fig. 15-1G). The Bowman probe is removed. The Jones tube is anchored by passing a 6-0 black silk double-armed suture several times around the tube just adjacent to its collar (Fig. 15-1G). Each end of the suture is passed through the skin of the medial canthus and tied over a cotton pledget to prevent the tube from sliding through the large ostium (Fig. 15-1H). A 6-0 black silk suture passed through and around the tube is another way of securing the tube.[3] The position of the tube is inspected within the nasal cavity. The tip should clear the septum by about 3 mm and extend into the nose about 2 mm.

The anterior lacrimal sac flap is then sutured to the anterior nasal mucosal flap with several 5-0 Dexon sutures. The periosteal incision is closed with 4-0 polyglactin 910 sutures, subcutaneous tissue is sutured with 5-0 Vicryl sutures, and the skin is then sutured with a continuous 6-0 black silk suture (Fig. 15-1H).

Six days postoperatively, the skin sutures are removed. Three weeks postoperatively, the suture anchoring the Jones tube is removed. The patient is instructed to irrigate the tube with sterile saline or dexamethasone phosphate ophthalmic solution, squirting a small amount of this solution over the medial canthal area and inhaling deeply through the nose. If the tube is functioning properly, the patient should be able to taste the irrigated fluid. Every 3 to 4 months, the tube is flushed with ophthalmic solution that is placed in a syringe and attached to a lacrimal needle. The needle is passed through the proximal tube, and the syringe contents are released. Every 8 to 12 months, the tube is removed, cleaned, and replaced. Also, if the tube is functioning poorly, it is possible that a different length tube is necessary. If the tube collar is too large, it is necessary to replace the tube with one that has a smaller collar diameter.

Routine Care of Jones Tube

Cleaning and replacement of Jones tubes is usually performed in the office. Topical proparacaine hydrochloride (Ophthaine) is applied over the eye. The collar of the Jones tube is grasped with the surgeon's fingernail or with the end of a lacrimal needle and is slid out of the CDCR ostium. The tube is cleaned with water directed over the collar as well as with water squirted through it with a lacrimal needle and syringe. At times, it is necessary to scrape off material that has accumulated on the outside of the tube. The CDCR ostium is then dilated with standard gold dilators (available through Gunther Weiss & Co.). There are two separate dilators that come with the Jones Pyrex tube set and each has dilators of different sizes on opposite ends.

Before dilation of the passage, proparacaine topical anesthetic is irrigated into the CDCR ostium. A lacrimal needle secured to a syringe containing proparacaine is inserted into the ostium, and proparacaine is irrigated into the fistula. The smallest dilator is then slid into the CDCR track. Then, progressively larger dilators are inserted until the largest dilator has been passed through the ostium and into the nasal cavity. The Jones tube is placed onto a Bowman probe, and the probe is passed into the CDCR ostium. The Jones tube is then slid into the dilated ostium with pressure on the collar by the surgeon's thumbnail. The proper position of the tube is then inspected at both the medial canthal and nasal cavity sites.

If it is necessary to replace the Jones tube with a new one, the size of the tube is determined as indicated in the Standard CDCR Technique section.

TECHNIQUE FOR REPLACEMENT OF JONES TUBE AFTER CDCR OSTIUM CLOSURE OR BECAUSE OF MISDIRECTED TUBE

If a Jones tube is lost, it should be replaced within several days to prevent the ostium from closing completely. This is especially true if the tube extrudes close to the time of the initial operation. However, should the ostium close completely or should it be necessary to replace the Jones tube in a different direction, this can be performed with a simpler technique than the original CDCR.

The operation can be performed using general or local anesthesia. If local anesthesia is used, the nasal cavity is packed with $\frac{1}{2}$ to 1 inch of continuous gauze saturated with 4 percent cocaine. Two percent lidocaine with epinephrine is injected subcutaneously over the nasal eyelids and medial canthal area. Topical tetracaine is applied over the eye. A lid speculum then separates the eyelids.

If there is a great deal of medial canthal granulation tissue or a hypertrophic caruncle, a small amount is excised 2 to 3 mm posterior to the skin-mucosal medial canthal junction. A 19-gauge needle is bent slightly and inserted 2 mm posterior to the skin-mucosal medial canthal junction, is directed 30 to 45 degrees inferiorly, and is passed until its tip meets the nasal septum. (Since a CDCR with bone removal has been performed previously, it is possible to direct this needle blindly into the lacrimal sac and bony ostium.) Several passages may be necessary to achieve the proper direction. A Von Graefe knife is then passed along the side of the needle and the needle is withdrawn. The knife then slices in a superior and inferior direction to enlarge the track. A No. 1 or 2 Bowman probe is passed along the shaft of the knife until it meets the nasal septum, and the knife is withdrawn. The Bowman probe is grasped with a hemostat at the position it entered the medial canthal tissue and is withdrawn. The distance from the probe tip to the hemostat is measured. A Jones Pyrex tube 3 to 4 mm shorter than this length is chosen. Usually, a tube with a 3- to 4-mm collar width is desirable.

Subsequently, standard gold dilators are used to enlarge the CDCR track progressively. The chosen Jones tube is then placed over a Bowman probe. The probe is passed into the dilated track, and then the tube is slid with pressure on its collar by the surgeon's thumbnail until the collar rests at the medial canthus. The nasal cavity is inspected to make sure that the tube enters the nasal cavity but clears the nasal septum by at least 3 to 4 mm. The tube is also irrigated with saline to ensure that fluid passes freely from the eye into the nasal cavity. Next, the tube is secured with a 6-0 silk suture wrapped twice behind the tube collar. The suture ends are then passed through the medial canthus and tied over a cotton pledget.

A MODIFIED GLASS TUBE FOR CDCR

The standard Jones glass tube used in a CDCR is at times subject to spontaneous displacement. Either medial migration into the surgically created fistula or lateral displacement and loss are possible. The problems are most frequent in patients who have had radiation therapy in the medial canthal area as treatment for tumors and also in patients who have sustained canthal trauma. In this group of patients, the tissues around the tube do not contract normally to lock the tube in position. Also, there is a group of patients with no obvious predisposition factors who have hypermobile tubes. In all these patients, loss or repeated malpositioning of the Jones tube can cause the procedure to fail. Gladstone and I[4] have developed a modified glass tube (available through Gunther Weiss, Inc.), which successfully eliminates this hypermobility problem in most cases. In addition, a special gold dilator has been developed for insertion of this new tube (also available from Gunther Weiss).

The standard Jones glass tube is 2.2 mm in diameter with a flange at the top (medial canthal end) that varies from 3.0 to 4.0 mm in width. The top flange helps prevent the tube from slipping into the ostium. At the nasal end, the tube gradually flares to a 2.8-mm diameter, which prevents lateral displacement of the tube in a majority of patients (Fig. 15-2A).

The tube Gladstone and I have developed has an additional 2.3-mm wide flange 4 to 6 mm from the top flange (Fig. 15-2B). The second flange anchors the tube in the fistula tissues and significantly decreases the tube's mobility.

To place this tube, a special gold-plated dilator is needed.[4] Standard gold dilators, which have diameters of 2.16 and 2.41 mm, do not adequately dilate the passageway to allow the 3.2-mm flange to pass easily into the ostium. A special dilator with probes measuring 2.67 and 2.92 mm is needed (Fig. 15-2C).

TECHNIQUE FOR PLACEMENT OF MODIFIED PUTTERMAN-GLADSTONE TUBE

After the initially placed Jones tube is removed, topical anesthetic is placed on the eye and injected with a lacrimal irrigating cannula into the existing CDCR fistula. To properly determine the length of the modified glass tube, a Bowman probe is placed through the ostium until it hits the nasal septum. The probe is then grasped at the medial canthus and withdrawn. This provides a measure-

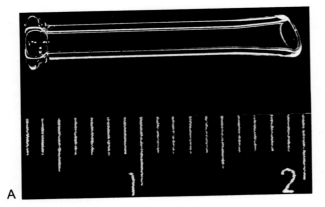

A

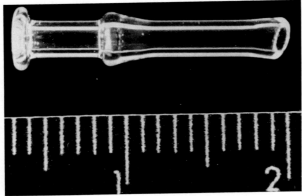

B

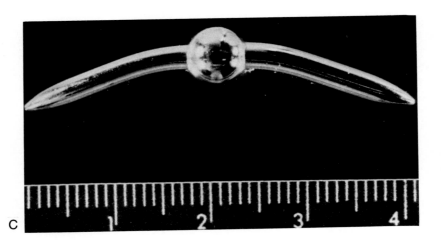

C

Fig. 15-2 (A) Standard Jones glass tube features a top flange of 3 to 4 mm, diameter of 2.2 mm, and gradual flaring out at the nasal end to 2.8 mm. **(B)** Modified glass tube has a second flange, 3.2 mm wide. It is placed 4 to 6 mm from the top flange. This significantly reduces the tube's mobility. **(C)** Special gold-plated dilator is used to insert the modified glass tube. Large-diameter ends allow the 3.2-mm flange to pass easily into tissue.

ment of the distance between the medial canthus and the nasal septum. Three mm is subtracted from this measurement to obtain the appropriate tube length.

Then, progressively larger dilators are inserted until the special 2.92-mm dilator is passed. (If the Jones tube has been recently lost, it is often necessary to begin with the smallest dilator.) The modified glass tube is placed over a Bowman probe, and the probe is passed into the ostium. This helps orient the surgeon as to the proper direction for insertion of the modified tube. The tube is then pushed into place by pressure from the surgeon's thumbnail. A mild to moderate resistance is felt when the 3.2-mm flange encounters the external opening of the fistula. This resistance is usually easily overcome, and the tube is advanced until the top flange is in a good position against the medial canthal tissues.

The position of the tube is then inspected within the nose. Ideally, the tube should protrude approximately 2 mm into the nose and clear the nasal septum by at least 3 mm. The length of the tube can be changed if these criteria are not met.

This technique has been performed in 14 patients, with successful retention of the tube in 12 patients. In these 12 patients, there was relief of symptoms associated with tube hypermobility.[4a]

Care of the modified tube is similar to that of the Jones tube. There is slightly more resistance to removing the tube for cleaning, but this has not been a problem.

COMBINED JONES TUBE-CANALICULAR INTUBATION AND CDCR

In patients with epiphora secondary to lacrimal pump dysfunction, obstruction of only one canaliculus, or common canalicular obstruction, it becomes difficult to decide whether to perform a dacryocystorhinostomy (DCR) or a CDCR. A DCR with excision of the obstructing canalicular tissue and temporary intubation of the lacrimal passages with elastic silicone tubing relieves epiphora in some of these patients. However, recurrent epiphora secondary to stenosis of the lacrimal passages frequently occurs and later requires a conjunctival DCR with placement of a Jones tube. If the Jones tube is inserted during the initial procedure, there will be some failures because the tube may shift or because patients are unwilling to care for the tube postoperatively or unable to tolerate the occasional need for tube replacement or adjustment. Because a conjunctival DCR frequently obstructs or destroys part of the distal or common canaliculi that was not previously obstructed, patients who cannot tolerate the Jones tube may suffer more epiphora postoperatively than preoperatively.

Epstein and I[5] developed a combined Jones tube CDCR with canalicular elastic silicone intubation that makes a second operation unnecessary and preserves the unobstructed canaliculi. When postoperative healing is complete, the elastic silicone tubing is removed and the Jones tube is plugged postop-

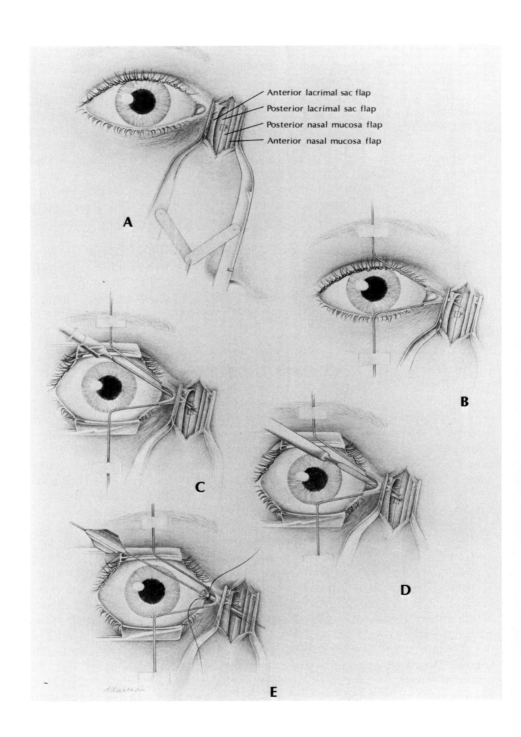

Anterior lacrimal sac flap
Posterior lacrimal sac flap
Posterior nasal mucosa flap
Anterior nasal mucosa flap

A

B

C

D

E

eratively. If the patient remains asymptomatic and the canaliculi can be irrigated freely to the nasal cavity, the Jones tube can be removed. However, if the symptoms recur, the plug can be removed and the Jones tube left in place to relieve symptoms without additional surgery.

The procedure is performed as follows. A DCR is performed according to standard techniques, whereby the posterior nasal mucosal flap is sutured to the posterior lacrimal sac (Fig. 15-3A).[1,2] The anterior tip of the middle turbinate is resected with a rongeur if it rises above the closed posterior flaps.

A punctum dilator is used to dilate the upper and lower lacrimal puncta, and a No. 0 Bowman probe is placed through the upper punctum and canaliculus into the common canaliculus and over the sutured posterior lacrimal sac-nasal mucosal flaps until it meets the nasal septum. A No. 00 or 1 Bowman probe is then placed through the lower punctum and canaliculus in a similar manner. An eyelid speculum is inserted between the eyelids to expose the caruncle. The Bowman probes are bent lateral to the puncta, and the ends are taped to the sterile head drapes (Fig. 15-3B).

The nasal half of the caruncle is excised with Westcott scissors. A 19-gauge needle is bent slightly and inserted 2 mm posterior to the skin-mucosal junction at the medial canthus and is passed over the sutured posterior nasal mucosal-lacrimal sac flaps (Fig. 15-3C). The needle is directed to avoid the intubated canaliculi by passing it anterior or posterior to the Bowman probes. A Von Graefe knife is passed along the side of the needle, and the needle is withdrawn (Fig. 15-3D). The knife then slices in a superior and inferior direction to enlarge the track. A No. 1 or 2 Bowman probe is passed along the shaft of the knife until it meets the nasal septum. The Bowman probe is grasped with a hemostat where it enters the caruncle and is withdrawn. The distance from the probe end to the hemostat is measured, and a Jones Pyrex tube 3 to 4 mm shorter than this length is chosen. A tube with a 3- to 4-mm collar width is desirable. The selected Jones tube is slid onto the probe, and the probe is again passed through the CDCR ostium until its collar rests at the medial canthus; the distal end is within the nasal cavity but at least 3 mm from the nasal septum (Fig. 15-3E). The Bowman probe is removed. The Jones tube is anchored by

---

Fig. 15-3 (A) Posterior flaps of nasal mucosa and lacrimal sac have been closed with a 5-0 Dexon suture. The anterior flaps remain open at this stage. (B) Bowman probes are placed through the upper and lower canaliculi into the common canaliculus and enter the new ostium between the anterior and posterior flaps. The Bowman probes are taped to the surgical drape to ensure stability. (C) A 19-gauge needle is passed 2 mm posterior to the skin-mucosal junction at the medial canthus, while the Bowman probes protect the common canaliculus. The needle may pass anterior or posterior to the probes. (D) A Von Graefe knife is passed through the previous tunnel and then is rotated inferiorly and superiorly to enlarge the tract. (E) A Jones tube placed on a Bowman probe is slid through the tract. A 6-0 black silk double-armed suture is wrapped around the Jones tube several times. (*Figure continues.*)

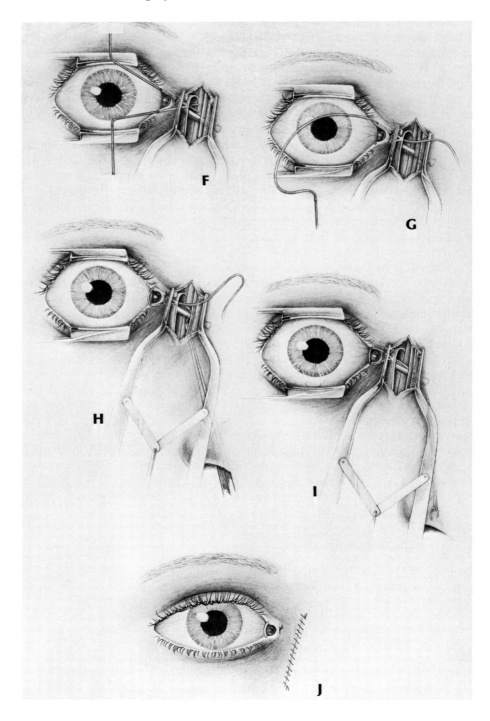

F

G

H

I

J

passing a 6-0 black silk double-armed suture several times around the tube just adjacent to its collar. Each end of the suture is passed through the skin of the medial canthus and tied to prevent the tube from sliding through the large ostium (Fig. 15-3F). A 6-0 black silk suture passed through and around the tube is another way of securing the tube.[3]

A Guibor elastic silicone tube with a Bowman probe cemented to each end is used to intubate the canaliculi. One end of the tube is passed through the upper punctum and canaliculus and over the closed posterior lacrimal sac-nasal mucosal flaps (Fig. 15-3G). The probe is withdrawn from the wound. A sterile ointment placed at the junction of the elastic silicone tube and the Bowman probe facilitates passage of the tube and prevents it from slipping off the metal probe. In a similar manner, the probe at the other end of the tubing is passed through the lower punctum and canaliculus. The metal probes are removed from the elastic silicone tubing.

Nasal forceps are passed through the nasal cavity until the tips are visible over the closed posterior lacrimal sac-nasal mucosal flaps. The tips grasp each end of the elastic silicone tube and pull them into the nasal cavity and out the external nostrils (Fig. 15-3H). A 4-0 polypropylene suture is passed around the tubes at the site where the tubes enter the nasal cavity from the lacrimal sac and where the tubes pass out of the external nostrils (Fig. 15-3I). These sutures prevent postoperative loss or migration of the tube. The long ends of the tubes are then cut so that they are flush with the external nostrils.

The anterior lacrimal sac flap is then sutured to the anterior nasal mucosal flap with several 5-0 Dexon sutures. The periosteum is sutured to periosteum with 4-0 polyglactin 910 sutures, subcutaneous tissue is sutured with 5-0 sutures, and the skin sutured with a continuous 6-0 black silk suture (Fig. 15-3J).

Six days postoperatively, the skin sutures are removed. Three weeks postoperatively, the suture anchoring the Jones tube is removed. After 3 months, the elastic silicone tubing is severed between the upper and lower puncta and slid out of the nose.

The patient begins using dexamethasone phosphate ophthalmic solution four times a day for $1\frac{1}{2}$ weeks and then twice a day for another $1\frac{1}{2}$ weeks. Next, the canaliculi are intubated with a lacrimal needle and irrigated with saline solution. If the saline passes easily to the nasal cavity and no significant canalicular obstruction is present, the Jones tube is plugged with a special poly-

---

Fig. 15-3 (*Continued*). (**F**) The Jones tube ultimately rests 3 to 4 mm lateral to the nasal septum. Each arm of the 6-0 black silk suture is passed on through medial canthal skin to anchor the Jones tube and is then tied. (**G**) An elastic silicone tube is passed through the upper canalicular system and out the lacrimal sac wound. The lower canalicular system is intubated with the other end of the metal probe. (**H**) With the metal probes removed, each arm of the tubing is brought into the nasal cavity and the nostril by grasping with nasal forceps. (**I**) A 4-0 polyester fiber suture conjoins the tubes in the ostium and in the distal nasal cavity to prevent migration. (**J**) Final appearance of combined CDCR with elastic silicone intubation.

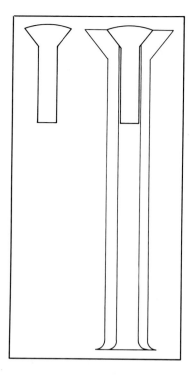

Fig. 15-4   Polyethylene Jones tube plug.

ethylene stent (Fig. 15-4). If the patient remains free of tearing with the Jones tube plugged, removal of the Jones tube is possible. However, if canalicular obstruction or epiphora recurs, the plug is removed and the Jones tube is left in place to drain the tears.

If the patient can tolerate the Jones tube, I believe that it should be left in place postoperatively, even if the normal lacrimal passages are preserved. If the Jones tube cannot be tolerated and the normal lacrimal passages are preserved, it can be removed and the physiologic lacrimal system will function adequately. The Jones tube should be plugged, mainly to determine whether the tube or the canalicular system is functioning primarily in the drainage of tears.

ACKNOWLEDGMENT

This chapter was supported in part by Core Grant 1792 from the National Eye Institute, Bethesda, Maryland.

EDITOR'S COMMENTS

Since the description of conjunctivodacryocystorhinostomy (CDCR) by Jones in 1961,[6,7] reports concerning the success rate have varied. Experienced lacrimal surgeons have published personal success rates as high as 86 percent,[8,9] while one review from a large hospital clinic found only a 40 percent success rate.[10] There are good reasons for these divergent experiences with CDCR, and they merit some discussion.

The concept of providing tear drainage through a small pipe, or Pyrex Jones tube, is straightforward, but implementation is quite difficult. This problem is compounded by the fact that very few patients need the procedure and few ophthalmologists will perform CDCR regularly. Consistent surgical success will only be possible if the surgeon has knowledge of nasal anatomy, training in surgical technique, and an adequate inventory of equipment. A large inventory of Jones tubes must be available, varying in length, shape (straight or curved), and collar size. Furthermore, success of the initial procedure only marks the beginning of a lifelong maintenance responsibility. Neglected Jones tubes will inevitably fail.

It has been reported that some patients will maintain a patent fistula after the late removal of a Jones tube,[11] and a mucous membrane graft is said to improve this approach.[12] Unfortunately, the editor has observed the prompt closure of a CDCR fistula when a tube was removed after ten years. This area is controversial, but the editor believes it is unwise to promise any patient that he or she will be able to discontinue use of the tube without risk of recurrent obstruction.

Candidates for CDCR must understand and accept the need for regular examinations and periodic tube manipulation. They must be prepared for the possibility of secondary surgery since granuloma formation, medial migration, nasal synechia, and other malpositions can occur.[13] Even drug toxicity has been reported.[14] Clearly the opportunities for failure are not uncommon, and long-term success will require consistent care from a qualified physician.

The problems with CDCR are analogous, in the editor's mind, to the challenge of contact lens fitting. A successful contact lens experience will depend upon patient selection, physician skills, and long-term follow-up. Success rates will vary widely in different settings.

The good news is that CDCR can be satisfying for both patient and surgeon. Candidates for CDCR have often experienced a number of previous surgical failures and appreciate the difficulty of their problems. They are most grateful when the Jones tube begins to function and provide good tear drainage. With proper care, the Jones tube can provide long-term relief.

REFERENCES

1. Putterman AM: Oculoplastic surgery. p. 2281. In Peyman GA, Sanders DR, Goldberg MF (eds): Principles and Practice of Ophthalmology. WB Saunders, Philadelphia, 1980
2. Jones LT, Wobig JL: Surgery of the Eyelids and Lacrimal System. p. 195. Aesculapius Publishers, Birmingham, Alabama, 1976
3. Putterman AM: Fixation of Pyrex tubes in conjunctivodacryocystorhinostomy. Am J Ophthalmol 78:1026, 1974

4. Gladstone GJ, Putterman AM: A modified glass tube for conjunctivodacryocystorhinostomy. Arch Ophthalmol 103:1229, 1985

4a. Mighori M, Putterman AM: A followup report of recurrent Jones tube extrusions treated with a modified glass tube. To be published.

5. Putterman AM, Epstein G: Combined Jones tube-canalicular intubation and conjunctival dacryocystorhinostomy. Am J Ophthalmol 91:513, 1981

6. Jones LT: An anatomical approach to problems of the eyelids and lacrimal apparatus. Arch Ophthalmol 66:111, 1961

7. Jones LT: Conjunctivodacryocystorhinostomy. Am J Ophthalmol 59:773, 1965

8. Welham RA, Guthoff R: The Lester-Jones tube: A 15 year follow-up. Graefe's Arch Clin Exp Ophthalmol 223:106, 1985

9. Lamping K, Levine MR: Jones' tubes: How good are they? Arch Ophthalmol 101:260, 1983

10. Lisman RD, Smith B, Silverstone P: Success rate of conjunctivodacryocystorhinostomy. Presented at the 17th Annual Scientific Meeting of the American Society of Ophthalmic Plastic & Reconstructive Surgery, Nov 8, 1986

11. Carroll JM, Beyer CK: Conjunctivodacryocystorhinostomy using silicone rubber lacrimal tubes. Arch Ophthalmol 89:113, 1973

12. Campbell III CB, Shannon GM, Flanagan JC: Conjunctivodacryocystorhinostomy with mucous membrane graft. Ophthalmic Surg 14:647, 1983

13. Pameijer JH, Henkes HE, Deblecourt PW: Experiences with the Jones tube in the Rotterdam Eye Clinic. Ophthalmologica Basel 171:353, 1975

14. Wood JR, Anderson RL, Edwards JJ: Phospholine iodide toxicity and Jones' tubes. Ophthalmology 87:346, 1980

16 | Endoscopy

John V. Linberg

Lacrimal surgery is peculiar in that the surgeon cannot directly visualize the anatomic result of a procedure, and results are generally evaluated in terms of function. In contrast, an ophthalmologist can usually inspect the results of other ocular procedures throughout the postoperative course because of the clarity of ocular media. While functional success is surely the most important objective for patient and doctor, visual inspection of an anatomic result provides an opportunity to evaluate surgical techniques and understand failures.

I first became involved with this dilemma as a fellow-in-training, while examining patients after dacryocystorhinostomy. I initially expected to observe a large and obvious intranasal ostium, since the opening created during surgery measures 10 to 20 mm. To my surprise and frustration, swollen mucosa prevented any view in the early postoperative period, and later no ostium was readily visible. Seeking the assistance of an otolaryngologist, I observed that even an experienced rhinologist had difficulty visualizing the DCR opening with head-mirror and speculum. It was at this juncture that I was introduced to nasal endoscopy, and enjoyed my first view of the intranasal DCR ostium.[1]

Over the subsequent eight years, nasal endoscopy has become routine in my evaluation of lacrimal disorders and has added a new dimension to my experience in lacrimal surgery. While the vast majority of lacrimal problems can be managed without endoscopy, this technique for nasal examination often removes the guesswork in difficult situations. Endoscopy has provided many opportunities for research, teaching, and improved patient care, and I recommend endoscopy to any serious student of lacrimal surgery.

INSTRUMENTATION

Endoscopy has become important in many medical subspecialties, and a variety of instruments are available in the general hospital setting. This fortunate circumstance often allows the lacrimal surgeon to try endoscopy without the initial expense of purchasing an instrument. The approach seems appropriate historically, since the first efforts at nasal endoscopy by Hirschmann were accomplished using a cystoscope designed by Nitze.[2,3]

Fiberoptic endoscopes offer the advantage of a flexible probe, and are required in many applications. However, image resolution is limited by the size of individual fibers that conduct the light, and brightness is sometimes marginal.[4] Other problems with fiberoptic endoscopes include expense, vulnerability to damage, difficulty with sterilization, and vagaries in control of the instrument's direction of view.[4]

Areas of interest in lacrimal surgery are accessible to rigid endoscopes with conventional solid optical elements. The advantages of these instruments include lesser expense, durability, and a brighter image with better resolution. Although my experience has been almost entirely with the Hopkins telescopic endoscope manufactured by Karl Storz, other designs and manufacturers are available, and I have no proprietary interest in any instrument. The emphasis given to the Hopkins telescope in this chapter is merely a result of my experience and is not meant to imply that other systems may not be equally useful.

A rigid rod lens telescope was developed by Professor H. H. Hopkins and bears his name.[5] Hopkins endoscopes are used in urology, laparoscopy, arthroscopy, and otorhinolaryngoscopy and are widely available. The rod lenses are cylinders of optical-quality glass with lens surfaces at each end. These rods are positioned so as to create air lenses between them. The rod lens design results in fewer air-glass interfaces than with conventional optical systems, producing a bright, clear image with little spherical aberration. While the image is carried by the solid rod lenses, illumination is provided by a bundle of fiberoptic strands that run along the periphery of the lens tube to the instrument tip. Dedicated systems for still photography,[6,7] video,[8] and cinematography[9] are commercially available, and "home-made" systems may also be fabricated.[10,1]

The Hopkins telescopic endoscope is available in three diameters (1.4 mm, 2.7 mm, 5.5 mm) and three viewing angles (0°, 30°, 70°). When the endoscope is introduced into the nose parallel to the septum, the structures of interest are on the lateral nasal wall. As a result, the 70° viewing angle (Fig. 16-1). is most useful for visualizing the DCR ostium[1,11] or the opening of the nasolacrimal duct under the inferior turbinate.[12,13] The nasal passages of most adults are large enough for the 5.5 mm diameter instrument, which provides the widest image. The smaller diameter instruments are useful in children or for looking under the inferior turbinate, a cramped area even in adults.[12,13]

TECHNIQUE

Nasal endoscopy is easily accomplished in an outpatient clinic setting under topical anesthesia, and sedation is not necessary. The examination should be entirely painless. Patients are naturally apprehensive at first sight of the chrome-plated probe, but they may be reassured that it has no sharp edges. It

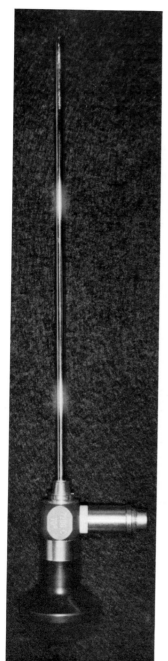

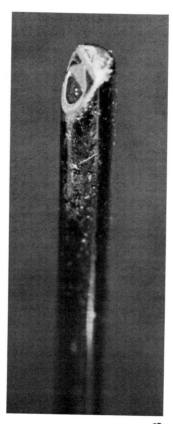

Fig. 16-1 (**A**) Hopkins rod lens telescope: 5.5 mm diameter, 70° viewing angle. (**B**) Magnified view showing blunt tip of endoscope.

A

B

is helpful to use the term "telescope" and let the patient look briefly through the eyepiece. If the first examination is performed gently after adequate explanation, subsequent evaluations can be accomplished quickly and with very little ado.

Before embarking on a discussion of the mechanics of endoscopy, the surgeon should consider the relationship between endoscopy and conventional nasal examination with a speculum. Ever since the division of otorhinolaryngology from ophthalmology, the nasal examination of lacrimal patients has been problematic.[14] Lacrimal disorders are generally regarded as the province of the ophthalmologist, but it is the otolaryngologist who receives training in nasal anatomy and examination. Some lip service is given to the concept that ophthalmology residents should receive instruction in nasal examination, but there has been little provision for this training. Chapter 3 is devoted to conventional techniques of nasal examination.

In the context of ophthalmology, it is important to understand that endoscopy is not a substitute for the conventional nasal examination. Indeed, endoscopy cannot be comfortably or successfully performed until after the standard nasal examination has been mastered. The endoscope must be introduced into the nose and directed to the area of interest without injury or pressure to nasal structures. The magnified and therefore limited field of view through an endoscope is confusing unless the landmarks of intranasal anatomy are familiar. Thus the conventional intranasal examination with headlight and speculum is a necessary first step in endoscopic technique.

Endoscopy can be performed without anesthesia, but the use of surface anesthetic agents does increase patient comfort. Four percent lidocaine hydrochloride applied with a nasal atomizer works well. Nasal decongestion with $\frac{1}{4}$ or $\frac{1}{2}$ percent phenylephrine hydrochloride will shrink nasal mucosa and facilitate manipulation of the endoscope. Neo-Synephrine should be avoided in cardiac patients, since a substantial amount of the drug can be absorbed.

Surgery, infection, allergy, and trauma all cause impressive edema of the nasal mucosa, but in most cases this obstacle can be overcome. Packing the nose with a cotton pledget moistened by 4 percent cocaine solution is very effective, and safe if the total dose is limited to 3 mg/kg. After a few minutes the first pack will open some space, and it can be replaced by a second packing higher in the nose. In this manner serial nasal packs will permit endoscopic examination of a dacrocystorhinostomy (DCR) ostium even a few hours after surgery.

Two areas are of principle interest in lacrimal surgery: (1) the site of a DCR ostium anterior to the middle turbinate, and (2) the opening of the nasolacrimal duct under the inferior turbinate (Fig. 16-2).

A good view of the DCR ostium is obtained using the 5.5 mm diameter Hopkins telescopic endoscope with a 70° view angle. The examiner introduces the rod through the nares with its axis parallel to the septum and at an angle of about 45° in relation to the frontal plane of the face (Figs. 16-2 and 16-3). The viewing port is directed laterally, away from the midline. The instrument passes in front of, and over, the anterior tip of the inferior turbinate. The

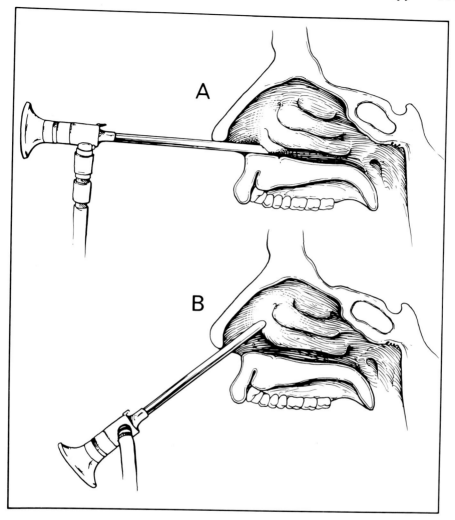

Fig. 16-2 Correct position of endoscope for visualization of **(A)** nasolacrimal duct ostium under inferior turbinate and **(B)** area of intranasal DCR ostium or Jones tube.

examiner guides the endoscope into the nose, using no force or pressure, and then immobilizes the instrument with both hands before viewing. A light touch is required because the instrument is long and can create considerable leverage within the nose. With some experience the examiner can position the endoscope for the desired view before using the eyepiece. This is helpful because once the examiner looks into the endoscope, there is no external frame of visual reference and the instrument tends to "drift."

The opening of the nasolacrimal duct under the inferior turbinate is more difficult to visualize because of limited space.[12,13] A smaller diameter (2.4 mm)

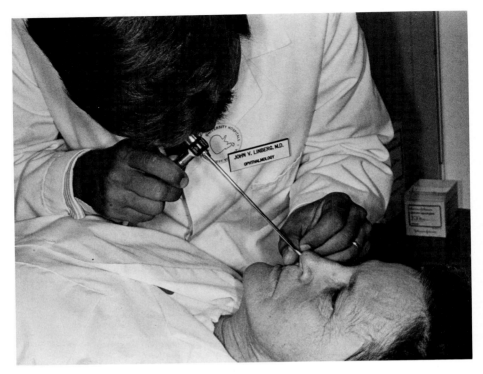

Fig. 16-3 Endoscopic examination of intranasal DCR ostium performed in the out-patient clinic using topical anesthesia. Note that endoscope is positioned in the sagittal plane, at a 45° angle to the frontal plane of the face. The instrument is gently inserted into the nose and immobilized with both hands before examination through the eyepiece begins.

instrument is introduced through the nares, along the floor of the nose, with the viewing port directed upward (Fig. 16-2B). Packing the area briefly with a cocaine-moistened pledget of cotton will again increase the available space and improve comfort.

Fogging of the endoscope tip by humidity within the nose can be a problem. Warming the probe in hot tap water before using it is helpful. Also, the patient can be instructed to inhale slowly through the nose and then exhale through the mouth during the examination. If mucus sticks to the endoscope viewing port, the instrument must be withdrawn and cleaned.

Once clinical observations have been completed and recorded, photographs may be taken. A flash generator and camera adaptor are commercially available. A standard single-lens reflex 35 mm camera with 100 mm lens will produce good still pictures. Photography is more difficult than direct viewing because the weight of the camera makes the endoscope unwieldy, and the image seen through the camera viewfinder is dim. Fortunately, the lens focus is set at "infinity" and no adjustment is required.

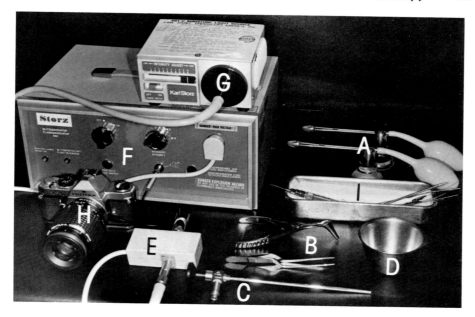

Fig. 16-4 Instruments for endoscopy arranged on a portable cart for clinic use. A, Atomizers with lidocaine hydrochloride 4 percent and phenylephrine hydrochloride $\frac{1}{4}$ percent. B, Nasal speculum and bayonet forceps for initial nasal examination using conventional techniques. C, Hopkins rod lens telescope. D, Container for hot water used to warm the endoscope tip and prevent fogging. E, Flash tube for photography. F, Flash generator for photography. G, Cold light source for endoscope examination. Fiberoptic light cord attaches to flash tube and provides continuous light for examination and positioning of endoscope prior to photography. H, Camera, a 35 mm SLR, with 100 mm macro lens. Adaptor on end of lens allows attachment of endoscope eyepiece. I, Tray for lacrimal irrigation or probing, which is sometimes performed simultaneously with endoscopy.

If the drugs, instruments, and equipment necessary for endoscopy are organized on a cart, then the examination can be performed with little loss of time or efficiency (Fig. 16-4).

CLINICAL FINDINGS

The intranasal ostium following successful DCR is remarkably consistent in appearance and location (Fig. 16-5).[1] The opening is situated just in front of the anterior tip of the middle turbinate, and typically measures less than 2 mm in diameter. Fluorescein instilled in the conjunctiva will rapidly appear at the ostium. If any doubt exists as to the identification of the surgical ostium, a Bowman probe may be passed through the canaliculus into the nose, and observed with the endoscope. The endoscopic view includes the middle turbinate

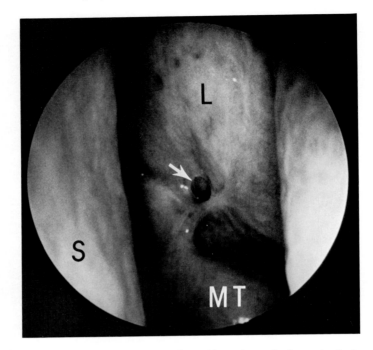

Fig. 16-5 Typical healed intranasal DCR ostium (arrow). Important structures for orientation are the septum (S), anterior tip of middle turbinate (MT), and lateral wall of nose (L). Diameter of ostium is approximately 2 mm.

and septum (Fig. 16-5), allowing the examiner to correctly identify the site of DCR surgery even if no ostium is present.

Occasionally the intranasal ostium will measure 3 to 5 mm, permitting a view of the recessed lacrimal sac mucosa (Fig. 16-6).[11] The irregular gray appearance of lacrimal sac mucosa is distinctly different from the thick, smooth, red mucoperiosteum of the nasal wall. Lacrimal sac mucosa will be seen to move laterally with each blink,[11] lending some credence to the concept of a lacrimal diaphragm proposed by Lester Jones.[15] However, patients have normal tear drainage after successful DCR in spite of the large DCR ostium, which obviously prevents any negative pressure gradient within the sac. These observations demonstrate that other mechanisms of lacrimal drainage physiology must be more important than the lacrimal diaphragm.

Given the large opening (10 to 20 mm) created during DCR, it is surprising and sometimes frustrating how quickly the opening shrinks after surgery. During the first postoperative week the ostium is covered with blood clot and mucus, making measurement difficult. At 2 weeks the view begins to clear, and usually the ostium has already shrunk to less than half of its operative size (Fig. 16-7). Within 2 or 3 months the ostium is reduced to an opening of a few millimeters (Fig. 16-8). The reduction in size is perhaps less surprising if we

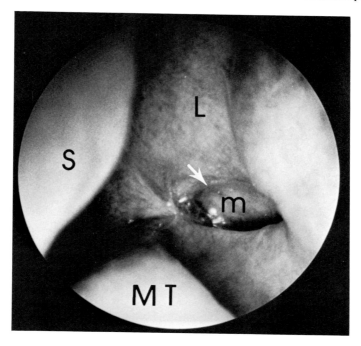

Fig. 16-6 Same view as in Fig. 16-5, but in a patient with an unusually large (3 × 6 mm) intranasal DCR ostium. The lacrimal sac mucosa (M) can be seen through the large ostium. During "real-time" endoscopy the movement of the lacrimal sac diaphragm can be observed with each blink.

Fig. 16-7 DCR ostium (arrows) two weeks after surgery, measures about 5 × 10 mm. A bridge of fibrous tissue (b) crosses the opening. The septum (S) is seen on the left.

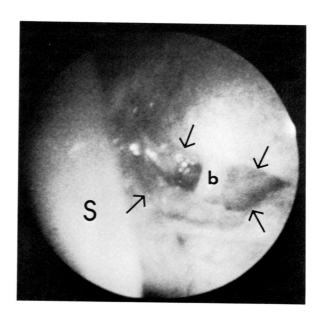

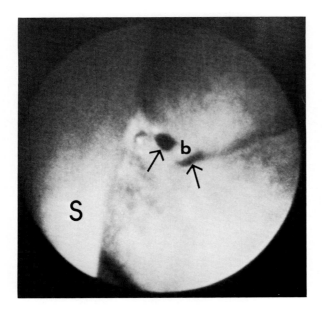

Fig. 16-8 Same patient as in Fig. 16-7, 9 weeks after uncomplicated DCR. Two small ostia are seen (arrows), approximately 2 mm in diameter, separated by a band of fibrous tissue (b). Septum (S) is seen on the left.

remember that the total daily output of the lacrimal glands is only 1.25 ml.[16] Clearly, an opening of 2 mm is perfectly adequate for the small volume of normal tear secretion, and patients with even small openings are typically free of epiphora.

A variety of stents, bolsters, packs, and sponges have been advocated for

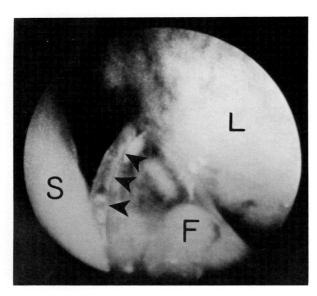

Fig. 16-9 DCR ostium 1 day after surgery. Fat (F) has prolapsed through the rhinostomy. Stents (arrows) have been placed. Septum (S) and lateral wall (L) of nose are marked.

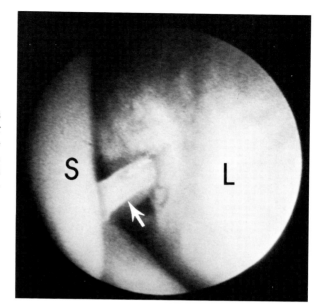

Fig. 16-10 Same patient as in Fig. 16-9 4 weeks after surgery. The prolapsed orbital fat is no longer seen, and an ostium is maintained by the stent (arrow). S, septum; L, lateral wall of nose.

DCR surgery. The 2 mm size of the final nasal ostium suggests that the small-diameter silicone tubes used for canalicular intubation are appropriate for DCR surgery,[1] and larger tubes are not required. Endoscopy provides some clues as to when these stents may be removed. Figure 16-9 was taken 1 week after a difficult DCR procedure, with prolapse of orbital fat into the surgical window. A stent is seen emerging from the fresh ostium. Four weeks later the nasal mucosa has closed the opening except for a fistula maintained by the stent, and orbital fat is no longer seen (Fig. 16-10). A functioning ostium remained open after removal of the stent, and its appearance was no different from that of uncomplicated DCRs performed without a stent. As demonstrated by this example, endoscopy can be used to verify when surgical edema and inflammation have resolved and healing is complete. Healing in the nasal mucosa is rapid, and prolonged use of stents is not necessary in most cases. The generally accepted practice of leaving stents in place for several months has probably resulted, at least in part, from the inability in the past to directly observe when healing has occurred.

Endoscopy will sometimes reveal small granulomas growing around the silicone stent at the intranasal ostium.[13] Similar granulomas occur around the eyelid puncta in some patients with stents,[17] and are probably an indication for stent removal (Fig. 16-11).

Silicone stents are best removed from the nose after the loop is cut at the medial canthal angle (Figs. 16-12 and 16-13). Unfortunately these tubes are sometimes difficult to locate in the nose with conventional examination techniques, especially if the knot becomes lodged under a turbinate. There is usually

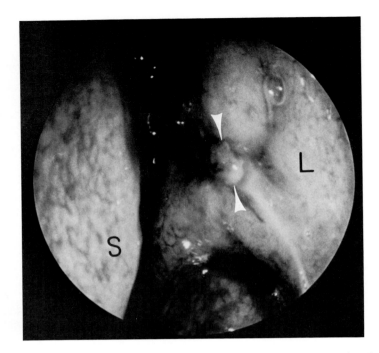

Fig. 16-11 Site of unsuccessful DCR with granuloma (arrows) obstructing the ostium. S, septum; L, lateral wall of nose.

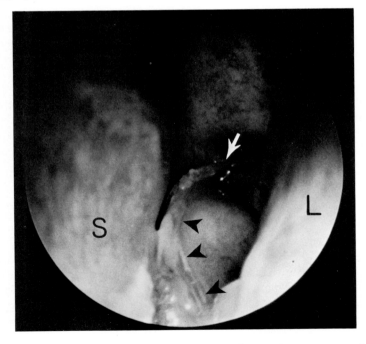

Fig. 16-12 View of silicone tubes (black arrows), in nasal passages, maintaining a DCR ostium (white arrow). S, septum; L, lateral wall of nose.

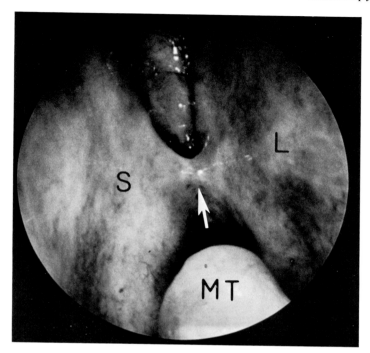

Fig. 16-13 Synechia (arrow) between septum (S) and site of DCR ostium, just above the anterior tip of the middle turbinate (MT). L, lateral wall.

little difficulty finding stents (Fig. 16-12) placed during DCR surgery, but stents placed in the nasolacrimal duct and knotted under the inferior turbinate can be troublesome. The "blind" manipulation of instruments under the turbinate often results in bleeding, pain, and edema. If the endoscope discloses that a stent has retracted up into the nasolacrimal duct, the nasal approach can be abandoned. If the stent is seen, it can be hooked under endoscopic visualization or, at least, instruments can be directed to the correct location.

Synechiae sometimes occur between the DCR ostium in the lateral wall of the nose and the septum, and may contribute to surgical failures (Fig. 16-13).[13] These adhesions result from inadvertent and unnecessary trauma to the mucosa of the septum. Postoperative edema usually produces apposition of septal mucosa and the DCR opening, and fibrous attachments will result if the septal mucosa is not intact. A nasal packing, properly positioned, will protect septal mucosa during the DCR dissection and is helpful for hemostasis. If a surgeon encounters frequent postoperative synechiae, a postoperative pack may be needed to prevent contact between septum and ostium. Synechiae should be removed during reoperation, and in this situation a postoperative packing will help avoid recurrence of synechiae. Endoscopic surgery has been described[13,18] and might be used for removal of synechiae.

The evaluation of DCR failures is an area in which endoscopy can be very

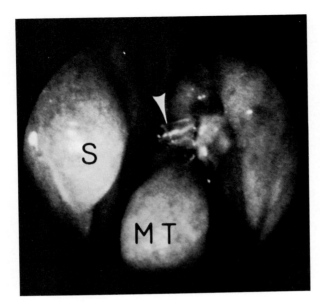

Fig. 16-14 Intranasal view of Jones tube (arrow) in good position. Note the excellent clearance between the end of the tube and the septum (S), above the middle turbinate (MT). This patient has an exceptionally wide nasal passage.

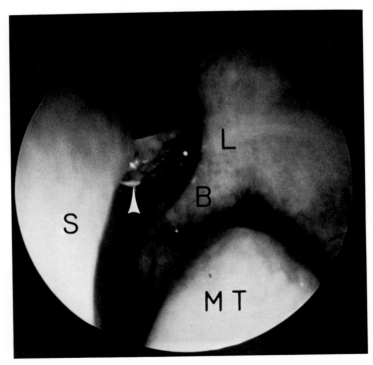

Fig. 16-15 Excessively long Jones tube is shown with tip (arrow) pressing against the septum (S). Tube emerges from the lateral wall (L) of the nose, just above the base (B) of the middle turbinate (MT).

useful. The distinction between closure of the nasal ostium and common canalicular stenosis is sometimes difficult to establish by probing or irrigation. The exact diagnosis is important because DCR reoperations are relatively easy and have a high success rate, whereas repair of common canalicular stenosis requires different techniques and has a guarded prognosis. If endoscopy shows an open ostium in the nasal mucosa and probing produces visible tenting of the lacrimal sac mucosa, a canalicular stenosis is present. If no intranasal ostium is seen and probing produces tenting of the nasal mucosa, closure of the DCR opening is the correct diagnosis.

Sometimes when epiphora persists after DCR surgery, the endoscope will disclose a normal, patent intranasal ostium. In these cases the physician's attention should be directed toward the possibilities of eyelid malposition, lacrimal pump failure, punctal stenosis, canalicular disease, or dry eye symptoms. We might assume that these conditions had been excluded before surgery, but individual cases can be confusing, and more than one factor may be contributing to epiphora. Direct observation is likely to reassure both patient and doctor that the operation has been successful, at least to the extent of establishing lacrimal sac drainage. The presence of a patent nasal ostium will prevent future

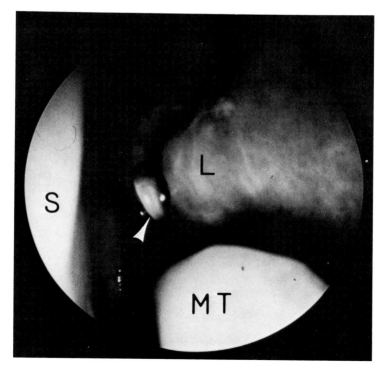

Fig. 16-16 Intranasal view of Jones tube (arrow) that is too short and barely projects through lateral wall (L) of nose. S, septum; MT, middle turbinate.

episodes of acute dacryocystitis even if tearing persists. With this reassurance, the patient is more likely to accept attention to the other aspects of lacrimal function.

The placement and maintenance of Jones tubes is described in Chapter 5, and the subject is mentioned here only in regard to the usefulness of endoscopy. The proper position of a Jones tube within the nose (Fig. 16-14) is critical to both comfort and function. Many patients requiring a Jones tube have a difficult nasal examination due to past trauma or previous surgery. In these cases, preoperative endoscopy will determine if there is adequate space for a properly positioned Jones tube, or whether nasal surgery will be required prior to the Jones tube placement. During surgery, the surgeon can use the endoscope to choose the correct length and position of a tube.

The endoscope is especially helpful in the postoperative care of Jones tubes, because visualization assists in the diagnosis and management of problem cases. As lid and intranasal edema resolve after surgery, a tube that initially seemed correctly placed may press against the septum (Fig. 16-15) and require replacement with a shorter tube. On the other hand, a short tube will occasionally be observed to recede into the nasal ostium (Fig. 16-16), with the threat of fistula closure. In these cases the indication for a longer replacement is clear

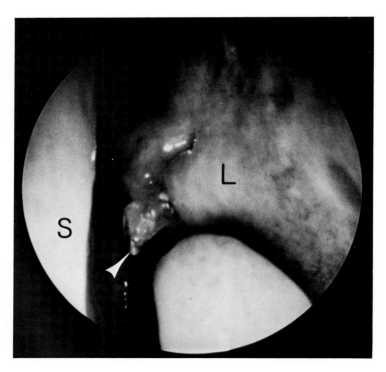

Fig. 16-17 Same patient as in Fig. 16-16, after replacement of Jones tube (arrow) with one long enough to clear the lateral wall (L) without impinging on the septum (S).

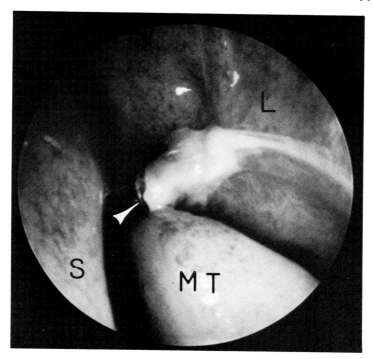

Fig. 16-18   Intranasal view of Jones tube (arrow) that is covered and obstructed by debris. This tube will function well once it has been removed and cleaned. S, septum; MT, middle turbinate; L, lateral wall of nose.

(Fig. 16-17). When a Jones tube fails to drain, endoscopy may demonstrate obstruction of the nasal end by mucous and cellular debris (Fig. 16-18). If the position is good, only a cleaning is required. The interval at which Jones tubes require cleaning is quite variable, and endoscopy facilitates maintenance of good function without excessive manipulation, by allowing a detailed inspection without removal.

In my experience, endoscopy has provided substantial assistance in the diagnosis and management of Jones tube patients. It is in this area that endoscopy has provided the greatest improvement in patient care.

SUMMARY

Endoscopy provides excellent visualization of the intranasal aspect of lacrimal surgery. The technique is simple, and easily performed in an outpatient clinic setting, using local anesthesia. The Hopkins telescopic endoscope, a commercially available instrument that is used in a variety of other medical subspecialties, is available in a general hospital setting. Photographic documentation is possible. These techniques can be valuable to patient care, research, and teaching.

ACKNOWLEDGMENT

This work was supported in part by an unrestricted departmental grant from Research to Prevent Blindness, Inc., New York, NY.

REFERENCES

1. Linberg JV, Anderson RL, Bumsted RM et al: Study of intranasal ostium external dacryocystorhinostomy. Arch Ophthalmol 100:1758, 1982
2. Hirschmann A: Uber Endoskopie der Nase und deren Nebenhohlen. Eine neue Untersuchungsmethode. Arch Laryng Rhinol 14:195, 1903
3. Nitze M: Eine neue Beobachtungs- und Untersuchungs-methode der Harnblase. Wien med Wschr 24:649, 1879
4. Jaumann MP, Steiner W: Endoscopy of the nose and nasopharynx. Endoscopy 10:240, 1978
5. Hopkins HH: Optical principles of the endoscope. Chapter 1. In Berci G (ed): Endoscopy. Appleton-Century-Crofts, New York, 1976
6. Hawke M: Endoscopic photography of the ear: An update. J Biol Photog Assoc 52:19, 1984
7. Katzenberg B: Annotated bibliography of endoscopy. J Biol Photog Assoc 52:25, 1984
8. Sommerlad BC, Hackett MEJ, Watson J: A simplified method of recording in nasal pharyngoscopy. Br J Plastic Surg 28:34, 1975
9. Rabinovitz ND, Stool SE: Endoscopic cinematography. J Biol Photog Assoc 52:15, 1984
10. Yanagisawa E: Videolaryngoscopy using a low cost home video system color camera. J Biol Photog Assoc 52:9, 1984
11. Tajima Y, Maruyana N, Ikegami M: Endoscopic observations on the internal surface of the lacrimal sac following dacryocystorhinostomy. Acta Soc Ophthalmol Jpn 76:1242, 1972
12. Cibis GW, Jazbi BU: Nasolacrimal duct probing in infants. Trans Am Acad Ophthalmol Otolaryngol 86:1488, 1979
13. Bosshard C: Endoscopy of the nose as an aid in lacrimal duct surgery. Klin Mbl Augenheilk 180:303, 1982
14. Jones LT, Boyden GL: The rhinologist's role in tear sac surgery. Trans Am Acad Ophthalmol Otolaryngol 34:654, 1951
15. Jones LT: An anatomical approach to problems of the eyelids and lacrimal apparatus. Arch Ophthalmol 66:111 1961
16. Moses RA (ed): Adler's Physiology of the Eye. CV Mosby, St. Louis, 1974
17. Anderson RL, Edwards JJ: Indications, complications and results with silicone stents. Ophthalmology 86:1474, 1979
18. Stammberger H: Endoscopic endonasal surgery—Concepts in treatment of recurring rhinosinusitis. 2. Surgical technique. Otolaryngol Head Neck Surg, 94:147, 1986

17 | History of Lacrimal Surgery

Roberto Javier Vásquez

The evolution of lacrimal surgery is a fascinating story. It began several thousand years ago with an empirical approach to problems of the lacrimal drainage system, and only recently has developed into a scientific approach with a firm anatomic and physiological basis. Early treatment of lacrimal disorders was not based on knowledge of the pathology, but was motivated by the need to relieve troubling symptoms. Radical cure of lacrimal disease was attempted by surgery, frequently after several vegetable and mineral remedies had been applied to the patient. The results accomplished by a few early surgical techniques remained practically unchanged for many centuries, as the following summary of early developments reveals.

The Code of Hammurabi, around 2250 BC, makes the first documented reference to the surgical treatment of a lacrimal fistula or a lacrimal sac abscess: "If a physician performs on a patient a deep cut with the operating knife or if he opens with the knife a nagabti and the eye is lost then the physician's hands should be cut."[1]

The ancient medical literature from Egypt, China, and India does not mention any surgical procedure for the lacrimal apparatus. However, the Greeks of the Alexandrian time clearly documented their methods for the treatment of the lacrimal abscess and fistula. Their surgical approach was empirical, but they had some anatomic knowledge.

Aulus Cornelius Celsus from Rome (25 BC to about 50 AD) treated the lacrimal fistula (aigilops) with excision, cautery, and burning.[1] The Syrian Archigenes of Apamea (1st century AD) mentioned three operations: (1) incision into the canthus followed by trephination of several small holes into the bone close to the nose, the application of caustic medication, and pouring of molten lead through a funnel; (2) baring of the bone and application of a branding iron;

315

and (3) incision and introduction of a small metal funnel that reaches the bone through which molten lead can be applied.[1]

Medical knowledge during the Roman Empire was derived from the work of earlier Greek authors. Galen of Pergamon (131 to 201 AD) probed the lacrimal punctum of animals with a hair.[1] Aetius from Amida, Mesopotamia (around 540 AD) performed excision of the lacrimal sac within the capsule and applied cautery.[1] Paulus from Aegina (around 668 AD) mentioned the three operations of Archigenes, but thought trephination of the bone unnecessary.[1]

With the decline of the Roman Empire, the Arab world became the repository for Greek medical knowledge, but added little to the development of lacrimal surgery. Ibn Sina from Bokhara (980 AD to 1037 AD) recommended the application of mongo bean (an Indian treatment) with a probe to the fistula. The same probe could be wrapped with wool, moistened with an astringent solution, and introduced into the fistula's depths.[1]

No significant advances in lacrimal surgery were made during the Middle Ages and the Renaissance. Ambroise Pare of France (b. 1510) used a metal shield to protect the eye during cauterization of the fistula.[1] Fabricius ab Aquapendente of Italy (1537 to 1619) devised a tube for the same purpose, and also advised the use of an enlarged incision.[1]

MODERN TRENDS

After centuries of minor, isolated developments, the modern era of lacrimal surgery began in the early 18th century. The innovations of Stahl and Anel, based on the anatomic contributions of Morgagni, Zinn, Rosenmüller, Vesal, and Fallopia, led to a rapid development of techniques and instruments for scientific lacrimal surgery. In some cases, the sudden increase in knowledge led to the simultaneous development of several techniques. Some of these techniques are still performed today, while others were tried for a brief time and discarded. Some have continued to evolve until the present day. This variable pattern of development makes it impossible to describe the modern history of lacrimal surgery in strict chronological order. Thus, we will discuss the development of each surgical procedure individually, bearing in mind that the procedures often overlap and that sometimes a minor modification in one technique has signified a great advance or provided the basis for a new procedure.

PROBING, DILATION, AND IRRIGATION OF THE LACRIMAL SYSTEM

Modern techniques of probing, dilation, and irrigation have had their roots in the work of earlier surgeons. Morgagni clarified the historical antecedents of this form of lacrimal surgery in 1723, pointing out that Galen was the first to probe the lacrimal punctum of animals with a hair. Morgagni recognized that the veterinarians of the 5th century had injected medications into the canaliculi using small tubules, and that Valsalva (1666–1723) had probed the lacrimal system from the punctum into the nose.[1]

In 1702, Stahl published a monograph that described how he treated the lacrimal fistula by introducing a violin string through the upper lacrimal punctum into the sac and then made an incision into it. A stent wetted in balsam was introduced and left for two weeks until no more pus appeared at the punctum. Compresses were used to complete the treatment.[1]

Anel developed a new lacrimal system probing method in 1713. He introduced a fine, blunt silver probe through the upper punctum, sac, and nasolacrimal duct. Through the lower punctum, he injected an astringent fluid with a fine-tip syringe. This maneuver was repeated daily until the fluid could easily reach the nasal cavity. The method generated conflicting opinions, encouraging many surgeons to follow him and others to experiment with different approaches.[1]

In 1715, Bianchi recommended probing and irrigating the nasolacrimal duct through the lower punctum, using a curved hollow probe.[1] De la Faye (1739) and De la Foreste (1753) performed this difficult maneuver, and Gensoul (1826) and Rau (1854) improved it.[1]

In 1734, Petit incised the lacrimal sac through the skin and then introduced a grooved probe through the entire nasolacrimal duct. A wick was inserted

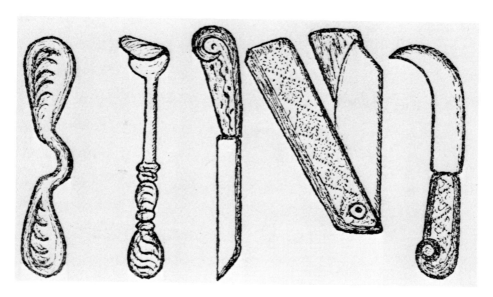

Fig. 17-1 Instruments used for skin incision and exposure of the lacrimal sac, from an English manuscript (1650–1680), following the technique of Petit. The patient was tied to the arms of a chair, and the head held by an assistant while the surgeon made an arcuate incision at the internal canthus over the lacrimal sac. (Ovio F: Storia dell'oculistica. Vol. 1. Cuneo, Edizioni Ghibaudo, 1950, p. 412.)

along the groove and replaced daily until the duct was healed, at which time the external wound could be closed (Fig. 17-1).[1]

In 1750, Mejean introduced a thread through the nasolacrimal duct and then wicks soaked in almond oil and green balsam (basilicon). A gold probe with a thread tied to an upper eyelet was pushed into the nose. The probe was removed and the thread cut off. Mejean then fastened a wick to the thread and pulled it into the duct, applying a new wick every day until the duct was healed. This procedure was still popular in the early 20th century (Fig. 17-2).[1]

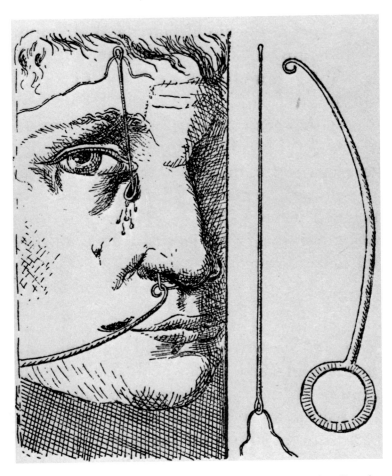

Fig. 17-2 Lacrimal pathway drainage by Benoit Mejean, 1753. An olive-tipped probe was introduced through the puncta, the fistula opening, or a cutaneous incision; a violin strand was attached to it through an eyelet. The probe was pulled from the nose with a hook. Note the similarity of the principle and instruments to the modern Crawford's method and intubation set. (Ovio G: Storia dell'oculistica. Vol. 1. Cuneo, Edizioni Ghibaudo, 1950, p. 413.)

In 1780, Blizard poured mercury through a fine tubule into the lacrimal puncta to cause mechanical dilation of the obstructed nasolacrimal duct.[1] Until the first decade of the 20th century, his method was still used by some ophthalmologists.

The next major development took place in 1857, when Bowman promoted the slitting of the canaliculus with a canalicular knife and dilation of the nasolacrimal duct with progressively larger probes, up to 1.5 mm in diameter, that were left in place for 15 minutes each. Treatments were performed daily, every other day, and then at longer intervals for a year, when the treatment was considered complete.[2] In 1863, Weber introduced several modifications to Bowman's technique. The superior canaliculus was slit with a canalicular knife; the nasolacrimal duct was dilated with thick probes (up to 2.0 mm in diameter); and, occasionally, the nasolacrimal canal was fractured. This was called the "rapid dilation method."[3] Agnew, in 1871, described the alternative of making an incision between the medial commissure and the caruncle, so that the lacrimal sac could be reached easily for drainage of the pus and probing. This incision avoided slitting the canaliculus or incision of the skin over the sac.[4] His innovation was attractive to many surgeons. In 1913, Verhoeff used a small triangular keratome to reach the sac. The keratome was introduced in front of the caruncle; the rest of the treatment followed Bowman's principles but used Theobald's probes.[5]

Ziegler, in 1910, performed the rapid dilation method with probes of his own design that had diameters of up to 4 mm. Years later he claimed that only 1 percent of his cases required repeated treatment (Fig. 17-3).[6,7]

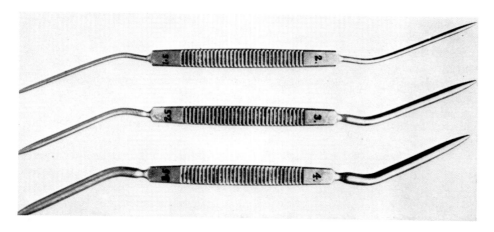

Fig. 17-3 Ziegler's lacrimal dilators introduced in 1912 for rapid dilation of the nasolacrimal duct. They were 40 mm long with diameters up to 4 mm. The probes were also used in intranasal DCR procedures. (Ziegler SL: A further note on rapid dilation in the radical treatment of lacrimal disease. JAMA 78:1701, 1922. Copyright 1922, American Medical Association.)

Golowin took rapid dilation to an extreme in 1923, performing traumatic dilation of the nasolacrimal duct using probes of 9 mm in diameter.[8] The rapid dilation method was still in vogue in 1928, when Brown used an expandable sea tangle probe.[9] The idea of expandable probes originated in the work of Critchett, who used *Laminaria* in 1864.[10]

CURETTAGE

Curettage of the nasolacrimal duct was introduced and used for only a brief time. During the final years of the 19th century, some European surgeons followed Mandelstamm, who performed this procedure; the technique was improved by Tartuferri.[7] In 1918, Thompson revived the curettage,[11] and in 1919, Green combined it with rapid dilation of the nasolacrimal duct.[12] Some years later the procedure was still advocated, but "only when there is proliferation in the lumen of the duct."[7] Today curettage has disappeared entirely.

GALVANOTHERAPY

With the intention of destroying the contents of the nasolacrimal canal and bypassing a stricture in the duct, Gorecki, in 1889, inserted a Bowman's probe into the canal as an anode while a platinum cannula was placed in the nostril as the cathode. Then, 2 mA of galvanic current were applied for 30 seconds. In 1908, Lotin applied 5 mA for 5 minutes through a silver wire in the fistula as the anode, placing the cathode in the nostril.[10] McEnery Brown reported his experience with galvanotherapy in 1910.[13] In 1931, Worms and Filliozat, as well as Defoug, revived the technique in Europe. In 1932, Weekers used currents of 700 mA for 2 to 3 seconds but without good results. In 1933, Spinelli reached the lacrimal sac through a skin incision, applied diathermy to the duct, and left a rubber tube in the duct for 12 days. In 1942, Morgenstern used 125 mA to bypass strictures of the duct, reporting good results with his technique.[14]

NASOLACRIMAL DUCT TUBULES AND STYLES

In order to maintain patency of a dilated nasolacrimal duct, many surgeons have experimented with tubules or solid styles. These devices have been placed temporarily or permanently, introduced through a sac incision or, rarely, through a slitted canaliculus. This technique has undergone many innovations, and intubation is widely used today for the treatment of congenital nasolacrimal duct obstruction.

In 1793, Ware suggested the placement of a nailheaded solid silver style into the nasolacrimal duct, to be left there for 4 to 6 weeks.[10] In 1801, Scarpa reported the use of a lead style (Fig. 17-4).[15] This was not free of complications, and at least one patient died of tetany.[1] In 1911, Smith introduced, through a

In 1889, Killian described an intranasal approach to resolve the problem of dacryostenosis. After resecting the anterior portion of the inferior turbinate, he inserted a Bowman probe as a guide in the nasolacrimal duct. He then opened the duct after removing the bony wall covering it.[46]

In 1893, Caldwell reported removing part of the inferior turbinate with an electric trephine until he had reached the nasolacrimal duct. He then followed the duct up until reaching a probe that had been passed through the canaliculus into the duct and thus established drainage.[47] Caldwell is credited as the first to attempt an intranasal approach to the tear sac.

In 1910, West resected a window in the nasal wall of the nasolacrimal canal and duct above the inferior turbinate, removing part of the lacrimal bone and superior maxilla.[48] This procedure was the basis of many variations that appeared in the following years.

In 1912, Polyak elevated a piece of nasal mucoperiosteum but did not save it. After a wide exposure of the lacrimal sac, he removed its entire nasal wall.[49] In 1914, Halle used a technique similar to Polyak's, reflecting back a flap of nasal mucoperiosteum before severing the sac from the nasolacrimal duct. He then returned the flap to its original position, cutting out a small hole for tear drainage. The purpose of the flap was to prevent the reflux of air through the canaliculi from the nose.[50]

Between 1910 and 1930, many ophthalmologists and otolaryngologists modified the endonasal approach. Some of them were Yankauer in 1912,[51] Bryan in 1912,[52] Khoronshitzky in 1914,[53] Hoffman in 1914,[54] Glogau in 1915,[55] Hanger in 1915,[56] Bookwalter in 1920,[57] Weiner and Sauer in 1920,[58] Koffler and Urbanek in 1925.[59]

In 1921, Mosher, previously a firm advocate of the intranasal approach, abandoned the technique after a tragic, complicated case. Instead he favored a combined external and intranasal approach, the so-called Mosher-Toti operation.[60] Despite early interest, fewer reports on the endonasal method appeared during the 1930s and 1940s. Most of these were small series of cases reported by otorhinolaryngologists. In 1937, Walsh and Bothman reported an 87.5 percent success rate in their 20-case series.[61] In 1942, Morgenstern used the intranasal approach to destroy the lacrimal sac mucosa by electrocoagulation.[23] The intranasal DCR is more appropriate for rhinologists than ophthalmologists. It never became popular, and has virtually been abandoned.

TRANSPLANTATION OF THE LACRIMAL SAC

In 1904, Speciale devised transplantation of the lacrimal sac using a cadaver, and then tested it in two patients without satisfactory results. Using a skin incision, he exposed the lacrimal sac and freed the lower end from surrounding tissues. He transected the sac as far down in the bony canal as possible, and elevated it. He then drilled a 9-mm opening through the nasal process of the superior maxilla, incised the underlying nasal mucosa, and inserted the lower free portion of the lacrimal sac through the rhinostomy. On his last patient he sutured the sac to the nasal mucosa. He published this operation in 1913.[62]

In 1911, Forsmark used the same approach but pulled the lower portion of the mobilized lacrimal sac into the nasal cavity with a suture. The thread was fastened in the cheek.[63] In the same year, Neumayer reported a technique similar to Forsmark's.[64]

In 1920, Burch introduced several modifications to Forsmark's technique. He first mobilized the sac from the lacrimal sac fossa up to the medial canthal tendon, and then mobilized the upper 5 to 6 mm of the nasolacrimal duct from the nasolacrimal canal (using Stevens tenotomy scissors and a flattened, blunt-tipped probe). He also made a bony window through the nasal process of the superior maxilla and resected the underlying nasal mucosa. He slit the nasal side of the nasolacrimal duct from its lower end upward a short distance into the sac, and then tucked the sac and duct through the bony opening. He introduced a soft rubber catheter or lead style through the canaliculus into the nose and left it for 1 week or more.[65]

In 1921, MacMillan placed the bony opening over the lacrimal bone and drew the lacrimal sac down into this opening by means of sutures attached in its lower end.[66]

Several variations of this idea appeared in the following years: Fasakas in 1924,[67] De Lieto Vollaro in 1929,[68] Del Barrio in 1929,[69] Rosengren in 1931[70] Stock in 1934,[71] and Stokes in 1935.[72] Gifford published one of the last reports on the operation and claimed an 80 percent success rate.[73] The most successful results were obtained when the rhinostomy was located in the ascending process of the maxilla. The procedure never became popular, and has not been reported since the late 1940s.

LACRIMAL PUNCTUM SURGERY

Localized stenosis of the punctum can sometimes be enlarged by dilation, but in other cases requires surgery. An early approach was dilation and simultaneous slitting of the canaliculus using Bowman's or Weber's technique (see p. 319). In 1858, Critchett used a three-snip procedure[10] and Viers still recommended it in 1955.[74] Jones condemned the procedure in 1962, arguing that it destroys the ampulla and the lacrimal pump.[75] Since 1954, Jones had been using a one-snip procedure in which a vertical cut, 2 mm long, is made in the conjunctival side of the horizontal segment of the canaliculus.[76] Later (1962) he changed the position of the cut to the vertical segment of the canaliculus.[75] In 1930, Haitz used a punch to treat punctal stenosis,[77] a method similar to the posterior lid excision reported by Hughes and Maris.[78] In 1977, Fein used applications of cautery around the ostium.[79]

The treatment of the dry eye syndrome sometimes requires the closure of the lacrimal punctum or canaliculus. This procedure was introduced in 1783 by Bosche, who performed it with caustic solutions prior to cataract surgery in patients with dacryocystitis. In 1891, Haab also recommended this method.[1] During the first half of this century the indications for the obliteration of the lacrimal punctum and/or canaliculi included prevention of ocular infection prior to intraocular surgery as well as cases of corneal or conjunctival disease thought to be influenced by infection of the lacrimal sac, filamentary keratitis, and keratoconjunctivitis sicca. The application of galvanocautery 5 to 6 mm inside the canaliculus or inside the ostium of the punctum was enough to achieve a permanent result.[80] Diathermy probes can also be used for this purpose.[81] In order to evaluate a patient's response to punctal occlusion, Beard performed a temporary ligature of the canaliculi.[10] The introduction of rods of gelatin,[82] chromic or plain catgut, and collagen,[83] plugs of silicone,[84] or the use of tissue adhesive (*N*-butyl cyanoacrylate),[85] are recent devices used for the temporary relief of the dry eye. Laser occlusion of the punctum has been used recently for a more permanent result, but no scientific report documents the procedure.

TREATMENT OF CANALICULAR STENOSIS

Dacryocystorhinostomy has a very high success rate in cases of epiphora secondary to the obstruction of the nasolacrimal duct. Stenosis located between the lacrimal lake and the sac is more difficult to repair.

Slitting of the canaliculus was performed by Bowman with his probes, and later by Weber with a canalicular knife, as we previously mentioned. This mutilating procedure, the stricturotomy, was still popular in the early 20th century but was gradually abandoned.

A number of other procedures have been developed in an attempt to treat canalicular stenosis more effectively. They are discussed below.

Canaliculodacryocystotomy

Canaliculodacryocystotomy was invented by Jones in 1954 to relieve strictures in the region of the internal common punctum, when the sac and duct are in good condition. He threaded a 22-gauge polyethylene tube through the lateral patent section of the canaliculus into the tear sac and down the nasolacrimal duct. Then he closed the lacrimal sac and sutured the flaps to the canaliculus.[76]

Canaliculorhinostomy

Arruga described canaliculorhinostomy in 1935 for cases in which the sac was absent or had to be removed. After performing a rhinostomy with a trephine, he introduced a probe into the lower canaliculus and cut the tissues covering the tip of the probe. He extended the incision vertically to obtain two lips that were sutured to flaps of nasal mucosa.[86] In 1979, Pashby and Rathbum reported good results with the use of a silicone tube for this procedure.[87]

Canaliculodacryocystorhinostomy

Canaliculoadacryocystorhinostomy is useful when the medial portion of the canaliculus or the common canaliculus is stenosed with or without compromise of the nasolacrimal duct. In 1953, after performing a DCR, Henderson bypassed the stricture in the common canaliculus using a polyethylene tube, leaving only 2 mm of the tube inside the sac.[88] In 1960, Jones advised the dissection of the canaliculi and the stricture in the common canaliculus. He performed a DCR and then excised the stricture. The remaining canaliculi were intubated using polyethylene tube and sutured to the sac wall.[89] In 1970, Tenzel reported the dissection of the stricture from inside the opened lacrimal sac.[90] More procedures followed; Werb used polyethylene tubes, and Quickert and Dryden used silicone tubes. Hurwitz has refined these techniques and clarified the indications, using a dacryocystogram for accurate diagnosis (see Ch. 14).

Reconstruction of damaged canaliculi is technically very difficult, and therefore surgeons have sought to establish new drainage pathways rather than salvage the abnormal canaliculi. During this century several modalities of surgical treatment appeared. Free grafts of labial mucosa or dermis, sutured over a tubular conformer, were placed between the lacrimal lake and the lacrimal sac through an incision at the caruncle. The first to use this method was Hoffman in 1904,[91] followed by Morax and Valiere-Vialeix in 1925.[92] Several modifications and reports on the procedure appeared in the following years: Jeandelize and Baudot in 1926,[93] Nizetic in 1936,[94] Thiel in 1942,[95] Guy in 1943,[96] Beiras Garcia in 1944,[97] Bargerter in 1947,[98] Tessier and Hervouet in 1951,[99] and Rycroft in 1951.[100] These free grafts gradually were abandoned because of their tendency to retract even when the conformer was left in place for long periods. Hoping to obtain a better graft viability, Roveda in 1952[101] and Burch Barraquer in 1953[102] used a pedicule graft of bulbar or cul-de-sac conjunctiva respectively.

Lacodacryocystostomy

Lacodacryocystostomy—anastomosis of the lacrimal lake to the sac—was introduced in 1937 by Zarzycki.[103] He sectioned the canaliculi remnants and, if they were completely obstructed, opened them with a conical probe. He then opened the lacrimal sac and united the two canalicular channels to the sac under the medial canthal tendon. After this, he sutured an advancement flap of bulbar conjunctiva to the posterior edge of the lacrimal sac mucosa. This procedure gained wide acceptance because of its simplicity. Several surgeons modified this procedure: Stallard in 1940,[104] Gomez Marquez in 1944,[80] and Valiere-Vialeix and Robin in 1953.[105] Because many cases were associated with an absent or severely damaged sac, Zarzycki's technique was often insufficient, and lacorhinostomy was the logical consequence. The pioneers of lacorhinostomy were Silva Costa in 1936[106] and Vila-Coro in 1942,[97] followed by Casanellas[80] and Belmonte Gonzalez in 1944.[107]

When the condition of the sac is good, a lacodacryocystorhinostomy can be performed. Introduced by Moulie in 1944,[108] this procedure was improved by Burch Barraquer[109] in 1968 as an alternative to the Jones conjunctivodacryocystorhinostomy. Burch used all of the available sac mucosa, cutting a long flap to form the posterior wall of the anastomosis with the bulbar conjunctiva. The nasal mucosa exposed by a wide osteotomy was fashioned into a long anterior flap that was sutured to conjunctiva.

Conjunctivodacryocystorhinostomy

In 1962, Jones[75] described a new procedure to be used when no functioning canaliculi are present. He completed a DCR up to the suturing of the posterior flaps of the nasal and tear sac mucosa (or lacrimal fascia, if the sac were missing). He then resected the caruncle and inserted a 23-gauge, 30-mm hypodermic needle from the lacrimal lake into the nose just anterior to the middle turbinate. Using the needle as a guide, he enlarged the passage with a cataract knife and inserted an 18-mm polyethylene tube. After 1 to 3 weeks, he substituted a Pyrex glass tube for the polyethylene one. In 1965, Weil, Sorana, and Cremona performed Jones' procedure but used an autogenous vein sutured to the nasal mucous membrane and conjunctiva.[110] In 1969, Reinecke and Carroll reported the use of a molded silicone tube instead of the Pyrex tube used by Jones.[111]

External Conjunctivorhinostomy

External conjunctivorhinostomy consists of implanting a synthetic tube (silicone and Pyrex) between the medial canthus of the nasal vestibule. The tube is implanted in a nearly vertical position through the soft tissues overlying the bony structure of the face. The technique was introduced by Murube del Castillo in 1966.[112] Other procedures designed to bypass the canaliculi include conjunctivobuccostomy,[113] which drains the lacrimal lake into the oral cavity, and conjunctivoantrorhinostomy,[114] which communicates with the antrum of the maxillary sinus.

REPAIR OF CANALICULAR LACERATIONS

Lacerations in the medial canthal area are often accompanied by transection of the canaliculus. Several devices and techniques have been developed for repairing these injuries. In 1948, Heinz used an indwelling horsehair as a stent to reconstruct the canaliculus.[10] Years later, Stallard recommended a strand of blue nylon for the same purpose, when the lower canaliculus was lacerated between the punctum and the medial canthus. He used a Rohrschneider's canaliculus cannula to pass the nylon strand retrograde through the upper canaliculus into the lacerated lower canaliculus. This was called the

Greaves' operation, and when it could not be accomplished, Stallard performed a retrograde intubation with nylon passed through an opening in the medial wall of the lacrimal sac into the lower canaliculus. When only a few millimeters of the lower canaliculus were occluded, he reconstructed the segment with a conjunctival flap, following a technique used by Meller.[115] In 1957, Jones used a 22-gauge polyethylene tube to reconstruct the canaliculus.[116] In 1962, Worst designed the "pigtail" probe, a spiral-shaped probe with a miniature hook in the tip, similar to the Rohrschneider's cannula. He canalized the upper and lower canaliculi with polyethylene tubing, tied between the two puncta, thus forming a closed loop.[117] The Worst probe frequently caused false passages and the hook destroyed tissue when the course of the instrument was reversed. Beyer modified the instrument in 1974, eliminating the hook and placing a French eye at the tip of the probe.[118]

In 1962, Viers introduced the use of malleable rods 10 to 12 mm in length and 0.6 mm in diameter, with a 4-0 black silk suture swaged to one end. The rod was passed through the punctum and canaliculus, bridging the severed edges. The wound was repaired and the silk suture emerging from the punctum was secured to the skin.[119] In 1974, Johnson used the silver wire from a #1 or 2 Bowman probe to stent the canalicular repair.[120] In 1984, Beyer-Machule used a silver wire inside a thin silicone sleeve, with a silicone plate that allowed fixation to the skin.[121]

LACRIMAL GLAND SURGERY

The extirpation, total or partial, of the lacrimal gland has been performed for epiphora and tumors. During the 18th century several surgeons performed this surgery: Daviel in 1741, Guerin in 1769, Demours in 1818, Travers in 1821, and Velpau in 1831.[1] The palpebral dacryoadenectomy was performed by Wheeler in 1915, in combination with a dacryocystectomy.[122] This approach was supported by Taiara and Smith in 1973, who reported that its effectiveness was enhanced by other procedures, especially Jones' conjunctivo-dacryocystorhinostomy.[123]

In 1845, Bernard used cauterization for ablation of the gland. Bettremiux used galvanocautery, and Streiber used a diathermy needle for the same purpose. These methods led to a significant inflammatory reaction. Tille destroyed the gland using titrated injections of 90 percent alcohol, repeated as necessary.[81]

The openings of the excretory ductules of the lacrimal gland can be obstructed by cauterization, but the result is said to be temporary, and therefore Friede[81] sectioned the ductules. This procedure was revived by Jameson in 1937.[124] The results were often disappointing, and the procedure eventually fell into disuse.

CONCLUSION

The developments described in this chapter include the most important aspects of the history of lacrimal surgery. Some procedures have survived the test of time and are widely used today, for example, the external DCR. Other procedures such as punctal occlusion are still evolving as new materials appear. Canalicular reconstruction is difficult, with success rates lower than for DCR. The alternatives to canalicular reconstruction—conjunctivodacryocystorhinostomy and external conjunctivorhinostomy—still seem to many ophthalmologists not the most clever solution. I hope that this historical review will help surgeons develop new ideas based on past experience, without repeating past errors.

ACKNOWLEDGMENT

This work was supported in part by an unrestricted departmental grant from Research to Prevent Blindness, Inc., New York, NY.

REFERENCES

1. Hirschberg J: The History of Ophthalmology. Vol. 3. JP Wayenborgh Verlag, Bonn, 1984
2. Bowman W: On the treatment of lacrymal obstructions. R Ophthalmol Hosp Rep 1:10, 1858
3. Weber A: Ueber das thranenableitungssystem. Anatomie der thranenleitenden wege. Klin Monatsbl Augenheilkd 1:63, 1863
4. Agnew CR: Practical suggestions for the treatment of lachrymal diseases. Am Practitioner 3:1, 1871
5. Verhoeff FH: Treatment of acute dacryocystitis. JAMA 60:727, 1913
6. Ziegler SL: The radical treatment of lacrimonasal disease by rapid dilation and allied measures. JAMA 54:2026, 1910
7. Ziegler SL: A further note on rapid dilation in the radical treatment of lacrimal disease. JAMA 78:1701, 1922
8. Meller J: Diseases of the lacrymal apparatus. Trans Ophthalmol Soc UK 49:233, 1929
9. Brown AL: A method of dilating the lacrymal duct by rapid dilatation with sea tangle probes—preliminary report. Arch Ophthalmol 57:397, 1928
10. Hughes SM: The history of lacrimal surgery. In Bosniak SL (ed): History and Tradition. Advances in Ophthalmic Plastic and Reconstructive Surgery. Vol. 5. Pergamon Press, Elmsford, NY, 1986
11. Thompson WR: The rational etiology and satisfactory treatment of dacryocystitis. JAMA 71:1727, 1918
12. Green J Jr: The treatment of dacryocystitis by curettage (Thompson): Supplemented by immediate rapid dilatation of the lacrimonasal duct. Am J Ophthalmol 2:723, 1919
13. McEnery Brown W: The treatment of the lacrimal sac. Ann Ophthalmol 19:259, 1910

14. Morgenstern DJ: Chronic tearing cured by reestablishment of normal tear conduction passages. Arch Ophthalmol 27:775, 1942
15. Burns RP: Eyelids, lacrimal apparatus and conjunctiva. Arch Ophthalmol 79:211, 1968
16. Sing DS, Garg RS: Polyethylene intubation of the nasolacrimal duct in chronic dacryocystitis. Br J Ophthalmol 56:914, 1972
17. Scarpa A: Saggio di Osservazioni ed Esperienze sulle Principalli Mallatie degli Occhi, Briggs J (trans). T Cadell and W Davies, Strand, London, 1806. Reprinted in The Classics of Ophthalmology Library. Gryphon Editions, Ltd, Birmingham, U.K., 1984
18. Smith P: On the use of lacrymal styles. Ophthalmic Rev 30:257, 1911
19. Quickert MH, Dryden RM: Probes for intubation in lacrimal drainage. Trans Am Acad Ophthalmol Otolaryngol 74:431, 1970
20. Anderson RL, Edwards JE: Indications, complications and results with silicone stents. Ophthalmology 86:1474, 1979
21. Blaskovics L: Zwei Falle von Tranensackeiterung, geheilt durch die Totische Operation. Z Augenheilkd 27:92, 1912
22. West JW: Die totale extirpation des tranensackel vonder nase aus mit Wiederherstellung des normalen abflusses in fallen von dakryocystitis. Z Augenheilkd 45:159, 1921
23. Morgenstern DJ: Intranasal drainage for cure of chronic tear sac infection. Arch Ophthalmol 27:733, 1942
24. Hogan MJ: Dacryocystorhinostomy. Trans Am Acad Ophthalmol Otolaryngol 52:600, 1948
25. Toti MA: Nuovo metodo conservatoire de cure radicale delle suppurazioni chroniche del sacco lacrimale (Dacriocistorinostoma). Clinica Moderna 10:385, 1904
26. Toti MA: The treatment of dacryocystitis by the formation of a fresh passage from sac to nasal cavity (dacryocysto-rhinostomy). Ophthalmic Rev 28:287, 1909.
27. Kuhnt H: Notiz zur technick der dacryozystorhinostomie nach Toti. Z Augenheilkd 31:379, 1914
28. Lowenstein A: Dakryozystorhinostomie nach Toti oder Eroffnung des Tranensackes von der Nase aus (West-Polyak)? Prag Med Wchnschr 39:489, 1914
29. Soria: Estudio historico y critico de la dacriocistorrinostomia. Arch Oftalmol Hispano-Am 21:104, 1921
30. Soria: Veinticinco anos de dacriocistorrinostomia 1919–1944. Arch Soc Oftalmol Hispano-Am 4:807, 1944
31. Ohm J: Bericht uber 70 Totische operationen. Z Augenheilkd 46:37, 1921
32. Mosher HP: The Mosher-Toti operation on the lachrymal sac. Laryngoscope 31:284, 1921
33. Dupuy-Dutemps L, Bourget: Cure de la dacryocystitie cronique commune et du larmoiment par la dacryocystorhinostomie plastique. Bull Acad Med Paris 86:293, 1921
34. Basterra J: Dacriocistorrinostomia. Arch Oftalmol Hispano-Am 26:385, 1926
35. Arruga H: Eine Veranderung in die Form des Trepans um die Durchbohrung des Knochens bei der Totischen Operation zu erleichtern. Klin Monatsbl Augenheilkd 82:239, 1929
36. Gutzeit R: Ein neues Knocheninstrumentarium zue Toti-operation. Klin Monatsbl Augenheilkd 84:92, 1930
37. Iliff CE: A simplified dacryocystorhinostomy. Trans Am Acad Ophthalmol Otolaryngol 58:590, 1954

38. Krasnov MM: Ultrasonic dacryocystorhinostomy. Am J Ophthalmol 72:200, 1971
39. Hallum AV: The Dupuy-Dutemps dacryocystorhinostomy. Am J Ophthalmol 32:1197, 1949
40. Abrahamson IA Jr, Stichel FL: Dacryocystorhinostomy: Report of a case with wire fistulization. Am J Ophthalmol 36:710, 1953
41. Romanes GJ: Dacryocystorhinostomy. Clinical report of fifty cases. Br J Ophthalmol 39:237, 1955
42. Bonaccolto G: Dacryocystorhinostomy with polyethylene tubing: Simplified technique. J Int Coll Surg 28:789, 1957
43. Veirs ER: Aids in restoring patency in obstructions of the lacrymal drainage system. Am J Ophthalmol 56:977, 1963
44. Mirabile TJ, Tucker C: Dacryocystorhinostomy with silicone sponge. Arch Ophthalmol 74:235, 1965
45. Gibbs DC: New probe for the intubation of lacrimal canaliculi with silicone rubber tubing. Br J Ophthalmol 51:198, 1967
46. Killian J: Diskussion zu Seiferts Vortrag, 6 Versamml. suddeutsch. Laryngologen, 1889
47. Caldwell GW: Two new operations for obstructions of the nasal duct with preservation of the canaliculi. Am J Ophthalmol 10:189, 1893
48. West JM: A window resection of the nasal duct in cases of stenosis. Trans Am Ophthalmol Soc 12:654, 1910
49. Polyak L: Ueber das Eroffnen des Ductus nasolacrymalis im vorderen Teile des mittleren Nasenganges. Z Augenheilkd 27:92, 1912
50. Halle F: Zur intranasalen Operation am Tranensack. Arch Laryngol Rhinol 28:256, 1914
51. Yankauer S: The technic of intranasal operations upon the lacrimal apparatus. Laryngoscope 22:1331, 1912
52. Bryan WMC: Submucous dacryocystorhinostomy for persistent dacryocystitis. Ann Ophthalmol 21:497, 1912
53. Khoronshitzky B: Die perkanalikulare Tranensackdurchstechung als Einleitung zur intranasalen Tranensackeroffnung und als selbstandige Operation. Arch Laryngol Rhinol 28:363, 1914
54. Hoffmann R: Ueber Dakryocystorhinostomie. Monatsschr Ohrenh 48:985, 1914
55. Glogau, O: A case of Dacryo-cysto-rhinostomy. Laryngoscope 25:28, 1915
56. Hanger FM: An intranasal operation without a guide for the cure of dacryocystitis. Laryngoscope 25:23, 1915
57. Bookwalter CF: Intranasal dacryocystostomy. Arch Ophthalmol 49:568, 1920
58. Weiner M, Sauer WE: New operation for the relief of dacryocystitis through nasal route. JAMA 75:868, 1920
59. Koffler K, Urbanek J: Eine Method der Vereinfachung der West-Polyakschen endonasalen Tranensackoperation. Z Augenheilkd 57:200, 1925
60. Mosher HP: Re-establishing intranasal drainage of the lachrymal sac. Laryngoscope 31:492, 1921
61. Walsh TE, Bothman L: Some results of intranasal dacryocystorhinostomy. Am J Ophthalmol 20:939, 1937
62. Speciale F: Sulla dacriorinostomia (secondo Toti). La Clinica Oculistica 13:1369, 1913
63. Forsmark E: Om dacryocysto-rhinostomien. Hygiea 73:1432, 1911
64. von Eicken C: Ein neues Verfahren zur Beseitigung von Stenosen des Tranennasenkanals. Verh Dtsch Laryngol 600, 1911

65. Burch FE: Conservation of the lacrimal sac. A method. Trans Am Acad Ophthalmol Otolaryngol 1:137, 1920

66. MacMillan JH: A new operation for the treatment of lacrimal obstruction. Am J Ophthalmol 4:448, 1921

67. Fasakas A: Neue Modifikation der Dakryozystorhinostomie. Klin Monatsbl Augenheilkd 73:426, 1924

68. De Lieto Vollaro A: Di un procedimiento personale di dacriocistorinostomia semplificata a modificazione del metodo fondamentale del Toti. Bollettino D'oculistica 8:561, 1929

69. Del Barrio A: Dacriocistorrinostomia y sus diversas tecnicas. Arch Oftalmol Hispano-Am 29:18, 1929

70. Rosengren B: En modifikation av Totis operation. Det oftal. Selskabis 1931, Forhandl. Dansk. Medicinisk Selkskab Hospitalstidende, Jorgensen & Co., Kobenhavn, Denmark, p. 24, 1932

71. Stock F: Ueber die Erfolge der Operation der Tranensackeiterung nach Einpflanzung des unteren Endes des Tranensacks in die Nase. Klin Monatsbl Augenheilkd 92:433, 1934

72. Stokes WH: Refinements in tear sac surgery. Nebr St M J 20:388, 1935

73. Gifford H Jr: Dacryocystitis. The transplantation operation. Arch Ophthalmol 32:485, 1944

74. Viers ER: The lacrimal system: Clinical applications. Grune & Stratton, New York, 1955, p. 48

75. Jones LT: The cure of epiphora due to canalicular disorders, trauma and surgical failures on the lacrimal passages. Trans Am Acad Ophthalmol Otolaryngol 66:506, 1962

76. Jones LT: Epiphora: Its causes and new surgical procedures for its cure. Am J Ophthalmol 38:824, 1954

77. Haitz E: Zur Behandlung der Tranenpunkstenose. Klin Monatsbl Augenheilkd 85:541, 1930

78. Hughes WL, Maris CSG: A clip procedure for stenosis and eversion of the lacrimal punctum. Trans Am Acad Ophthalmol Otolaryngol 71:653, 1967

79. Fein W: Cautery applications to relieve punctal stenosis. Arch Ophthalmol 95:145, 1977

80. Arruga H: Ocular Surgery. 3rd Ed. McGraw-Hill, New York, 1962

81. Dohlman CH: Punctal occlusion in keratoconjunctivitis sicca. Ophthalmology 85:1277, 1978

82. Foulds WS: Intra-canalicular gelatin implants in the treatment of keratoconjunctivitis sicca. Br J Ophthalmol 45:625, 1961

83. Schwab IR: Keratoconjunctivitis sicca. p. 54. In Abbott RL (ed): Surgical Intervention in Corneal and External Diseases. Grune & Stratton, Orlando, FL, 1987

84. Freeman JM: The punctum plug: Evaluation of a new treatment for the dry eye. Trans Am Acad Ophthalmol Otolaryngol 79:874, 1975

85. Patten JT: Punctal occlusion with N-butyl Cyanoacrylate tissue adhesive. Ophthalmic Surg 7:24, 1976

86. Arruga H: La curacion del lagrimeo en los casos en que habia sido extirpado el saco lagrimal. Soc Oftalmol Barcelona, 1935

87. Pashby RC, Rathbum JE: Silicone tube intubation of the lacrimal drainage system. Arch Ophthalmol 97:1318, 1979

88. Henderson JW: Management of strictures of the lacrimal canaliculi with polyethylene tubes. Arch Ophthalmol 44:198, 1950

89. Jones BR: The surgical cure of obstruction in the common lacrimal canaliculus. Trans Ophthalmol Soc UK 80:343, 1960

90. Tenzel RR: Canaliculodacryocystorhinostomy. Arch Ophthalmol 84:765, 1970

91. von Hoffman H: Paper read at the Tenth International Congress of Ophthalmology, Lucerne, Switzerland, B 41, 1904

92. Morax V, Vialeix V: Reconstitution des voies lacrymales par des greffes dermoepidermiques. Ann Ocul 162:161, 1925

93. Jeandelize P, Baudot R: Refection d'un canalicule lacrymal par greffe dermoepidermique. Bull Soc Ophtalmol Paris 4:363, 1926

94. Nizetic Z: Ueber die Dakryorhinostomie nach Arruga. Klin Monatsbl Augenheilkd 99:314, 1937

95. Thiel R: Zur widerherstellungschirurgie der tranenwege. Klin Monatsbl Augenheilkd 108:576, 1942

96. Guy LP: Surgical construction of lacrimal passage. Arch Ophthalmol 29:575, 1943

97. Beiras Garcia A: Contribucion a la cirugia de las vias lagrimales "Lacorrinoplastia". Arch Soc Oftalmol Hispano-Am 4:26, 1944

98. Bargerter A: Zur Zehandlung der Tranenrohrchenstenose. Ophthalmologica 114:195, 1947

99. Tessier R, Hervouet D: Conjontivo-rhinostomie par epithelial inlay. Bull Soc Ophtalmol Fr 64:580, 1951

100. Rycroft BW: Surgery of external rhinostomy operations. Br J Ophthalmol 35:328, 1951

101. Roveda JM: Dacriotunelizacion. Arch Oftalmol B Air 27:32, 1952

102. Burch Barraquer M: Contribucion a la cirugia de la epifora por lesion canicular. Arch Soc Oftalmol Hispano-Am 13:357, 1953

103. Zarzycki P: La lacodacryocystostomie. Bull Soc Ophtalmol Paris 49:9, 1937

104. Stallard HB: Operation for epiphora. Lancet 2:743, 1940

105. Valiere-Vialeix V, Robin A: Le traitement de l'obliteration canaliculaire par la lacodacryostomie; reintervention dans les echecs par obliteration de la bouche anastomotique. Bull Mem Soc Fr Ophtalmol 66:53, 1953

106. Silva Costa: Canal conjuntivo-pituitario. A Folha Medica, 1936

107. Belmonte Gonzalez N: Lacorrinostomia. Arch Soc Oftalmol Hispano-Am 4:33, 1944

108. Moulie HB: Lacodacriocistorrinostomia en un solo tiempo. Arch Oftalmol B Air 19:466, 1944

109. Burch Barraquer M: Laco-cisto-rinostomia. Arch Soc Oftalmol Hispano-Am 28:331, 1968

110. Weil BA, Sorana JE and Cremona EG: Conjuntivo-dacrio-cisto-rinostomia mediante autoinjerto de vena. Arch Oftalmol B Air 40:246, 1965

111. Reinecke RD, Carroll JM: Silicone lacrimal tube implantation. Trans Am Acad Ophthalmol Otolaryngol 73:85, 1969

112. Murube del Castillo J: Operacion contra la epifora en dacriocistectomizados. Arch Soc Oftalmol Hispano-Am 26:834, 1966

113. Verin P, Valdy A, Benjelloun D, Maurin JF: Suppleance chirurgicale des canalicules par la greffe arterielle ou la dacryo-buccostomie. Bull Mem Soc Fr Ophtalmol 89:169, 1977

114. Bennett JE, Armstrong JR, Jones RE, Schiller F: Conjunctivoantrorhinostomy: a gravity drainage operation utilizing the maxillary sinus, with report of two cases. Arch Ophthalmol 62:248, 1959

115. Stallard HB: Eye Surgery. 4th ed. John Wright and Sons Ltd, Bristol, U.K., 1965, p. 277

116. Jones LT: Epiphora. Its relations to the anatomical structures and surgery of the medial canthal region. Am J Ophthalmol 43:203, 1957
117. Worst JGF: Method for reconstructing torn lacrimal canaliculus. Am J Ophthalmol 53:520, 1962
118. Beyer-Machule CK: A modified lacrimal probe. Arch Ophthalmol 92:157, 1974
119. Veirs ER: Malleable rods for immediate repair of the traumatically severed lacrimal canaliculus. Trans Am Acad Ophthalmol Otolaryngol 66:263, 1962
120. Johnson CC: A canaliculus wire. Am J Ophthalmol 78:854, 1974
121. Beyer-Machule CK: Lacrimal stents. p. 171. In Bosniak SL (ed): The Lacrimal System. Advances in Ophthalmic Plastic and Reconstructive Surgery. Vol. 3. Pergamon Press, Elmsford, NY, 1984
122. Wheeler JM: Removal of the lachrymal sac and accessory lachrymal gland. Int J Surg 28:106, 1915
123. Taiara C, Smith B: Palpebral dacryoadenectomy. Am J Ophthalmol 75:461, 1973
124. Jameson PC: Subconjunctival section of the ductules of the lacrimal gland as a cure for epiphora. Arch Ophthalmol 17:207, 1937

Index

Page numbers followed by f represent figures; those followed by t represent tables.